thirteenth edition

NURSING
IN
SOCIETY

a historical perspective

JOSEPHINE A. DOLAN, M.S., R.N.

Professor of Nursing, University of Connecticut

W. B. SAUNDERS COMPANY   1973

Philadelphia • London • Toronto

W. B. Saunders Company: West Washington Square
Philadelphia, Pa.   19105

12 Dyott Street
London, WC1A   1DB

833 Oxford Street
Toronto 18, Ontario

Nursing in Society — A Historical Perspective   ISBN   0-7216-3132-0

Print No.   9   8   7   6   5   4   3   2   1

Dedicated

To My Loved Ones

Preface

The thirteenth edition of this textbook is being published in the hundredth anniversary year of the graduation of the first school of nursing in the United States. This book is designed to meet the need for a concise yet systematic history of nursing for those who wish to orient themselves to this field of endeavor without perusing extensive and detailed documents. To meet this objective this book has been written for the student of nursing, the busy practitioner of nursing and other members of the health team as well as persons interested in the evolution of health fields.

The fascinating story of the evolution, emergence and expansion of nursing from a simple practical skill to a complex profession has been compressed into thirteen chapters. Nursing is depicted against the societal setting and the cultural and scientific background of the history of mankind. Nursing history is linked to social history, and the new title of the book is a reflection of this relationship as are the chapter titles.

The story of nursing is recounted not as the chronological reporting of events and personalities but as an interpretation of the response of nurses to the needs of people for regaining or retaining health as well as for care during sickness. From the farthest reaches of time, in the most primitive settings, the nurturing efforts and independent role of the nurse in response to survival needs were directed toward keeping people healthy as well as comforting the sick. The development of this wellness-illness component of nursing is woven throughout the chapter contents. Religious influences played a significant role in emphasizing the plight of the sick and poor and the need for human dignity, in elevating the status of women and in stimulating the emergence of dynamic nurse leadership. These recruits to nursing were socially skilled, intellectually endowed and as knowledgeable scientifically as the times permitted.

There has been an attempt to orient the reader to the recurring issues of the present by recounting the recognition of these problems by nurses in the past as well as their successes in wrestling with similar perplexing situations. A selective process had to be utilized in the interest of accomplishing a concise presentation of this important field. The author recognizes the important contributions of many past and present individuals and groups whose achievements it has not been possible to include.

In a book of this size, an attempt to cover all important contributions is necessarily curtailed. Thus, only certain highlights of each period can be presented. The chapters have been rearranged to produce a more logical sequential development. There is a greater emphasis on the emergence of the role and function of the nurse and the delivery of nursing services, especially in the last one hundred years.

Extensive revisions have caused deletion of some material with replacement by more significant data in focusing on present-day nursing. Many new illustrations enhance the visual presentation and serve as an elaboration of the content.

The explosive force of constantly advancing scientific knowledge and the electrifying influence of quick communication of new discoveries and developments have changed the frontiers of civilization. Recorders and interpreters of history can describe only briefly the most important aspects of human development in one small volume.

It is hoped that this book will increase understanding of the relationships of the physical, biological, psychological, social, cultural and spiritual aspects of life to nursing as a humanistic science and will permit the student to see the correlation between these and the role of the nurse.

Grateful appreciation is due to the many persons who have generously assisted in the location of new material and in reading, criticizing and preparing the manuscript for publication.

I sincerely hope that with all its limitations this book will elicit an appreciation and pride in the heritage of nursing.

JOSEPHINE A. DOLAN
Storrs, Connecticut

Contents

CHAPTER 1

The Genesis of Nursing

Care of the Sick in Primitive Cultures

Nursing as an art to be cultivated and a profession to be followed is modern; nursing as a practice originated in the dim past where some mother among the cave dwellers cooled the forehead of her sick child with water from the brook. . . .

Sir William Osler[1]

The task of identifying and describing the evolution of the role of nursing in the history of mankind is truly monumental because our primitive ancestors left no record of their art of nurturing except for the indisputable fact of the survival of the human race. *Nursing has been essential to the preservation of life.*

Let us pause and envision the first scene in the history of mankind. The setting is a primitive one where families live in close proximity for protection. Community living is essential for survival. The period of this setting is timeless. It could be as ancient as the Paleolithic Age or as modern as our own era. It is as old as the very first family and yet as current as this very day in some part of the world, even in our own country. For some communities in today's world have not advanced beyond the Stone Age methods of living and of caring for the sick. The fight for life and survival has been carried on down through time and in many places has not been affected by civilizing influences.

The care of the sick in primitive cultures today is not necessarily the same as that of prehistoric people; however, isolation from progress may present a similar frame of reference for judging the earliest and most elementary methods of caring for the sick.

All through time there have been basic needs essential to the maintenance of life, and the concern for these has formed the basic components of nursing.[2]

Survival needs assume primary importance and are physiological in nature. These *primary* physical needs are for oxygen, water, food, rest, exercise, elimination, procreation and shelter.

There are *secondary* needs which are influenced by social and cultural pressures and are psychosocial. These needs are reflected in human behavior—need for love, security, self-esteem and accomplishment.

The provision of these basic needs differed in quantity and quality. It was often a challenge to obtain enough clean and noncontaminated water; suitable food for physical growth; adequate noninjurious clothing; shelter from the elements and protection from the ravages of disease; love, warmth and human dignity; the opportunity for rest, relaxation and recreation, with the satisfaction of faith in a religion for emotional and spiritual growth; a sense of belonging, and someone to care about a person as well as for a person.

Throughout history the *major problems of community health* have been:

---

[1]Osler, William: *Aequanimitas.* Philadelphia, Blakiston Co., 1932, p. 156.

[2]Henderson, Virginia: *Basic Principles of Nursing Care.* London, *I. C. N.*, pp. 9, 10.

1. To obtain water and food of good quality and in sufficient quantity.
2. To control and improve the physical environment by proper sanitation and prevention of pollution.
3. To prevent transmission of disease.
4. To provide health care.
5. To cope with the perplexing problems of pain, bleeding, shock and infection.
6. To relieve disability and poverty.

Primitive peoples provided the necessities of life by persistent effort and ingenuity, through trial and error. The crudest implements were used to obtain food, clothing and household needs. The wise woman selected such natural objects as seeds, nuts, leaves, roots, herbs and bark from trees, and devised ways of extracting the medicinal ingredients from these raw materials.

Intuitively she found foods for as balanced a diet as possible. She even discovered that certain foods contained poisonous ingredients and investigated until she was adept at withdrawing the deleterious substance from the staple items in the diet. During this process, she ascertained that certain foods caused vomiting or diarrhea; this knowledge then formed a part of her folk healing. The values of folk remedies, herbs and plant lore have been passed on through the ages. Sometimes the information remained accurate, but at times weird ingredients were added and the information became inaccurate. The woman became adept in the management of her home and family and added to her abilities in caring for the needy, the application of loving compassion and tender protection.

ROLE OF THE NURSE

From the time of the first *mother* down to the present day, we find women protecting children and caring for elderly and sick members of the family. They helped their neighbors during periods of illness. Nursing evolved as an *intuitive* response to the desire to keep people healthy as well as to provide comfort and assurance to the sick. The essence of this desire was reflected in the caring, comforting, nourishing, cleansing components of commitment to the patient. Simple procedures for the care of the sick were adopted; skills in practicing these remedies were improved; knowledge of the efficacy of these treatments spread from one community to another and was passed down from one generation to another.

Tenderness, concern, love and hope were expressed in the simple remedies, such as rubbing a painful area or aching body with soft motions, applying heat or cold and concocting herbal therapy. Herbal teas and ointments were compounded from products of nature and recipes were treasured by families through the years. Empirical practices in nursing evolved.

Many baffling problems needed to be studied and solved; among them was the dilemma of the cause of sickness. External causative factors of trauma or illness, such as a fall that resulted in a noticeable bruised area, could be seen or understood; however, man was baffled and bewildered by sudden illness. The sudden ache inside his body, the paroxysms of sharp and throbbing pain, the inability to retain his food, the lack of sight, the muscular spasms, the loss of movement of one side of his body with concomitant loss of vocal expression were incomprehensible and were considered by man to be supernatural in cause.

PRIMITIVE THEORIES OF DISEASE

Primitive disease concepts appeared to be associated with the following areas:

1. *Sorcery*

A sorcerer had the ability to use magical ritual formulas to compel the supernatural forces to produce injury, disease and even death in another person. This power over another was associated with the ability to "hex" or to cast an evil spell. As a consequence the fear-ridden body of the victim reflected physiological disorders. In many cultures children were considered to be particularly susceptible.

2. *Magic*

There were two types of magic — *homeopathic* (imitative) magic and *contagious* magic. Homeopathic assumed that things that resembled each other were the same. An image was made of one's enemy and this was injured in the belief that consequently the victim would be injured.

Contagious magic assumed that things once in contact were always in contact and therefore what was done to one affected the other. It was felt that a person should never permit himself to become dissociated from any part of his body because of the danger of someone's gaining control of him and working his occult powers on him.

In many cultures the shaman or root doctor was believed to possess countermagic.

3. *Breaking a Taboo*

A person was believed to be automatically punished if he broke that which was considered to be "taboo." The cultural acceptance of this fate was so strong that a person often wasted away for no apparent reason.

4. *Intrusion of a Disease Object*

Illness was believed to be induced by the bodily entrance of some small object. Its removal was accomplished by sucking, and the medicine man then removed it from his own mouth. Where the power of suggestion seemed to have motivated the illness, the sight of an object's being removed had a miraculous effect on the victim.

5. *Bodily Invasion by a Spirit*

The demonic theory of disease emphasized the possession of the body by the devil or other evil spirits which caused physical and mental distress, disease and even death.

6. *Loss of the Soul*

The soul could be enticed to leave the body by an evil spirit or a sorcerer. During its wanderings, an injury could have happened to it and prevented its return. A soul-catching ceremony would then be required to effect its return.

7. *Dreams*

The influence of dreams seemed to cause sickness. The elements of the dream acted as a suggestive mode of behavior. It has been believed that the soul left the body during periods of dreaming.

Empirical practices were now combined and supplemented with *occult* practices. The causes of illness were believed to be beyond nature as man observed it; the causes were supernatural and were visible signs of *malevolent gods*. Indeed these gods struck a person with such force and suddenness that this person frequently became paralyzed and unable to speak. This condition was referred to as a stroke. Fear of the unknown has been terrifying to people throughout time. In a desperate search for a solution to these problems there evolved the *theory of animism,* which explains that everything in nature is alive with invisible forces and endowed with supernatural powers.

Good spirits brought blessings; evil spirits (demons) brought trials, tribulations, sickness and death.

It was imperative that a solution be found by which the body could be freed from the influences of evil spirits. The solution seemed to revolve around the aspects of *submission, sacrifice* and *supplication.* Submission has resulted in the attitude of "what cannot be cured must be endured." Sacrifice involved animal and sometimes human victims. Children, the physically and mentally handicapped and the aged were the unfortunate ones selected to placate irate evil spirits. Supplication was expressed through prayer.

Primitive Measures

Primitive peoples searched for a means of protection from these malevolent forces. *Amulets* were those articles that, when worn or carried, protected the wearer from evil influences, black magic and disease. *Talismans* were objects that would bring good luck. Primitive medicine stood midway between magic and religion. As the magic lore increased, it became much too burdensome to administer, and a special person was designated to master these skills. Thus, the medicine man emerged.

ROLE OF THE MEDICINE MAN

Sympathy and necessity were the motivating forces that impelled the person who came forward to answer cries of need. This person was called a *shaman.* The shaman, also referred to as the *medicine man* or *witch doctor,* assumed a solemn supervisory relation to disease and its cure. He was called upon in critical emergencies to share his wisdom and skill in detecting the reason for the sickness; in prescribing a treatment; in performing surgery; or in conducting religious rituals to eject the evil spirits from the body of the patient (Fig. 1–1). He was a man of mystery, a man apart from the group, one who had endured a long, toilsome and physically and mentally exhaustive course. He had mastered ventriloquism and magic tricks, had a comprehensive knowledge of herbs and knew the precise details of ritualistic treatment.

The shaman handled disease almost entirely through psychotherapeutic maneuvers. His chief objective was to frighten the evil spirit out of the body of the sick person. He did this by dressing himself in skins of animals and equipping himself with a large gro-

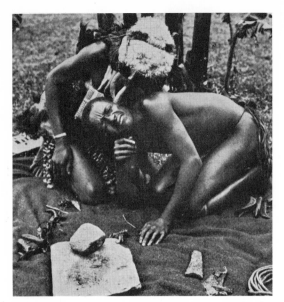

Figure 1–1. Medicine man drawing out the evil influence by means of a sucking tube.

tesque mask and some implement, such as a rattle or a drum, capable of creating an annoying noise.

His therapy was a fear or shock technique to rid the body of evil spirits. The technique appealed to all the senses. Emotional stress caused by anxiety, fear and hopelessness can produce chemical changes within the body so that the techniques of the medicine man frequently did help his patient.

The medicine man's treatment might be summarized as follows:

Refuse the sick person rest and quiet to encourage the evil spirit to depart from the person's body by:

1. Startling the evil spirit with a frightening mask, blood-curdling yells and deafening noises.
2. Jolting the evil spirit by shaking, biting, pinching, kicking and pummeling the patient.
3. Ferreting the evil spirit out with obnoxious odors.
4. Driving out the evil spirit by giving the patient vile-tasting concoctions to drink. These included purgatives and emetics.
5. Annoying the evil spirit by alternatively plunging the patient in baths of hot and cold water.
6. Enticing the evil spirit to enter an animal (kept at the side of the sick person for that purpose) or an inanimate object, such as a figurine.
7. Pacifying the evil spirit by making sacrifices (usually animal).
8. Placating the evil spirit by using amulets.
9. Resorting to objects with magical powers such as *fetishes* (Fig. 1–2). The fetish was a primitive carved figure that was

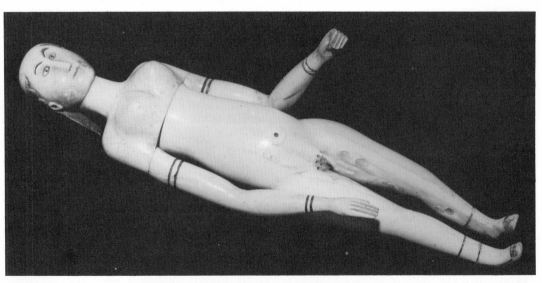

Figure 1–2. Walrus carving (fetish). Hair or bits of clothing inserted at junction of upper part of doll. Shaman directs ceremonial to doll for relief of patient. (Courtesy of Howard Dittrick Museum.)

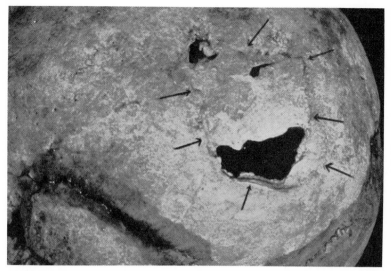

Figure 1–3. A trepanned skull from eastern Arkansas. Arrows indicate original extent of operation. Healing process can be seen.

presumed to carry supernatural power. It was treated frequently as an idol and deified.

10. Encouraging the evil spirit to come out of the body by chanting a rhythmic incantation.

When the evil spirit remained within the person and the symptoms had not subsided, the shaman resorted to an operation called *trepanation*.[3] Trepanning consisted of boring a hole into a person's skull by means of a sharp stone in order to permit the imprisoned devil, demon or evil spirit to escape (Figs. 1–3 and 1–4). This was performed to relieve headaches, or to alleviate other conditions, such as epilepsy. The patient did not always survive the treatment.

Even when a woman in labor was ready to deliver her baby, techniques were used for scaring the baby from her body. Horses galloped toward a mother who had been strapped to a tree, or a woman stood with her legs stretched apart and a lighted fire was

placed between her legs in the hope of hastening the delivery process.

In some primitive communities a woman in labor and preparing for the delivery of her child was required to remain alone and assist herself. Presumably the activities of daily living helped keep her musculature in good condition and permitted a relatively easy delivery. Occasionally the woman who most recently delivered a baby, although not neces-

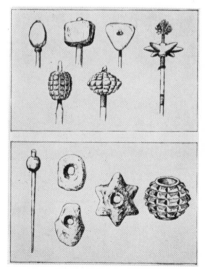

Figure 1–4. Stone mace-heads from the South Pacific (above) and from America (below), used in connection with trepanation.

---

[3] "Trepanation, the making of an opening in the skull with sharpened flint or shark's tooth, is now considered an obsolescent term; the modern surgeon prefers the term trephining, the cutting out of a cranial disk. The object of trepanation was to give the demon confined within the skull a chance to escape; the object of trephination is to remove intracranial pressure. Since trephining stems directly from trepanning, and the ancient and modern operations are fundamentally identical, medical historians cling to the elder word." Robinson, Victor: "Trepanation after Lister." *Ciba Symposia, 1*:192, 1939.

sarily the most experienced person, aided the mother during the birth process.

Primitive nursing and the care of the sick by the medicine man were not peculiar to the Stone Age; they have persisted to the present day. Louise Stinetorf[4] in *White Witch Doctor*, portrays a more recent interpretation of primitive nursing and care of the sick. One can picture the homemade implements and instruments as the author describes the use of splinters of bamboo or thorns as scalpels. Miss Stinetorf stresses the sparing use of pain-relievers and anesthetics:

To the primitive mind all sickness is caused by devils and no devil leaves such a nice comfortable abode as a human body willingly. It fights to the last against being evicted. Such a titanic struggle is bound to rip a man to pieces inside and hurt him exceedingly. The bigger and stronger the devil, the worse the struggle to get him out, and consequently the greater the pain, the prouder the person is after it is all over.

Miss Stinetorf indicates that vile-tasting and unpalatable medications seemed to be received with greater appreciation by the patient and greater faith was placed in their efficacy.

At one time, Miss Stinetorf developed malaria. After she recovered, she was informed that her native attendants had debated the merits of performing a trepanning operation on her:

We knew that the spirits of the Great Mother Forest were calling to you, and we debated among ourselves as to whether or not we should break open your skull and set your spirit free so that it might answer them.[5]

An interesting comparison of the professionally prepared person versus the medicine man is presented by Miss Stinetorf:

Natives say medical practices are superior to those of the ordinary witch doctor. Fewer of the patients die, fewer of those who live are deformed, all of them suffer less from the treatments, and it is pleasant not to be afraid of him as a person.[6]

PRIMITIVE TREATMENTS

Primitive man cured his minor troubles through empirical techniques (Fig. 1–5). It

---

[4]Stinetorf, Louise: *White Witch Doctor.* Philadelphia, Westminster Press, 1950, pp. 70–71.

[5]*Ibid.*, p. 183.
[6]*Ibid.*, p. 176.

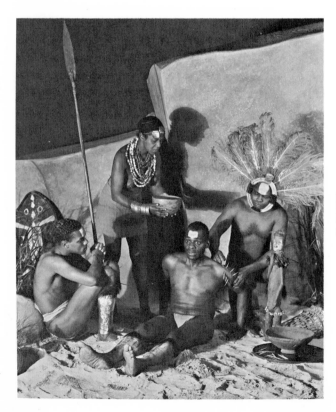

Figure 1–5. The shaman inserts thin, sharply pointed slivers of wood to close a wound. Then leaves are placed over this to serve as bandages. Note the carved wooden figurine at the patient's side. (Courtesy of Davis & Geck Co.)

was felt that affliction of the mind or body should not be separated and that the body (natural spirit) and soul (vital spirit) must remain together within a person's body to achieve good health. When the soul left the body, illness or death could result. Hallucinations, delirium or shock was feared because it was felt at such times that the vital spirit or soul had been stolen and was wandering. Special carved bone charms were used by *soul catchers* to entice the lost soul back into the body.

An example of a soul-catching ceremony has been presented by Guthrie.[7] The scene is carried out in the presence of many members of the community, who form a circle around the patient. Amidst the flicker of the firelight, while in a trance, the soul catcher sends forth his soul to find and cajole the wandering soul of the sick person to return. A description of the event is chanted and when the soul returns, it is prevented from further peregrinations by the tying of a palm leaf around the victim's wrist.

Sympathetic magic was also employed in the selection of medicines that resembled the hoped-for cure for the affliction being treated. For example, the bark of the willow tree,

[7]Guthrie, Douglas: *A History of Medicine.* London, Thomas Nelson & Sons Ltd., 1945, p. 5.

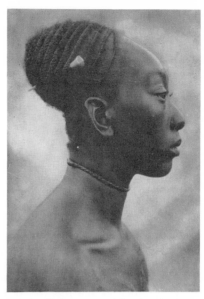

Figure 1–6. Deformation of head and scarification of chest of Mangbetu woman of the Congo. (Courtesy of American Museum of Natural History, New York.)

which is agile and supple, was used to relieve the stiffness of a person suffering from arthritic problems. The medicine was found successful, and later chemical analysis revealed that the bark is an excellent source of salicylate, the important ingredient in aspirin.

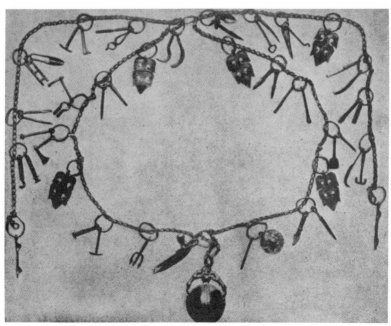

Figure 1–7. A charm bracelet of the fourth century A.D.

Currently, medical scientists have been analyzing the ingredients of the brews of witch doctors in the hope of discovering important life-prolonging drugs. Many ancient remedies may offer new hope in some of our baffling diseases. It has been well known that some of the commonly used medications were obtained from extracts of plants.

Culturally Approved Mutilations

In primitive communities many of the culturally approved mutilations were detrimental and injurious to health. These included deformation of the head (Fig. 1–6) and feet, application of bands of metal to stretch the neck and the insertion of pieces of wood, ivory or metal to enlarge the lips and ear lobes. The practice of cutting the skin and either burning names or rubbing ashes into the scarification has been revived in our own day.

When we ponder the beliefs, customs and rituals employed in the care of the sick and in the preservation of health in the primitive communities, we find evidence of their presence today. From the earliest families, primitive and highly civilized, to the families of to-day, primitive as well as highly educated, we note the use of superstitious practices. Such practices still involve the use of the fetish, amulet, talisman and charm. Our present-day amulets include horse chestnuts carried to ward off rheumatism, a bag of camphor worn around the neck to prevent influenza, horseshoes, rabbits' feet, four-leaf clovers and charm bracelets (Fig. 1–7). The carrying of charms and amulets counteracts the undesirable effects of such things as black cats, broken mirrors, walking under ladders, Friday the thirteenth and hexes, and also the "evil eye" influences.

Robinson has stated, "Intellectually we are but a stone's throw from the Stone Age; and emotionally we are still living there."[8]

In retrospect, nursing has always responded to the human need for survival. The independent role of the nurse was reflected in the ability to keep people healthy as well as bringing comfort and well-being to the sick. The wellness and illness component of nursing was provided for individuals and families most frequently in their homes.

---

[8]*Op. cit.*, p. 10.

REFERENCE READINGS

Baker, W., and Risse, M.: "Delusions of Witchcraft: A Cross-Cultural Study," *British Journal of Psychiatry, 114*:(1968) 963–972.

_____: "Clinicopathologic Conference, Case Presentation," *Johns Hopkins Medical Journal, 120*:(1967) 186–199.

Bessey, Maurice: *Magic and the Supernatural*, London, Spring Books, 1966.

Douglas, Mary (Ed.): *Witchcraft: Confessions and Accusations*, London, Tavistock Publications, 1970.

Galvin, James and Ludwig, Arnold: "A Case of Witchcraft," *Journal of Nervous and Mental Disease, 1933*: (1961) 161–168.

Gillin, John: "Magical Fright," *Psychiatry, 11*:(1948) 387–400.

Gillin, John: "The Making of a Witch Doctor," *Psychiatry, 19*:(1956) 131–136.

Haggard, Howard W.: *Devils, Drugs and Doctors*, New York, Harper and Brothers, 1929.

Hill, Douglas: *Magic and Superstition*, London, Hamlyn Publishing Group, 1968.

Lomas, Peter: "Taboo and Illness," *British Journal of Medical Psychology, 42*:(March 1969) 33–9.

Middleton, John (Ed.): *Magic, Witchcraft and Curing*, New York, The Natural History Press, 1967.

Payne, George H.: *The Child in Human Progress*, New York, G. P. Putnam's Sons, 1916.

Redgrove, Stanley: *Bygone Beliefs*, London, William Rider and Son, Ltd., 1920.

Rosenthal, Ted., et al.: "Social Strata and Perception of Magical and Folk-Medical Child-care Practices," *Journal of Social Psychology, 77*:(1969) 3–13.

Simmons, Leo W.: *The Role of the Aged in the Primitive Society*, New Haven, Yale University Press, 1945.

Snell, John: "Hypnosis in the Treatment of the 'Hexed' Patient," *American Journal of Psychiatry, 124*:(September, 1967) 311–316.

Williams, Joseph J.: *Voodoos and Obeahs—Phases of West India Witchcraft*, New York, Dial Press, 1933.

CHAPTER 2

Influence of Ancient Cultural Practices on Health Care (Part I)

After the prehistoric period, with its indefinite records and lack of documentation of daily living activities, writing was invented, a calendar was devised and history was recorded for posterity to scrutinize.

The care of the sick in primitive groups was the first scene in the theater of life, but we are aware that ancient cultured groups existed side by side with the primitive ones, just as they do today. To assist in studying the contributions of the ancient cultures, let us turn our attention to Biblical presentations and archeological findings.

Archeology brings man's record of existence to view and permits scrutiny of the past. History has been recorded through time in hieroglyphic inscriptions, cuneiform tablets, papyri, books, documents and case histories. Art work has played an important role in the presentation of data. Scenes change because of the differences in social and ethnic styles, but creative thinking is observed and ingenious solutions to crucial problems are evident.

Ethnologists have noted that, with the development of each race and nation, the healing arts have either occupied a position of importance or been conspicuous by their absence in the life of each community.

A complete setting for the first glimpse of man and his progress down through the centuries should begin with an appreciation of the creation of the world in which man was to live, as well as an awesome reverence for the creation of man.

Man and the universe were made to exist in the profound execution of the plan of Creation. This awe-inspiring fact continues to mystify humanity, but its reality is witness to

the fact. The Bible relates: "The heavens show forth the glory of God, and the firmament declareth the work of His hands."[1]

The Biblical scholars have indicated that God had given man a perfect body—free from sickness, infirmities and old age—and that removal of the perfection from each body leads to sickness, suffering, old age and physical death. Study of the evidence of the antiquity of disease in skeletal remains has resulted in the emergence of the science of *paleopathology*.

There is no exact date of the beginnings of human history. It is curious how small a portion of the habitable globe was the site of all those human activities, the record of which constitutes ancient history.

For centuries Egypt had been considered the earliest site of civilization until energetic and curious archeologists in the 1840's began excavating the mounds of dirt in Mesopotamia. In these folds of earth were buried important treasures. What was found in this fertile strip of land between the Tigris and the Euphrates rivers has established Mesopotamia as an earlier cradle of civilization.

Community living changed from tribal groups to empires and, thence, into urban settlements. Some cities have thrived; others have faded into obscurity. Many of our problems—overcrowding, slums, high crime rates, gradual inadequacy of water supply, disease outbreaks and economic losses—plagued ancient peoples. What role did disease play in the disappearance of these ancient civilized groups?

---

[1] Psalm *18*:2.

9

Water gradually became the vehicle for the spread of disease because of its use for drinking, bathing, washing clothes, swimming, religious rituals and disposal of human and animal waste.

THE SUMERIANS

When the Sumerians moved into the land between the Tigris and Euphrates, they had developed not only a system of writing but also a set of laws and a mature culture.

Sumerian artifacts unearthed by archeologists reflect the nature of their daily living and yield evidence of their advanced craftsmanship, their medical skill, and their burial customs, which shed light on the individual of five thousand years ago (Fig. 2–1).

The excavation of the grave of Queen Shubad unearthed a rich array of funerary gifts made of gold, silver and copper; the queen's headdress and jewels were exquisite. Outright murder occurred at the burial of the Queen; all of her ladies-in-waiting, servants, soldiers and her court harpist were murdered while standing in position at her bier so that they might accompany the Queen in death. The scene is an example of planned, compulsory human sacrifice. A soporific was probably used to assist in achieving a painless suffocation.

Temples of Healing

As the concept of animism became an accepted one, man attempted to placate and to worship evil spirits as gods. He built *temples* to them hoping to please them so that disease and misfortune would be eradicated. With this movement the medicine man became a *priest-physician* who worked in the temple. Medicine as a field of endeavor now began the evolution from witchcraft to craft.

The world's oldest known medical prescriptions, scratched on a 4000-year-old clay tablet, were translated in 1953 (Fig. 2–2). The ancient physician wrote on both sides of the tablet with a reed stylus sharpened to a wedge-shaped edge. Unfortunately, the tablets do not contain the names of the diseases for which the remedies were prescribed. The translators of the cuneiform script on the clay tablets report that it was unusual that the ancient doctor did not resort to magic spells or incantations. It is quite remarkable that this oldest page in medical history yet discovered is so completely free from magical elements.

THE BABYLONIANS

Babylon, a Mesopotamian city believed to have been founded in the late third millennium B.C., was the center of the empire of

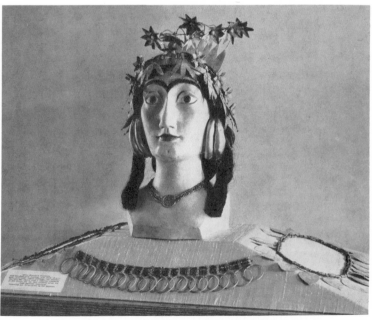

Figure 2–1. Woman's headdress from the Great Depth Pit in Ur. (Courtesy of the University Museum, Philadelphia.)

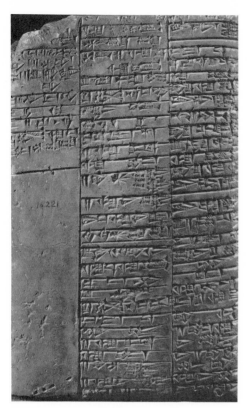

Figure 2–2. The oldest known medical prescriptions written in cuneiform script on clay tablet. (Courtesy of the University Museum, Philadelphia.)

Babylonia. Under Hammurabi, *ca.* 2000 B.C., Babylon became an important city and the capital of the kingdom. The society was divided into a quasi-feudal type with the upper stratum made up of wealthy landowners, merchants and priests; the middle class consisted of less wealthy merchants, peasants and artisans; the lowest class was comprised of slaves. The religion of the Babylonians centered around the worship of Bêl, later called Marduk, who was identified with the planet Jupiter. Marduk was described as a cruel god who exacted human blood, frequently children's, in return for his favor. The temple priests were made eunuchs. Handicapped members of society were used as sacrificial victims. The poor were threatened with brutal punishment for the smallest offenses; occasionally the punishment meted out to them was to be dismembered on the altar of Bêl.

Hammurabi, the king of Babylonia, has been remembered for his *Code of Law*, a compilation of the oldest preserved codes of ancient law (Fig. 2–3). The Code of Law was somewhat humanitarian and tried to prevent the defrauding of the helpless and to reduce the cost of medical care. Fees to be charged to a "gentleman" and those to a "slave" were presented clearly:

> If a doctor has treated a man for a severe wound with a lancet of bronze and has cured the man, or has opened a tumour with a bronze lancet and has cured the man's eye, he shall receive ten shekels of silver.
> If it was a freedman, he shall receive five shekels of silver.
> If it was a man's slave, the owner of the slave shall give the doctor two shekels of silver.

The startling aspect of the Code was that the governing body replaced the individual as the avenger of injustice and malpractice. The penalties were severe and resulted frequently in cruel physical punishment. Doctors were responsible to the government; in fact, the Code of Hammurabi regulated the physician's conduct:

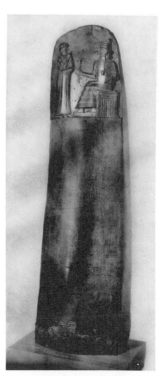

Figure 2–3. Stele of Hammurabi, which is exhibited at the Louvre in Paris. Hammurabi is receiving the laws from the sun god; below this is the code in cuneiform. (From cast at Oriental Institute Museum. Courtesy of Oriental Institute, University of Chicago.)

If a physician has treated a free-born man for a severe wound with a lancet of bronze and has caused the man to die, or has opened a tumour of the man with a lancet of bronze and has destroyed his eyes, his hands one shall cut off.

One is impressed with this undesirable aspect of the Code; the retributive nature of the punishment follows literally "an eye for an eye."

The doctor as priest-physician occupied a prestigious position, but the surgeon, because he worked manually, occupied a much lower rank and it was he who was subject to the malpractice punishments of the Code.

The Bible inveighed against the punitive emphasis of this code.

Abraham, a descendant of Noah, was a contemporary of Hammurabi and grew up in Ur of Chaldea, a Babylonian city.

Babylon was destroyed by the Assyrians under Sennacherib and its real splendor belongs to the later period of Babylonia, after the city was rebuilt. The brilliant color and luxury of Babylon became famous during the rule of *Nebuchadnezzar* (*ca.* 605–562 B.C.). He was responsible for the construction of the Hanging Gardens of Babylon, one of the seven wonders of the world and a most outstanding architectural achievement (Fig. 2–4). A continuous supply of water was furnished by a chain pump that forced the water through the arches and thereby irrigated the famous medicinal herb gardens.

Medical treatment in Babylonia was primitive. The notion persisted that illness was caused by sin and by displeasure of the gods. Disease (dis-ease) was inflicted as a punishment for sinning. The person was unclean and needed purification. Temples became the centers of medical care (Fig. 2–5). The Babylonians also inaugurated a quaint custom of bringing the sick person out into the busy market place. Here, all who passed inquired about the disease and if the passerby or a relative or friend had similar symptoms, he prescribed a cure. Thus were the diagnosis and treatment handled. This practice may have been necessary because of a shortage of

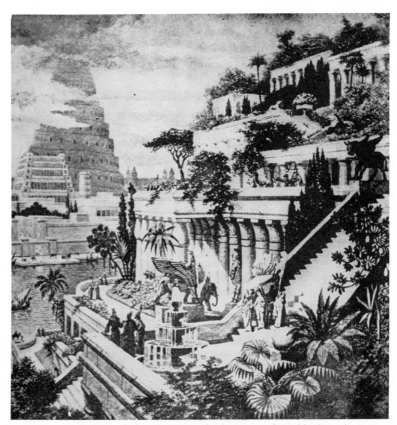

Figure 2–4. The Hanging Gardens of Babylon containing the famous medicinal herb gardens. (Brown Brothers.)

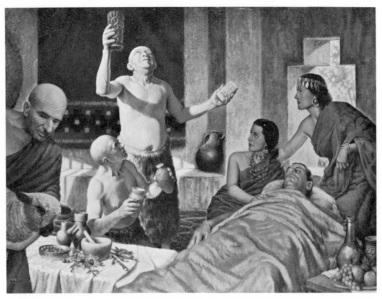

Figure 2–5. An artist's conception of a Babylonian sickroom. The role of the nurse as she assists the patient is portrayed. (© 1951 by Parke, Davis & Co.)

doctors. Principal methods of treatment consisted of ridding the human body of the demons of disease by incantations and by the application of certain herbs. Medicines continued to be vile-tasting concoctions. Many disgusting ingredients were taken internally in the hope of ejecting the evil from the sick person's body.

Ancient Babylonian medical texts, recorded on clay tablets, presented first a description of the symptoms of the disease, followed by the prescription and directions for compounding the medicine and finally an incantation to the gods.

An animal was kept at the side of the patient in the hope that the demons would take

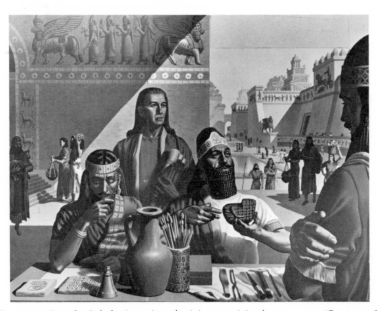

Figure 2–6. Representation of a Babylonian priest-physician practicing hepatoscopy. (Courtesy of *Lederle Bulletin.*)

up their abode within its body; then the animal, the scapegoat, was sacrificed. It has been mentioned that sacrifices to the gods were frequent and often cruel; human beings were offered on occasion.

Prognosis, or the probable outcome of the disease, was controlled by the art or practice of divination. This was carried out by *hepatoscopy,* or the inspection of the liver of sacrificial animals (Fig. 2–6). From hepatoscopy the Babylonians learned the structure of the liver and the gallbladder, and their clay models are excellent anatomical specimens.

In Ezekiel *21:21,* one reads "For the king of Babylon stood at the parting of the ways, at the head of the two roads to use divination: he made his arrows bright, he consulted with images, he looked into the liver."

Why the liver? Because it was felt that the liver was the source of blood and the residence of the soul. By inspecting the liver, the priest-physician could communicate with the mind of God.

In spite of the magico-mystical practices of medicine, the records of obvious *clinical observations,* one of the bases of scientific thought, cannot be ignored. An early Babylonian case study reports:

The sick one coughs frequently, his sputum is thick and sometimes contains blood, his respirations give a sound like a flute, his skin is cold but his feet are hot, he sweats greatly and his heart muscle is disturbed. When his disease is extremely grave his intestines are frequently opened . . .

In the sickroom scene in Figure 2–5 note the team approach to patient care with the nurse figure assisting the patient while the physician directs his colleague, the pharmacist, to concoct the medicine. Observe the nursing, pharmaceutical, medical and spiritual care of the sick.

THE PERSIANS

The Persians were a group of Iranian tribes, which Cyrus the Great (600?–529 B.C.) welded into a nation. He defeated the Median suzerain Astyages in 550 B.C. and became leader of the Medes and Persians. The conquests of Cyrus were further extended from Egypt to the borders of India under the leadership of Darius the Great (558?–486 B.C.).

The religion of the Persians centered around the teaching of the prophet Zoroaster who preached that Ahura Mazda was the creator of the world, the source of light and the embodiment of good, engaged in constant struggle with Ahriman, the spirit of darkness and evil. Zoroastrianism is still practiced in Iran and in India by the Parsees, who are descendants of the Persians.

The oldest medical records of the Persians are found in the few surviving books of Zoroaster. Many of the ideas about medicine and sanitation were adopted from their neighbors. It is clear that belief in the demonic theory of disease was practiced. The most reliable cure was the recital of invocations for spiritual assistance.

The Zoroastrian bible, the *Avesta,* contained the ceremonial rules relating to the natural laws of birth and death. One of these concerned itself with abortion. To destroy life was to destroy the highest form of creation, and the punishment was the same as for murder.

Principles of public health and sanitation were stressed in Zoroastrian medical laws and practices. For instance, in order not to contaminate earth or water, after a person's death his body was fastened to the roof of a special high tower called "Tower of Silence." Birds picked the bones, which dried out and then dropped down into the pit below, and in this way decomposition was prevented. Anything that had become contaminated was purified by being washed with the urine of a bull.

The Persians, who regarded music as an expression of the good will of Ahura Mazda, were said to have cured various illnesses by the sound of the lute.

Three types of practitioners emerged from the medical centers: those who healed with the knife, those who healed with herbs and those who healed with holy words. The latter had the most prestige, and the surgeons had the least.

Rules were established to test the skill of candidates before they were permitted to practice. The surgeon had to perform his first three operations on non-Zoroastrians. The Code of Zoroaster resembled the Code of Hammurabi and evidently was modeled on it. Fees were determined according to the status of the patient.

It is with the Achaemenid kings, from about 550 B.C., that Persian history begins. The most famous of these kings were Cyrus the Great and Darius III.

In 330 B.C. Alexander the Great defeated the Achaemenids, demolished the palace of Persepolis and destroyed most of the Zoroastrian literature.

THE ANCIENT EGYPTIANS

The ancient empire of Egypt occupied the long, narrow valley lying on each side of the Nile. It was a rich, fertile area nourished by the annual floods that inundated the area and deposited valuable silt. Grain was grown very early in the valley of the Nile, causing Egypt to be referred to as the "breadbasket of antiquity." The importance of grain in the valley is seen in the Biblical story of Joseph and his dream interpretation.

The Egyptians exhibited careful planning to meet certain community needs and avert public health problems. They built irrigation canals and granaries for the proper and provident storage of food. Famine and malnutrition have plagued many peoples throughout history.

An early public health measure was the building of water storage basins for irrigation purposes in the Nile Valley (Fig. 2–7). The stored water was found to be an important safeguard in eliminating the transmission of many diseases.

The place where the ancient Egyptians left us their best efforts in the area of communication skills is in the *pyramids.* Scrutiny of these pyramids has helped us to understand the burial customs, the philosophy and the religious beliefs of the Egyptians. They believed that at the termination of physical life the soul continued to exist through all eternity. There was another world, another life beyond the earth and sky, peopled with the dead. Each person brought with him to this new world the essential earthly possessions that he required for daily living, including a dwelling, food and drink, clothing and even servants. In the earliest periods, it was the custom of the Pharaoh, or a very socially prominent person, to require his servants and slaves to be sacrificed to accompany him in death so that he could arrive in the new life with his household retinue. In later periods this practice was replaced with the use of representational wall paintings. These murals provide an unusually clear photograph of living in this period, and often also indicate disease conditions that were prevalent (Fig. 2–8).

The body had to be prepared carefully and preserved against destruction so that the wandering soul could return to it. Thus the practice of *mummification* or *embalming* became necessary (Fig. 2–9). In the *house of death,* an establishment away from civilization, the elaborate process of embalming was carried

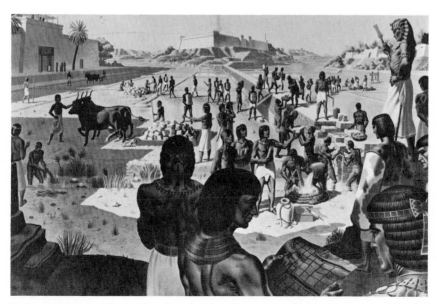

Figure 2–7. Representation of the construction of an Egyptian water storage basin. (Courtesy of *Lederle Bulletin.*)

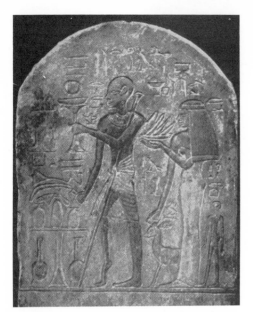

Figure 2–8. Portrayal of a case of poliomyelitis on an Egyptian tombstone.

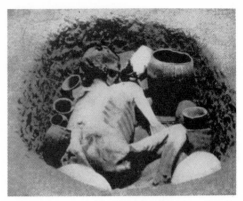

Figure 2–10. Prehistoric Egyptian grave. The corpse was buried in a squatting position (sleeping position) such as is also frequently found in many prehistoric European graves.

out by people specially skilled in this field. Special oils, ointments and herbs were used and the vital organs were removed and placed in canopic jars. Though this was an

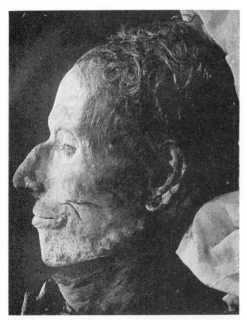

Figure 2–9. The head of the mummy of Ynaa, father-in-law of King Amenhotep III, found in the Valley of the Kings. (C. W. Ceram: *Gods, Graves, and Scholars.* Alfred A. Knopf, 1952.)

elaborate procedure, it was a routine one and had no connection with scientific advancement. Dissection or observation for medical purposes was not practiced, and the fields of anatomy and pathology were not developed as a result of the process of embalming.

What do we learn by studying the mummified bodies? It must be kept in mind that the very dry climate of Egypt acted as a natural embalming agent so that many bodies have been found in shallow graves preserved without the benefit of the artificial embalming process (Fig. 2–10). Looking at these and at the carefully preserved bodies in the tombs we see definite evidences of the diseases that were prevalent at the time. Rare skill is seen in their art of bandaging and in the efforts of their dentists and surgeons.

The position of the *doctor* in ancient Egypt is an interesting one. He, as did the aspirants to all the learned professions, received his preprofessional and professional preparation at the *temple* of the prevailing deity. The practitioners of the professions were usually members of the lower classes of priesthood; religion and medicine were closely related. Patients came to the temple to intercede with the gods and were treated by the medical practitioners (Fig. 2–11). During the treatment the priest-physician appealed for assistance from the gods and suitable tribute was offered to them.

The *medical area* of the temple is thought to be somewhat comparable to a large outpatient clinic, with the doctors examining

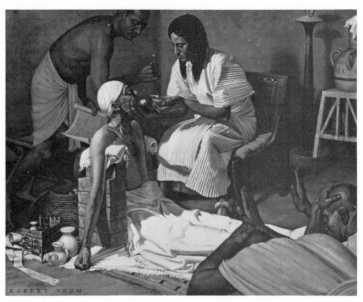

Figure 2–11. Representation of a sickroom scene in an Egyptian temple. An ingenious method of giving the medication that has been prepared in accordance with directions on a papyrus scroll. (© 1957 by Parke, Davis & Co.)

and the medical students observing. There were medical specialists at this time, as Herodotus the famous Greek historian writes: "Medicine is practiced among them on a plan of separation; each physician treats a single disorder and no more: thus the country swarms with medical practitioners, some undertaking to cure diseases of the eye, others of the teeth, others of the head, others of the intestines, and some of those which are invisible [internal]." The physician in charge of the intestines gave the enemas and purges. Trepanning operations were performed by the specialist of the head and these were done for medically sound reasons. The physician was also dentist and pharmacist.

One of the most outstanding physicians was *Imhotep*, chief physician to the court of King Djoser (or Zoser), *ca.* 2700 B.C. Imhotep acquired fame also as an architect through the construction of the great pyramid for the king at Sakkara. Later Imhotep was deified and ranked with the gods as the Egyptian god of medicine.

Medical records of ancient Egypt have been of immense value in understanding Egyptian medical care. One of the most important and best preserved is *Papyrus Ebers* acquired by archeologist George Ebers in 1875 and now located in the University Library in Leipzig. This is supposed to have been written originally about 2500 B.C. and recopied about 1550 B.C. It contained approximately 700 prescriptions for all kinds of diseases, arranged in sections according to the different organs to be treated.

The *Edwin Smith Surgical Papyrus* is another famous papyrus scroll and is actually a surgical text. It categorized the diagnoses, treatments and prognoses of types of injuries and fractures according to each region of the body. One of the earliest known references to surgery (Fig. 2–12) has been found in this papyrus. The treatment of a tumor and abscess has been presented as "an ailment which I will treat with the fire drill." The fire drill or fire stick was an Egyptian device for kindling fire. It provided the surgeon with a convenient means of procuring a hot point to apply to an inflamed area.

The other member of the trilogy of illustrious papyri is the *Hearst Medical Papyrus*, which seems to have been a general practitioner's formulary. The medical papyri reveal a high level of clinical observation.

The impression left by Egyptian culture on civilization has been a profound one, due partly to the thousands of years of its existence and partly to the archeological excavations of the evidence of this existence.

In summary, Egypt has contributed more to prove the antiquity of disease than any

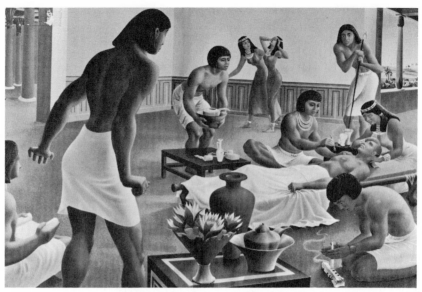

Figure 2–12. An artist's conception of an operation that might have taken place in Egypt about 2500 B.C. Note the emotional support and assistance given to the patient by the nurse figure. (Courtesy of *Lederle Bulletin*.)

other country up to this time, because of its natural climate and its religious and funerary customs that combined to preserve the dead. Data have been gathered by examination of skeletal remains, by laboratory tests and x-ray, by scrutiny of artistic endeavors and by analysis of the medical and surgical papyri.

Bones showed signs of malformation and infection. The Egyptians were cognizant of many disease conditions, such as tuberculosis, arteriosclerosis and parasitic infections. Fractured bones were splinted with care.

THE ANCIENT HEBREWS

The best source book on the history of the Hebrews is the Old Testament of the Bible. The oldest traditions of the Hebrew people are found in Genesis beginning with the genealogy of Shem (eldest son of Noah), the birth of Abraham and the presentation of the patriarchal history.

The historical thread of the ancient Hebrews has been noted in the Babylonian, Assyrian and Egyptian cultures. After Abraham's divinely inspired flight from Babylonia to Egypt and thence back to Canaan, a solemn covenant was made between God and Abraham, who was to be the father of a people chosen to preserve the worship of one God. This covenant, which was renewed with Moses on Mount Sinai

500 years later, contained privileges and such obligations as the necessity to circumcise every male child of Abraham's descendants. Jewish liturgy speaks of "Thy Covenant which Thou has sealed into our flesh." It is interesting to note that a sharpened stone was the instrument used by Abraham to circumcise himself.

The outstanding contribution of the ancient Hebrews to the cultural heritage of the world was their religion. This religion of one true God, Yahweh, made them unique among all their contemporaries. His guidance and divine revelation was apparent in the men sent by God to guide His people: "From the time when your fathers left the land of Egypt until this very day I sent you all my servants, the prophets, early and late."[2] This constant, divine guidance kept their religion alive despite the ever-present attractions of the polytheistic influences of the Hebrews' neighbors.

Moses was one of these divinely motivated "servants." He was born in Egypt at a time when the presiding Pharaoh was alarmed at the disproportion in population between the Egyptians and slaves (captives from conquests of hundreds of years) on the one hand, and between Egyptians and freemen, such as the Hebrews, on the other. The

[2]Jeremiah 7:25.

Pharaoh commanded that the Hebrew birth rate must decrease. The first suggestion was to engage the men in a building project at which they were whipped and treated cruelly, becoming physically exhausted. When this proved unsuccessful, midwives were ordered to kill all Hebrew male offspring. Since this attempt at wholesale genocide failed, an order was issued to drown all Hebrew male babies in the river.

It was as a result of this order that at birth Moses was placed in the river in a waterproof reed basket and withdrawn from the water by the Pharaoh's daughter who raised him as her son in the best Egyptian tradition of the time.

He received a superior education for his era. Although his learning was obtained in a pagan atmosphere, his mother, who had been selected as nursemaid for him, inculcated in him the religious beliefs and traditions of his Hebrew family heritage.

Moses responded obediently to God's command to lead His people out of bondage but met with stubborn opposition from the Pharaoh. It was not until the tenth plague killed the first-born of each Egyptian family that the Pharaoh reluctantly released the Israelites.

Moses did not have a peaceful pilgrimage on this trip out of Egypt and onward toward the Promised Land. The Israelites complained constantly and vacillated between their religion and the practices of their polytheistic friends, including the worship of idols and carrying amulets as the Egyptians had done.[3] On Mount Sinai, God gave to Moses the *Ten Commandments* and the First Commandment was an injunction against this practice of worshiping false gods (Fig. 2–13). Yet, before Moses reached the foot of the mountain, the people had cajoled his brother Aaron into collecting all their golden jewelry to construct a golden calf or bull, which they promptly idolized. In fury and disappointment, Moses smashed the newly acquired Ten Commandments against a rock. A newly hewn set was kept in the Ark of the Covenant.

The Israelites were promised by God when they left Egypt that if they would obey His Commandments, He would protect them from disease.[4]

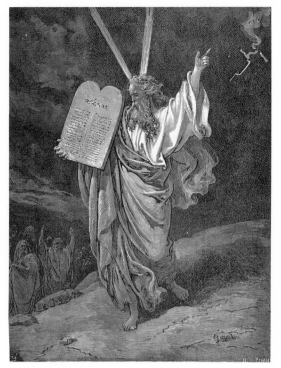

Figure 2–13. Moses comes down from Sinai.

If thou wilt diligently harken to the voice of the Lord, thy God, and wilt do that which is right in His sight, and wilt give ear to His commandments, and keep all His statutes, I will put none of these diseases upon thee, which I have brought upon the Egyptians; for I am the Lord that healeth thee.

The Ten Commandments embody the most important set of rules for ethical human relationships and provide an excellent frame of reference for mental health.

The Hebrews, realizing the need for strong unified action, believed that they were ready to establish a monarchy. The judge and prophet Samuel carried out the necessary plans. Saul was crowned king. He was successful at the beginning of his reign and then became subject to periods of melancholy and depression. David, a young shepherd and a gifted harpist, soothed Saul with relaxing music (Fig. 2–14). This is an early example of music therapy. Saul took his own life when he was unsuccessful in battle, and David succeeded him as king.

David, a personable young man, was admired and honored. The new capital, Jeru-

---

[3]Reference to the prohibition of carrying amulets is noted in *Genesis 31:30–35.*

[4]*Exodus 15:26.*

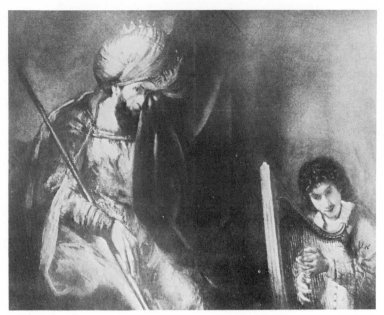

Figure 2–14. David playing before Saul to soothe and quiet him. Painting by Rembrandt van Rijn.

salem, was called the City of David. This brilliant leader was succeeded by his son, Solomon, whose famous temple replaced the portable tabernacle housing the Ark of the Covenant.

Mosaic Health Code

Many rules and regulations were propounded in regard to social and religious customs and health and sanitary practices. These are compiled in what is called the *Mosaic Code.* This code presents a systematic, organized method of the prevention of disease. It included principles of personal hygiene relating to such things as rest, sleep, hours for work and cleanliness, and included especially rules for women concerning menstruation and child bearing. Principles of public hygiene and sanitation are noted in the rules for the selection and inspection of food and for the slaughtering of animals for food, in the regulation of diet and disposal of excreta and garbage, and in the diagnosis and reporting of communicable diseases with concomitant isolation, quarantine and disinfection.

Moses did not include any Egyptian or Babylonian medical innovations in his code. It is remarkably scientific. He directed that

when a patient had a communicable disease, such as leprosy, the patient was to be *isolated* from the community.[5]

The rules for prevention of the spread of intestinal diseases (cholera, dysentery and typhoid fever) required that a spade be used to cover excretions after defecation.[6]

The difference between what was clean and what was unclean was delineated very clearly. Moses provided detailed instructions on the correct way to cleanse one's hands. Repeated washings in running water with a time lapse for drying in the sun were recommended.

A startlingly sound scientific injunction is the one related to circumcision. It identified the safest time to perform such an *operation,* ". . . and he that is eight days old shall be circumcised."[7]

The knowledge of the importance of animals in the transmission of disease is portrayed vividly in the story of the capture of the Ark of the Covenant by the Philistines who brought it to the temple of their god, Dagon.[8] Not only does the story describe the epidemic of bubonic plague, but it emphasizes

---

[5] Leviticus *13*:46.
[6] Deuteronomy *23*:12–13.
[7] Genesis *17*:12.
[8] Samuel *1*:5–6 (also called I Kings).

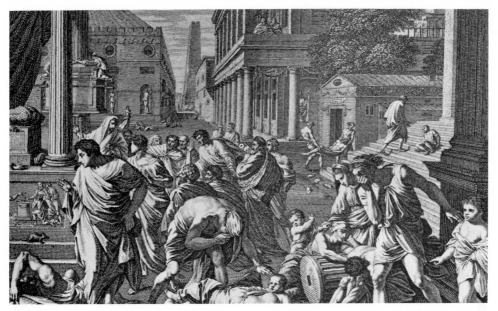

Figure 2–15. The Plague of Ashdod, by Poussin. The picture portrays the sudden onset and fatal nature of bubonic plague. Note the presence of rats.

the place of rodents as carriers of the disease (Fig. 2–15).

Sanitary legislation has been shown in the accounts of the cases of leprosy in which the afflicted were inspected, isolated and reinspected before being readmitted to the community. Diphtheria was one of the most dreaded diseases and when it occurred the horn (shofar) was blown to warn the community of this calamity.

The high priest was priest-physician and health inspector whom the Hebrew people were admonished to honor. Persons excluded from the community because of disease were compelled to secure permission from the priest-physician before returning; the cured leper was addressed by these words: "Go and show yourself to the high priest."

Each culture has left some evidence of the diseases with which it was visited, but the Bible has furnished as graphic a picture of the afflictions of this period as the Egyptian wall paintings and mummies presented. In addition to leprosy and diphtheria, dysentery, dropsy, apoplexy and mental illness have been mentioned; some of the treatments prescribed were circumcision, the use of fig poultices, artificial respiration and the use of music as therapy for mental illness.

The Bible presents an interesting description of the foods, food preservation and treatments of the ancient Hebrews. Grapes and figs were consumed as fresh products, preserved by drying, consumed as grape juice and drunk as wine after fermentation. Olives were a source of food and the oil was used both as food and medicine. Oil and wine were first-aid remedies. Food restrictions were clearly delineated. The methods of cooking revealed good health principles because they used boiling or roasting.

An early experiment in nutrition was recorded when Daniel requested the steward to feed him and his friends vegetables rather than the rich diet of the king. Daniel and his friends became "better in appearance and fatter in flesh."

The Hebrews appreciated the value of milk because their description of the promised land involves one "overflowing with milk and honey."

Houses of hospitality, forerunners of the later inns, hotels and hospitals, were plentiful. The Hebrews were exemplary in the practice of hospitality, for visiting and caring for the sick was a religious duty. A nurse's role included midwifery.

Today, many Jews adhere to the traditional practices laid down so carefully for them in this ancient period. Their fundamental laws of moral and physical conduct are found in the *Torah,* the Hebrew name for the first five books of the Old Testament, which are called the Pentateuch. The Torah, containing the written law, and the *Talmud,* embodying the complications of oral law, have been the accepted authority for Orthodox Jews everywhere.

The significance of the family as a social and religious unit is stressed today as it was in the time of Moses. The Biblical story of Ruth is an inspiring picture of family life. Ruth, a Moabite, married the son of a Hebrew couple and after her mother-in-law was bereft of her entire family, including Ruth's husband, Ruth extended to her this example of filial devotion:

Entreat me not to leave thee
Or to return from following after thee:
For whither thou goest
I will go;
And where thou lodgest
I will lodge:

Thy people shall be my people
And thy God my God. . . .

In summarizing the contributions of the ancient Hebrews, we recognize the gift of a deep spiritual, monotheistic faith, the basic concepts of bacteriology with the identification of that which is clean or unclean, isolation techniques to prevent the spread of communicable diseases, the prevention of many diseases because of adherence to the dietary regulations and the public health laws of the Mosaic Code.

The contributions of the first great civilizations reflect a high degree of empiricism, scientific observations in the clinical role of the doctors, obvious problem solving in the development of equipment to make patients more comfortable, and the inception of the field of public health, but no identifiable nurse or organizations of nurses other than the continued role of the individual capable, compassionate nurse figure—the mother.

REFERENCE READINGS

Albright, W. F.: *The Archaeology of Palestine.* Baltimore, Penguin Books, 1951.

Breasted, James H.: *The Conquest of Civilization.* New York, Harper & Brothers, 1938.

Elgood, Cyril: *A Medical History of Persia.* London, Cambridge University Press, 1951.

Everyday Life in Bible Times. Washington, D.C., National Geographic Society, 1967.

Grosvenor, Gilbert, et al.: *Everyday Life in Ancient Times.* Washington, D.C., National Geographic Society. (Many excellent illustrations.)

Heaton, E. W.: *Everyday Life in the Old Testament.* New York, Charles Scribners' Sons, 1956.

Leake, C. D.: *The Old Egyptian Medical Papyri.* Lawrence, University of Kansas Press, 1952.

McMillen, S. I.: *None of These Diseases.* Westwood, N.J., Fleming H. Revell Co., 1963.

Moodie, Roy Lee: *Paleopathology, An Introduction to the Study of Ancient Evidence of Disease.* Chicago, University of Illinois, 1923.

Morton, Henry: *Women of the Bible.* New York, Dodd, Mead & Co., 1941.

Oursler, Fulton: *The Greatest Book Ever Written.* New York, Doubleday & Co., 1951.

Renault, Mary: *The Bull from the Sea.* New York, Pantheon Books, 1962.

Renault, Mary: *The King Must Die.* New York, Pantheon Books, 1958.

Smith, C. Raimer: *The Physician Examines the Bible.* New York, Philosophical Library, 1950.

Steuer, R. O., and Saunders, J. B. de C. M.: *Ancient Egyptian and Cnidian Medicine.* Berkeley & Los Angeles, University of California Press, 1959.

Thorwald, Jürgen: *Science and Secrets of Early Medicine.* New York, Harcourt, Brace, and World, Inc., 1963.

Waltari, Mika: *The Egyptian.* New York, G. P. Putnam's Sons, 1949.

Weinreb, Nathaniel: *The Babylonians.* New York, Doubleday & Co., 1953.

Wells, Calvin: *Bones, Bodies, and Disease.* New York, Frederick A. Praeger, 1964.

Woolley, Leonard: *History Unearthed.* London, Ernest Benn Ltd., 1963.

CHAPTER 3

Influence of Ancient Cultural Practices on Health Care (Part II)

THE ANCIENT AMERICANS

The coming of the Santa Maria, Pinta and Nina to our shores prompted historians to write books about the "New" World, but they were actually additional chapters in the overall history of the Americas. We have become cognizant of the fact that highly developed cultures had flourished in the Western Hemisphere before Columbus, before the Spanish conquistadors and even before the arrival of the Norsemen. Hermann states that "it may be assumed with some certainty that highly evolved cultures flourished on the soil of the New World from 2000 to 1000 B.C., but that is all we do know for sure."[1]

There are still many questions to be answered by historians and archeologists. Until these questions are answered, attention is focused on only three of the rediscovered cultural groups that existed in Central and South America: the Mayas, Incas and Aztecs.

The *Mayan* Indians were supposed to have occupied the Yucatan peninsula from about 2500 B.C. to about 1600 A.D., but the earliest certain date is 320 A.D. Rediscovery of their ancient cities began in 1839. Archeological investigation has revealed that the people were skilled in astronomy, art and mathematics, and produced an excellent calendar.

Yucatan, the center of the Mayan culture, and Guatemala are unbelievably rich in ruins. Pyramids and other architectural feats are being extracted from primeval jungles. The curious hieroglyphic inscriptions on the

Mayan ruins have not been deciphered completely, but many legends have been recounted of the early customs of the people. One of these explained that in times of stress, processions of people wended their way to the Sacred Well of Sacrifice. Their objective was to placate the irate gods with offerings of beautiful maidens and captive youths. At the termination of the ceremonies, the maidens were thrown into the Sacred Well, and the youths killed on the sacrificial blocks.

Mayan religious practices centered around human sacrifice. One form of sacrifice was the removal of the hearts of adults, and in another children were sacrificed. The ceremonies were presided over by either the high priest or members of the priesthood. In addition to this duty, the priests were also soothsayers, medical advisors and herbalists.

The custom of skull deformation was common among the Mayas (Fig. 3–1). Four or five days after birth, children were placed face downward and one board was tied to the back of the head and one to the forehead. These were bound tightly together so that the head was compressed upward. The Mayan stone cutters depict this condition and show the receding forehead that forms a continuous line with the nose (Cf. Fig. 3–2).

Little is known about Mayan medical practices, although one custom involved the medicinal use of *sweat baths*.

The *Aztecs* were an aggressive, war-like group ruling central Mexico at the time of the Spanish Conquest.

Mexico City stands on the remains of the Aztec kingdom. Not far from the city, the Pyramids of the Sun and Moon can be viewed;

[1]Hermann, Paul: *Conquest by Man.* New York, Harper & Brothers, 1954, p. 188.

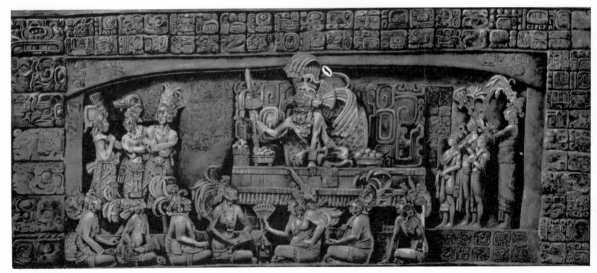

Figure 3–1. A Mayan relief that shows a chief or high priest conducting a conference. The natural setting and realistic expression are executed superbly. Note the hieroglyphs forming the border and the deformation of the heads of the members. (Courtesy of University Museum, Philadelphia.)

these pyramids of ancient America functioned as temples for religious ceremonies.

One religious practice of the Aztecs required human sacrifice in an atrocious form. At the climax of a ceremony the living heart was excised from the bodies of a thousand or more victims. When Cortés asked Montezuma's permission to visit one of the temples,

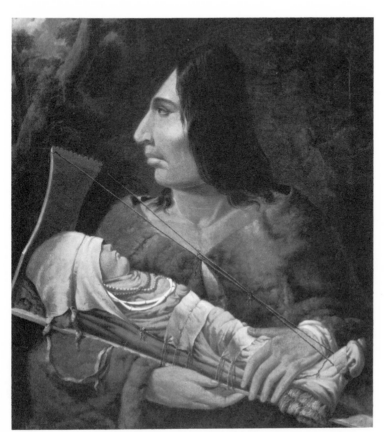

Figure 3–2. "Caw-Wacham" by Paul Kane (1810–1872). Note deformation of the mother's head and the technique employed to reshape the head of the baby. The board used for reshaping is concealed under the chamois that is tied to the frame of the cradleboard. (Courtesy of The Montreal Museum of Fine Arts.)

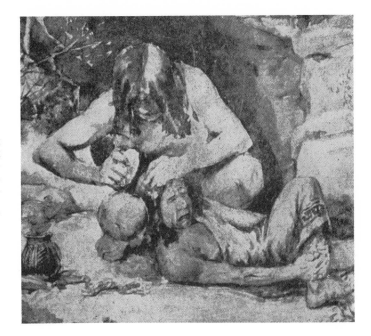

Figure 3–3. An ancient Peruvian trepanning operation. In the sketch a hole is being made in the skull into which the oil, heating in the clay pot, will be introduced. To produce sedation, the operator applies coca juice into the affected area from the coca leaves that he chews. (Courtesy of R. L. Moodie. Reproduced from *Paleopathology*.)

he observed the block on which these sacrificial victims were slaughtered with an obsidian or volcanic glass knife.

The Aztecs had great faith in sweat baths and many sweat houses, or "temascals," have been found.

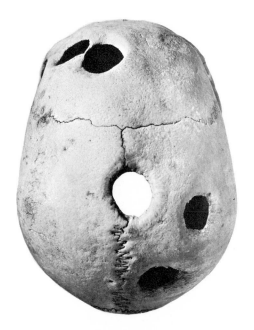

Figure 3–4. A trepanned skull from Peru. (Courtesy of Peabody Museum of Yale University, New Haven.)

The *Inca Empire* was located in Peru. The Incas were skilled engineers and provided themselves with a remarkable system of roads and suspension bridges; they also left evidence of medical prowess. Their outstanding medical technique was trepanning; they were noted also for their skillful cranial bandaging (Figs. 3–3, 3–4 and 3–5).

The many physical afflictions with which man was seized at this time were attributed to the displeasure of the gods. Tribute to the gods took the form of a pottery or stone effigy ("huaco") of the sick person (Fig. 3–6). Many of these effigies have been found and, along with skeletal remains, assist us in understanding the pathological conditions which prevailed in Central and South America.

Remarkably creative case studies have been preserved in these clay figurines, which have resulted in a unique artistic record of patient care. These figurines may well have been used as teaching models to assist a person learning the skills of patient care. They may have been brought to a teaching medical clinic where a diagnosis could be determined (Fig. 3–7). Because of the terrain of the country, bringing the patient to the clinic was not feasible, but bringing a teaching model was an acceptable solution.

Beds seemed to be individual in design, with canopies for protection from the sun, elevations for protection from the ground, and separations in the webbing of the frame-

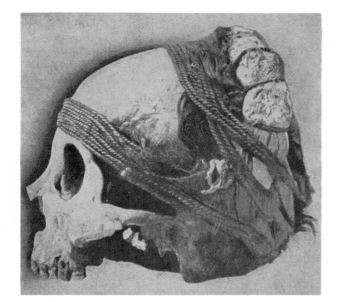

Figure 3–5. An old Peruvian skull showing a trepanation bandage. This specimen is now in the San Diego Museum of Man.

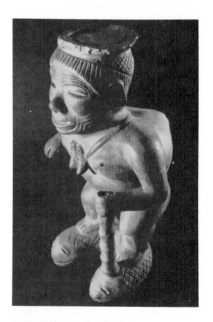

Figure 3–6. Clay figurine depicting disease among pre-Columbian Indians of Central and South America. (Courtesy of Howard Dittrick Museum, Cleveland Medical Library Association.)

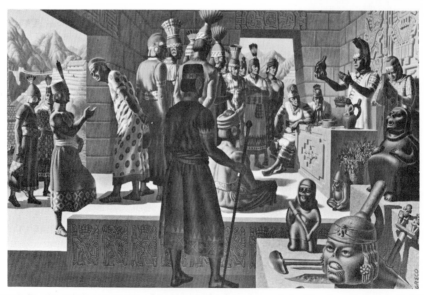

Figure 3–7. An artist's conception of an Inca medical teaching clinic. (Courtesy of *Lederle Bulletin*.)

work of the bed to permit the passage of excretions.

The usual posture for delivering babies was in the squatting position and many clay figurines verify this.

Diseases were prevalent and many marked evidences have been observed. Treatments abounded, including bloodletting, cupping or sucking, massage, sweating, splinting, setting of bones, tooth extracting, amputation, suturing, bandaging, poulticing, and trepanning.

Displeasure of the gods was an accepted concept of the cause of disease. Shamans were active as medicine men. The magic rite of transference of disease to animals was part of the care of the sick.

Herbs were administered for emetics, laxatives, purges, diuretics and for the relief of respiratory distress. Poisons were known and used. Cobwebs were utilized, very much as they were by the ancient Egyptians, to encourage coagulation of blood in wounds.

Cupping was the sucking or drawing out of a foreign object by the use of a hollowed out horn. Many of these treatments were performed only by the medicine man.

The use of sweat baths or sweat huts held a prominent place in the mores of the various groups of American Indians. Methods of achieving the objectives of the bath varied with each group. Most frequently it consisted of pouring or sprinkling water over very hot stones that were enclosed within an airtight structure or hut.

Some groups incorporated the use of aromatic substances in the procedure; others beat their bodies with bunches of twigs to stimulate the circulation of the blood and hasten the sweating process. Many Indians terminated the bath with a quick plunge into cold water or by rolling in the snow.

The sun god was worshiped by ancient American groups, especially the Iroquois, Aztecs and Incas. The therapeutic value of heat as well as light may have been recognized.

Several colorful customs persist; one of these embodies art in the therapeutic plan of *sand painting*. Medicine men have been skilled in the creation of these intricate designs, which were made specifically for an individual and a special occasion. They were most useful in the ceremony for the healing of an illness (Fig. 3–8).

The medicine man gathered many varieties of colored sand and crushed minerals. He carried out his plan by the skillful maneuvering of his thumb and forefinger, which permitted a trickle of sand to follow the predetermined pattern of the painting. Strange but beautiful pictures developed on the natural-colored sand background. They had great religious significance and the medicine

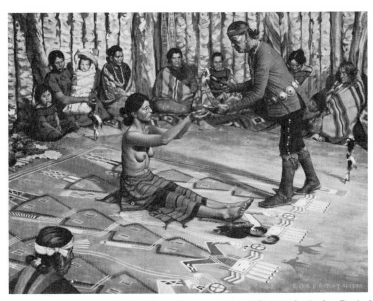

Figure 3–8. Artist's representation of a healing ceremony. (© 1957 by Parke, Davis & Co.)

man endeavored to seek healing through this painting.

In addition to the sand painting, a technique of hypnotherapy was integrated into the healing ceremony. The shaman sought to excite the senses. The picturesque sand painting appealed to the *sense of sight;* the ritual of the prayerful chant energized the *sense of hearing* (similar to a primitive lullaby); the feathers touched to the patient's body stimulated the *sense of touch;* the sweet-smelling herbs placed in the fire released an incense that was directed to the *sense of smell;* and herbs given to be consumed spurred the *sense of taste.*

During the ceremony the patient was the center of attention: he absorbed this loving attention. Faith on the part of patient, shaman and participating friends was an important ingredient in this ceremony.

These colorful designs were made on the floor of a hogan or a specially built medicine hut. At termination of the elaborate ceremony, the medicine man destroyed the paint-

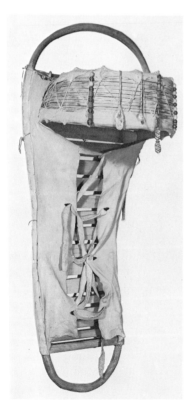

Figure 3–9. Apache baby carrier or cradleboard. Note bead and feather charms to ward off evil spirits. (Courtesy of Museum of the American Indian.)

ing, gathered the sand and scattered it to the four corners of the earth.

Another interesting custom has been the use of *cradleboards* (Fig. 3–9). Navajo babies have two types of cradles. The first is a canopy cradle or "face cover," which is a protective shield from dust and other disturbing elements. When the baby appears to be able to survive, a second and more durable cradleboard is built by the father. Because of the Navajos' superstitious nature, it was customary not to make preparations for a new baby until the need was assured.

There are many styles of cradleboards. The father may use one flat board, two boards strapped together or slats attached to a frame. Blankets are tucked inside the outer animal skins that are laced and into this the baby is tied securely and comfortably. Cradleboards can be plain or ornate, can be free of ornamentation or have articles to ward off evil spirits in the form of beads, silver or turquoise charms or animal feathers and tails.

The cradleboard is made to be carried on the back of the mother or propped against a sturdy object. This places the baby on eye level with the members of the family who sit around on the floor of the hogan. This seems to establish his presence as part of the family and increase his feeling of security.

On the Indian reservations in the United States today, many of the primitive customs are still practiced, although some have been prohibited by the United States government. For example, in 1883 the government forbade the practice of torture that accompanied participation in the Sun Dance. In some areas of the United States, snake cults flourish, but are looked upon with disfavor when the followers of the cult are severely or fatally poisoned.

In July, 1955, the responsibility for Indian health was transferred from the Bureau of Indian Affairs to the U.S. Public Health Service in the Department of Health, Education and Welfare. Thus, more doctors will be available to care for a people still very much intrigued by the prestige of the medicine man and his practices.

CONTRIBUTIONS OF THE ANCIENT CHINESE

China, the fabled middle kingdom, is one of the oldest and most innovative cultures in world history. Its artistic and technological achievements span a period of several millennia. The exact origin of the Chinese peoples remains a mystery because of the absence of accurate records predating the Shang dynasty, *ca.* 1776–1122 B.C.

The three early religions in China had an influence on the development of patient care. *Taoism* and *Confucianism* were indigenous to China; *Buddhism* was imported from India. Underlying these religions has been China's *primitive folk religion.*

Taoism, dating from the sixth century B.C., combined magic and mysticism and emphasized the value of charms in combatting the demons of disease. Usually these charms were written on paper, burnt and the ashes administered in tea, hot water or some medicinal liquid. Then other charms were distributed around the house and carried on the person's body. Later Taoists, searching for the elixir of life and the transmutation of base metals into gold, adopted the study of *alchemy.* In its truer significance, alchemy became the chemistry of the Middle Ages, and from this medieval science modern chemistry grew.

After Confucius' time (551–479 B.C.), every aspect of Chinese culture and society carried the stamp of his teaching. *Confucianism* stressed solidarity of the family, respect for elders, veneration of scholars and village government by elders. It encouraged the already existing belief in *ancestor worship,* which, carried to extremes, handicapped scientific investigation by preventing the dissection of bodies and resulted in a lack of knowledge of anatomy, physiology, pathology and surgery. It was not until 1913 A.D. that legal permission was granted for the performance of autopsies in China.

Progress in medical thinking had been thwarted by the worship of ancient physicians. In fact, as late as 1734 A.D. all court physicians and medical college officials were required to be present at a sacrificial ceremony at which the following prayer was recited:

Great are the virtues of the ancients. They established the art of medicine to relieve suffering humanity. On this day we offer these animals as sacrifice. May the merciful gods drive away all disease, protect our bodies and grant peace to the country![2]

---

[2]Wong and Wu: *History of Chinese Medicine.* Shanghai, China, National Quarantine Service, 1936, p. 185.

Buddhism presented a negative approach to the healing art. It taught that sin was the cause of disease and was sent by the gods. Thus, one was not encouraged to cure an affliction. In some oriental countries a devout Buddhist will not eat milk or eggs. The killing of animals or anything with potential for life such as eggs is sinful. Dogs and monkeys roam the streets and wards of the hospital unimpeded. Lice are removed from the body with care but not killed. Begging is encouraged because this aids a person in working out salvation for a better next life and thus rehabilitation is not an accepted plan for patient care. Buddhists offer to Buddha a golden replica of the diseased part of the body and place it at the statue of Buddha in the Temple. In Thailand the temple elephant is sacred.

These three religions were superimposed on the fundamental Chinese primitive beliefs in universal animism. Basic to the Chinese healing arts have been the usual superstitious practices of sacrificial offerings, frightening evil spirits by beating gongs and shooting off firecrackers and the acceptance of the most bitter medicines offered by the Chinese medicine man.

The *yang* and *yin* theory established some scientific basis for disease. The yang was the male principle, positive, desirable, active, fiery and full of life in contrast to the yin, or female principle, negative, cold, weak, dark and lifeless. Life consisted of the interaction of these principles. When they were in equilibrium one was healthy; when there was an improper balance one suffered discomfort and disease.

It is obvious that the undesirable aspects of this theory were associated with the female. This was in keeping with the traditionally subordinate social position of the Chinese female.

Many female babies were abandoned at birth and the project of rescuing them was undertaken by Christian missionaries. Notable among these was *Candida,* who, together with her grandfather, the Prime Minister, was converted to Catholicism in the sixteenth century by Jesuit priests. Candida bought a large estate and used it to lodge and care for the abandoned infants. She and many like her cared for these unwanted children.

An undesirable Chinese custom was the practice of foot deformation, or the binding of the feet of female babies.

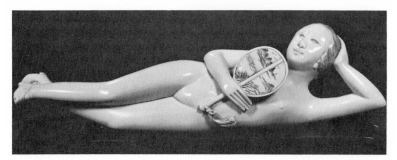

Figure 3–10. A carved ivory figurine upon which the female patient marked where she had pain. Note the foot deformation. (From author's collection.)

It was against Chinese custom for a woman to be undressed in the presence of a physician, nor might he examine her. Ivory or alabaster figurines were kept in the homes of the higher class. The Chinese medicine man carried with him a less ornate one for patients who did not possess one. The point of discomfort was marked on the figurine and carried to the physician for his diagnosis and recommended treatment (Fig. 3–10).

The influence of the *evil eye* on babies was a source of worry for parents; therefore, male babies were given female names and dressed as girls in the hope that evil spirits would be less interested in afflicting the baby.

Very little mention has been made of the counterpart of the hospital in ancient China. Wong and Wu list the founding of so-called

Halls of Healing by 651 B.C.; Berdoe[3] indicates that the absence of such institutions was because the Chinese people would consider themselves remiss in their duty to family and relatives if they did not take care of them at home.

The founder of Chinese medicine is considered to be the legendary emperor *Shên Nung,* said to have been responsible for careful investigation of medicinal herbs (Fig. 3–11). He was supposed to have experimented on himself, thus discovering a large number of drugs, including poisonous ones. The results of his research were allegedly compiled in the *Pen Tsao* or the Herbal.

---

[3]Berdoe, Edward: *The Origin and Growth of The Healing Art.* London, Swan, Sonnenschein & Co., 1893, p. 130.

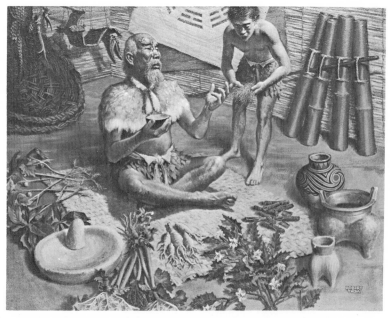

Figure 3–11. Shen Nung and pharmacy in ancient China. (© 1951 by Parke, Davis & Co.)

Huang-ti, the legendary Yellow Emperor, has been credited with having written *Neiching,* the canon of medicine. According to the Neiching there were four steps in determining a diagnosis: observation, auscultation, interrogation and palpation (look, listen, ask and feel). Palpation referred mainly to examination of the pulse, which was of prime importance. The Chinese were skilled at understanding the pulse and its variations in health and disease.

Both the Pen Tsao and the Neiching were done in lacquer upon strips of bamboo or palm leaves and exhibited the ideographic tadpole characters analogous to Egyptian picture writing.

Among the most celebrated Chinese physicians of the Han dynasty (206 B.C.–221 A.D.) were: *Ts'ang Kung,* first century B.C., who kept records of personal observations that have been considered remarkable case histories; *Chang Chung-ching,* second century A.D., who left important records and suggestions for medical treatment; and *Hua T'O,* second century A.D., a renowned surgeon who discovered and used anesthetics for the operations he performed. Surgeons, however, were not considered on so high a plane as physicians.

Historians agree that the Chinese were ingenious in developing the field of medical therapeutics. Moxa, cupping, cautery, massage and puncture were practiced as far back as the Stone Age. Wong and Wu say that the Neiching stressed "When the seat of the trouble is in the muscles employ puncture; in the blood vessels, use moxa; in the tendons, apply cautery."[4] In making punctures "needles" were used. These were originally made of flint, but later were changed to metal as a result of improvements in the manufacture of instruments in the Copper and Bronze Ages. These needles have been found in the country districts where another custom has been noted, using broken pieces of pottery instead of scissors in cutting the umbilical cord of newborn babies. Needling occupied a rather important position in ancient times. It developed into the art of acupuncture. This highly specialized branch of Chinese medicine has been considered a universal

---

[4] *Op. cit.,* pp. 2–3.

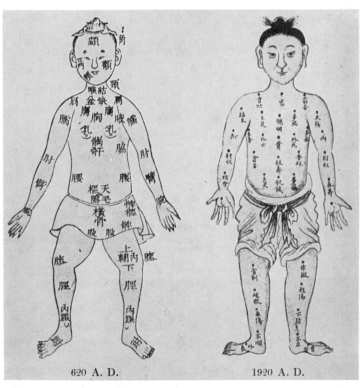

620 A. D.   1920 A. D.

Figure 3–12. Chinese acupuncture diagrams. (Courtesy of Dr. E. V. Cowdry.)

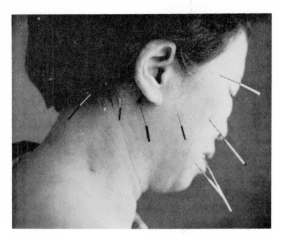

Figure 3–13. Acupuncture being used to relieve facial paralysis.

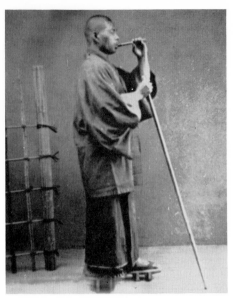

Figure 3–15. Blind man who performs massage blowing whistle as he goes through the street to announce his presence. (Courtesy of Peabody Museum of Salem, Mass.)

panacea. *Acupuncture* has consisted of inserting needles for an inch or so with a twisting motion into a designated area (Fig. 3–12). The old method of acupuncture has been refined to a new method of therapeutic acupuncture which consists of hand manipulation of the needles with an up-and-down and concurrent twirling motion between the thumb and index finger. (See Figures 3–13 and 3–14.) In addition, there has been an increased acceptance of acupuncture as a form of anesthesia. Research is being conducted to determine the possible existence of some anatomical structure which would explain the traditional channels or meridians which were first described in written and diagrammatic form many centuries ago. Western medicine has been integrated with the traditional arts of acupuncture and herbal therapy in present-day China. What may be the first use of acupuncture for anesthesia in the United States is described in a letter to the editor of the *Journal of the*

American Medical Association reporting on anesthesia for a tonsillectomy.[5]

Massage evolved out of the natural impulse to rub, soothe and stroke an injured or painful spot. The Chinese developed this ability to an extraordinary degree and used a modern vocational rehabilitation method of employing blind masseurs (Fig. 3–15).

Moxa, a very painful form of counterirritation, involved the application of ignited cones of mugwort to the skin. The smoldering fire burned the skin gradually, causing blisters to form.

Specific medicines and treatments were devised for prevalent diseases (Fig. 3–16). Leprosy has been known from earliest times

---

[5] Liu, Wei-Chi: Acupuncture anesthesia: a case report. J.A.M.A., *221*:87–88, July 3, 1972.

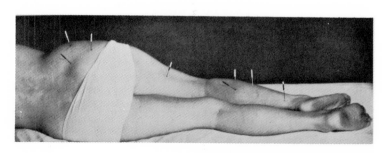

Figure 3–14. The position of the patient and insertion of acupuncture needles for the treatment of sciatica.

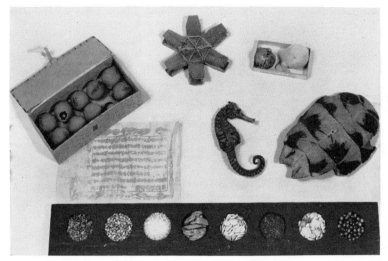

Figure 3–16. Exhibit of Chinese drugs. (Courtesy of Peabody Museum of Salem, Mass.)

and chaulmoogra oil has been used in its treatment. Medicinal seaweed, rich in iodine, was mixed with bouillon to combat goiter. Animal organs such as liver and thyroid glands were used. The poppy gave up its precious content of opium because of the careful scrutiny of the Chinese. The herb, Ma Huang, was found to possess an important alkaloid, ephedrine. An ingenious method of extracting the potent medicinal value of herbs and drugs was accomplished in the *Chinese medicine cooker*. The herb or drug was placed in the center section of the cooker and around it was banked live charcoal; the heat released the beneficial properties.

Opium and its derivatives have long been used to relieve pain. Widespread drug abuse plagued China until well into the twentieth century. In recent years the Chinese Communists have sought, with much success, to eliminate the social use of opium and other narcotics.

Toads were used in the formation of plasters and were applied to carbuncles, boils, ulcers, sites of dog bites and inflammations of all kinds. The secretion of toads contains adrenalin.

"Spirits of hartshorn" (ammonia water) was another contribution of the Chinese. Originally, spirits of ammonia was obtained by the destructive distillation of the horns and hoofs of animals.

The most famous herbal medicine is ginseng, a plant so rare and highly valued

that it has been reported as selling for more than $4000 a pound.[6] It can be distinguished from similar vegetation only by its glow in the dark.

Other medicines that have remained popular through the centuries include ingredients of crickets, toad tears, snakes, horns of a special rhinoceros from India or Nepal, lizards, seahorses, tigers' bones immersed in wine and many other substances.

The shell of the tortoise has been used for purposes of divination down through the centuries. The hollow undersurface was brushed with ink and turned upside down (convex side downward) over a flame until the ink coating dried and crackled into line patterns. These were interpreted by those who had special abilities to read the message of the spirits.

Another form of divination, which was consulted to determine the prognosis of a patient's condition, was the *witch ball* (Fig. 3–17). This is an intricately carved ivory Cantonese magic ball that reveals rare beauty and an ingenious and skilled craftsmanship. As many as 12 ivory balls fit inside one another, and the stars, constellations and astrological influences are incorporated into their design. By inspecting this work of art, a prognosis was made.

---

[6] Durdin, Peggy: "Medicine in China: a revealing story." *New York Times Magazine*, February 28, 1960, p. 76.

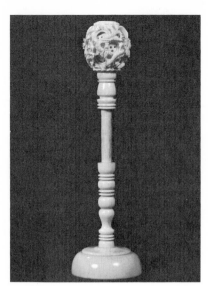

Figure 3–17. A carved ivory witch ball used for divination. (From author's collection.)

People in the East also recognized the value of moist heat. Hot mineral baths as well as burying patients up to their necks in hot sand packs were popular.

Drugs were carried in an *inro*, a box consisting of several compartments or sections, each of which contained vials of medicine

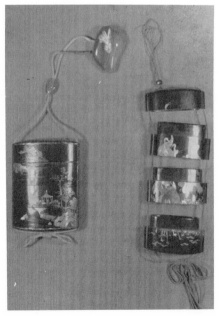

Figure 3–18. Two Inros — medicine boxes — one opened to show the drug compartments. (Courtesy of Peabody Museum of Salem, Mass.)

(Fig. 3–18). These were fastened to the belts of the medicine men.

Smallpox was described in the third century A.D. and a method of *vaccination* was devised. Smallpox scabs were ground into a powder and blown through bamboo tubes into the nostrils. Frequently the undergarment of a child afflicted with smallpox was worn by a healthy child for two or three days. Concomitant with the scientific advancement of smallpox vaccination was the superstitious practice of a child wearing a very ugly mask to ward off the deity of smallpox.

In studying the contributions of the ancient Chinese we are aware of the paradox of a deeply superstitious yet highly gifted and civilized culture that gave us valuable knowledge of drugs as well as other acceptable medical treatments. Many of these Chinese medical practices were adopted by the Koreans, the Japanese and other Orientals.

China's vast body of traditional medical lore is among the most ancient. Today, Chinese doctors have revived an increasing number of the ancient medical practices.

CONTRIBUTIONS OF THE ANCIENT HINDUS

The triangular subcontinent of India has been host to civilization for thousands of years. Natural barriers of mountains and seas have isolated India from the rest of the world and encouraged the growth of an indigenous culture.

As early as 2000 B.C. tribal Aryans from the Iranian plateau settled on the plains of India. They either subjugated the natives or drove them out into the mountains and desert plains, and by 1500 B.C. these settlers had established themselves in the valley of the Ganges.

Between 1000 and 800 B.C. there was a struggle between the ruling class and the priestly caste for supremacy in India. Thence evolved the idea of Brahma, the eternal spirit, and the religion of *Brahmanism* (also called Hinduism) which affirms the doctrine of the transmigration of the living soul, namely, its passage into the body of a higher or lower form after physical death according to past conduct. Hinduism is the most widely accepted of the religions of India. In common practice, worship or devotion is directed to one or more of the deities comprising the Trimūrti or divine Triad: Brahma, source and giver of life; Vishnu, the preserver; and Siva, the destroyer.

The territory of the Jumna and Ganges Rivers is sacred to the Hindus, and every twelve years on certain days selected by astrologers, the faithful come to these rivers to bathe and wash away their sins. When one feels the approach of death, it is that person's greatest desire to go or to be taken to Benares, a city on the Ganges, to participate in this religious bathing. At death, the bodies are placed on funeral pyres in Benares, cremated, and the ashes sprinkled on the Ganges.

Since this religion has advocated ancestor worship and reverence for animals, especially cows and monkeys, it has been a sacrilege to eat products from these animals. From earliest times, hospitals were built to care for animals.

The oldest scriptures of Hinduism are the Vedas (*ca.* 1500 B.C.) written in Vedic, the parent language of Sanskrit; these are the historical documents of India and are also of religious significance. The Hindus say that these four books, Rig-Veda, Yajur-Veda, Sama-Veda and Atharva-Veda, were given to Brahma originally. The Rig-Veda (*ca.* 1500 B.C.) contains suggestions for medical treatment by the use of herbs and incantations.

Two of the best-loved Hindu scriptures have been the Bhagavad-Gita (Song of God) and the Upanishads, a group of poetic dialogues on metaphysics written after the Vedas and largely commentaries on them. The Upanishads endeavored to impart knowledge of ultimate reality.

Temples have been of importance in the life of the people of the East and they have been masterpieces of artistry. Contemplation and meditation have occupied much attention and there have been many followers of the monastic way of life.

Yoga has been a method of "yoking" of an individual's soul to the Supreme Being. This mystical experience of spiritual detachment from one's surroundings has involved certain exercises. Bodily purity, attained by purgation and bathing, is followed by concentration of thought on one subject with the purpose of excluding worldly diversions. The values of certain yoga postures, breathing exercises, breath control and concentration as well as relaxation have been noted by health authorities in recent years.

Siddhartha Gautama (*ca.* 566?–483 B.C.), the son of a northern Indian warrior-king, attained enlightenment (*ca.* 531 B.C.) and as Buddha ("the enlightened") introduced a new religious philosophy which came to be known as Buddhism. This religion offered a chance to escape the all-pervading self-denial of Brahmanism by calling on believers to extinguish the falsehood of worldly desire, thus opening the road to the "passionless peace" of Nirvāna. *King Asoka* of India (269–237 B.C.) became a convert to Buddhism, but he was unsuccessful in fostering its acceptance on a permanent basis. He has been credited with the construction of hospitals, especially for pilgrims.

There were two renowned physicians in ancient India, Charaka and Susruta. Both of these men collected medical information into a compendium or samhita. *Charaka,* in the second century A.D., presented in a clear, understandable fashion the ethical standards required for those who cared for the sick. Volume I, section xv of his samhita emphasized that the men who were assistants should be "of good behavior, distinguished for purity, possessed of cleverness and skill, imbued with kindness, skilled in every service a patient may require, competent to cook food, skilled in bathing and washing the patient, rubbing and massaging the limbs, lifting and assisting him to walk about, well skilled in the making and cleansing of beds, readying the patient and skillful in waiting upon one that is ailing and never unwilling to do anything that may be ordered." There was a realization of the need for a skilled person to be at the patient's side.

Susruta, who lived about the fifth century A.D., described diseases, medicinal plants, procedures relating to surgery and some 121 different surgical instruments. Among those mentioned were scalpels, lancets, scissors, saws, needles, forceps, catheters and syringes. Hindu surgeons were familiar with amputation, cauterization (with boiling oil and pressure), delivery by cesarean section, and the removal of cataracts and brain tumors (Fig. 3–19). They were especially skilled in such plastic surgery as skin grafting and rhinoplasty (or nasal reconstruction). The need for this latter type of surgery arose out of the custom of amputating the nose as a form of punishment. According to Susruta, a

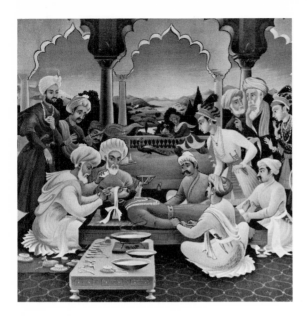

Figure 3–19. Artist's representation of Hindu surgeons performing a trepanation on King Bhoja of Dhar. A brain tumor was removed and the patient survived. Patient had been sedated or under the effect of tranquilizers. (Courtesy of *Lederle Bulletin*.)

surgeon would cut a leaf of a tree to the size of the missing nose, apply this pattern to the cheek and cut a piece of skin of the same size. This tissue was then sewed to the stump of the nose. To facilitate breathing a tube was inserted into each nostril (Fig. 3–20).

Susruta also described the plastic surgery operation for the correction of an ear lobe deformity. Plastic surgery was carried out by specialists who belonged to a caste of potters known as Koomas. They were skilled at reconstruction and used their hands as sculptors and pottery makers did; thus the public associated them with these working groups.

The method of teaching students of surgery is presented most interestingly by Garrison:

Realizing the importance of rapid, dexterous incision in operations without anesthesia, they had the student begin by practising upon plants. The hollow stalks of water-lilies or the veins of large leaves were punctured and lanced, as well as the blood vessels of dead animals. Gourds, cucumbers, and other soft fruits or leather bags filled with water, were taped or incised in lieu of hydrocele or any other disorder of a hollow cavity. Flexible models were used for bandaging and amputations and the plastic operations were practised upon dead animals. In so teaching the student to acquire ease and surety in operating by "going through the motions," the Hindus were

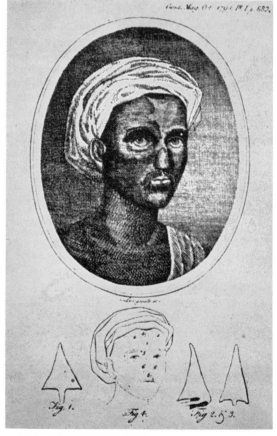

Figure 3–20. Indian rhinoplasty showing details of the technique of nasal reconstruction.

pioneers of many recent wrinkles on the didactic side of experimental surgery.[7]

Another reason for this careful practice might have been the fine a doctor was compelled to pay if he caused injury to a patient.

Many diseases such as diabetes and tuberculosis were described, as were the transmitters of certain diseases, such as rats in plague and mosquitoes in malaria. To forestall the spread of malaria, Marco Polo described the Hindus' use of mosquito netting. Vaccination was employed to prevent smallpox, and the narcotic effects of certain drugs such as hyoscyamus and cannabis indica in surgical anesthesia were noted.

There has been a resurgence of interest in the Ayurvedic medicine and many aspects of this type of medical care have been taught with so-called modern scientific methods. Several herbs that have been mainstays in the medical regime of the medicine man have become modern discoveries in other parts of the world. One such remedy prescribed by ancient Hindu medicine men for hysteria and nervousness was the plant rauwolfia from which is extracted the modern drug reserpine, popularly known as a tranquilizer.

By 1774 Great Britain had established colonial preeminence in India, having checked French aspirations to that end during the preceding decades. Many of the native customs were forbidden by the British and gradually disappeared because of legislation. Several of these customs pertain to women. The Sarda Act, passed by Indian Legislature in 1930, penalizes marriages unless the wife is 14 years of age, although child marriages from the age of eight are noted. Another recalcitrant custom is known as *purdah;* this is the practice of keeping women in seclusion and serves to retard social, physical and mental development. *Suttee,* or the burning of a widow on her deceased husband's funeral pyre, as well as the practice of throwing infants into the Ganges, has been forbidden.

It is in the area of teaching methods and surgery that the ancient Hindus left their greatest contribution to medicine.

THE ANCIENT GREEKS

Many of the ancient empires had disintegrated. Clinging to tradition, they failed to introduce innovation and improvements of old methods, such as agriculture, into their societies. An infusion of new ideas was needed to release stored energy and channel it into constructive ways of improving the health of society.

The Greeks took the important step forward and provided leadership in many creative aspects of life, including art, philosophy, medicine and the biological sciences.

The records of ancient Greece are deeply intertwined with such legends as one finds in Homer's *Iliad* and *Odyssey.* A combination of facile pen and vivid imagination was believed responsible for these epic poems until the German archeologist Heinrich Schliemann (*ca.* 1876) excavated the site of ancient Troy and brought a sense of reality to the well-known tales.

The Olympic games furnished a unifying force because producing participants with healthy bodies was the aim of every family in Greece.

A pantheon of gods and goddesses furnished the Greeks' religious motivation, and a profound veneration for these gods was noted from earliest history. *Apollo,* the sun god, was the *god of health* and his son, *Asklepios,*[8] who may have been a human and deified after death, has been considered the *god of medicine.*

Asklepios has been represented as holding the staff of the traveler intertwined with the serpent of wisdom. The present-day medical symbol, the *caduceus,* is patterned after this representation. Two of the daughters of Asklepios are deities: *Hygeia,* the goddess of health (Fig. 3–21), and *Panacea,* the goddess of medications. The identifications of these two goddesses proved that the Greeks had recognized the need for keeping people healthy. This health maintenance was separate from medicine as was the area concerned with the preparation of medications.

The Greeks had implicit faith in the gods and before making important decisions consulted them at one of the Oracles. The shrine of Apollo at *Delphi* was one of the most famous Oracles. The gods were supposed to communicate their answers in one of four ways: delivered orally by priests and priestesses; made known by signs; presented in

[7]Garrison, Fielding: *An Introduction to the History of Medicine.* Philadelphia, W. B. Saunders Co., 1929, p. 72.

[8]Asklepios is the oldest spelling. Asclepius is found more frequently than is the Latin form, Aesculapius.

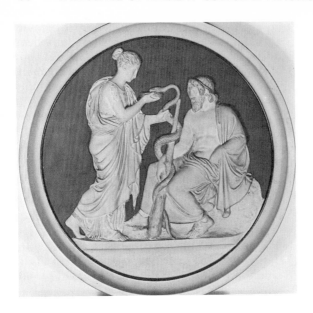

Figure 3–21. Aesculapius and Hygeia. This plaque is a copy of one by Thorwaldsen made in 1810. It represents Hygeia offering some food to her father's serpent. (From author's collection.)

the form of dreams; or communicated directly with spirits.

Asklepios gave his counsel in the form of dreams, which were interpreted in turn by the priests in the temple. One of the chief temples erected in his honor was *Epidaurus,* a famous medical center of Greece, which was similar to a very fashionable present-day health resort. The temple was an architectural masterpiece, built on a high hill with a magnificent view. The grounds afforded scenic walks, an outdoor theater, gymnasia and baths of invigorating mineral waters. On arrival, the patient sacrificed an animal to Asklepios, received a purifying bath in the mineral spring followed by massage, and then went to sleep on one of the porches, surrounded by sweet odors and

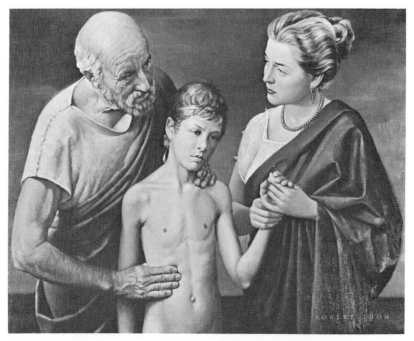

Figure 3–22. Hippocrates: Medicine becomes a science. (© 1958 by Parke, Davis & Co.)

soothing music. Then he was supposed to drift into the *incubation* or *temple sleep.* The dream was to contain Asklepios' counsel, which was then interpreted by the temple priests. The followers of this cult were called *Asklepiads.* Pregnant women and patients with incurable diseases were not admitted to the temples for medical assistance.

Artists and sculptors presented the human body in action. They emphasized the muscles in motion under the skin. They aimed at perfection, removing imperfections from view; however, the preserved stone slab votive offerings that hung on the temple wall were exceptions. These replicas of aspects of illnesses indicate cures and were left by grateful patients.

It is paradoxical that in these unscientific surroundings there emerged a distinguished leader who extricated the care of the sick from magic and superstition and imbued it with a scientific spirit. This leader, born on the island of Cos in the year 460 B.C., belonged to a renowned Asklepiad family and was referred to by Aristotle as "the great Hippocrates" (Fig. 3–22). *Hippocrates* deserves his title of *"Father of Medicine."* By stressing that there is a *natural cause* for diseases, he liberated the care of the sick from the influences of the mythical deities and magic; by teaching *accurate observation* of the sick and keeping careful records of treatment he laid a foundation for clinical medicine; by reporting unsuccessful as well as successful methods of treatment, he presented a modern scientific approach; by emphasizing the importance of constant and skilled care at the patient's bedside he prepared the way for the position of the professional nurse (he dismissed the slave and insisted on his medical students observing and administering bedside care); by instructing at the bedside, he demonstrated the value of clinical instruction by precept and by example; by practicing the high ethical principles embodied in the Hippocratic Oath he laid the cornerstone of an excellent moral code for medicine.

Hippocrates' care of the sick was *patient-centered,* and he used the scientific method in the solution of the problems of his patients.

He emphasized treating the whole person. In endeavoring to do this, he indicated that disease was not inflicted by the gods but was a condition related to the laws of nature and that a physician must understand, in addi-tion to the specific illness, the person who was ill and the surroundings from which he came. In describing Hippocrates' regimen for patient care, Plato had written "To heal even an eye, one must heal the head, and indeed the whole body."

Hippocrates' contribution of the clinical case history became one of the most important tools of scientific patient care. He coupled the information about the person who was ill with details of the patient's environment and the results of the complete examination in his analysis of the needs of the patient. The plan for care that Hippocrates outlined was direct and concise.

In a period when intellectual skills took precedence over manual skills, Hippocrates combined the two successfully to achieve good patient care.

This great teacher of clinical medicine, using a scientific approach to the solution of medical problems, also reported his lack of success in order to assist others in avoiding similar mistakes, "I have written this down deliberately believing it is invaluable to learn of unsuccessful experiments and to know the causes of their failures."

Thales, who was born about 640 B.C., was the first of the great Greek philosopher-scientists. He stressed that although one must find solutions to problems, one must also discover the principles on which these solutions are based.

Aristotle, another famous natural scientist and an Asklepiad, contributed to the field of medicine. His inspiration came in the areas of botany, zoology, physiology, embryology and comparative anatomy, and he taught by dissecting animals.

In the *Iliad,* mention is made of the presence of army surgeons on the field of battle. First aid was administered and the art of bandaging was depicted on one famous antique vase that shows Achilles bandaging the wounded arms of Patroklos (Fig. 3–23). Homer may well have been a surgeon with one of the regimental armies. His descriptions reveal an extensive medical orientation if not a skilled practitioner's background.

Description of Disease

Some of the Greek words for symptoms of disease in Hippocrates' day were still in use many centuries later. The word cynanche,

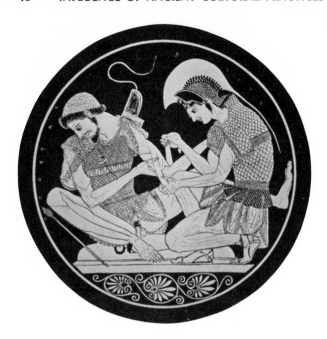

Figure 3–23. Vase painting (ca. 520–510 B.C.). Achilles bandaging arm of his friend Patroklos. Arrow at left may have been removed from wound. (Courtesy of Metropolitan Museum of Art.)

in the form kynanche, was used to identify the difficult swallowing, and often suffocation, that accompanied a diphtheritic throat. For example, cynanche was recorded as the cause of George Washington's death.

It has been reported that the doctors merely looked at George Washington's throat. When Hippocrates inspected a throat, however, he recorded the following observations: "in cases of ulcerated tonsils, the formulation of a membrane like a spider's web is not a good sign." He states further that "ulcers on the tonsils that spread over the uvula alter the voice of those who recover." Obviously some patients recovered from diphtheria but suffered the accompanying diphtheritic paralysis that resulted in a raspy voice. This is another example of the combination of clinical observation and reason on the part of Hippocrates.

The Role of Environment in the Spread of Disease. Thucydides gives a stirring account of an epidemic in Athens during the Peloponnesian War. The occurrence of epidemics has been well documented. Diphtheria and malaria were two of those described. Greek physicians associated the outbreaks of malaria with swamp areas, but felt that the fever of malaria was due to the consumption of the swamp waters.

Hippocrates emphasized the role of environment in the spread of disease in his work on *Airs, Waters and Places*. Rosen reports that for two thousand years this was the basic epidemiological text.[9] It remained an important document until the late nineteenth century when the sciences of bacteriology and immunology made their appearance. Hippocrates understood the role of climate, soil, water, mode of life and nutrition as factors of endemicity. He noted that certain diseases were always present and therefore *endemic;* however, other diseases flared up at certain periods and involved large numbers of people. Thus, an *epidemic* ensued.

Humoral Theory

The theory of the four elements—fire, air, earth and water—was advanced at this time. Bodies were thought to be composed of varying quantities of these four elements; when a state of equilibrium prevailed, health resulted. These four elements also corresponded to the four necessary qualities of heat and cold, moisture and dryness. This theory became the basis of the *humoral theory,* which governed the thinking of medical leaders for centuries.

Hippocrates stated that *health* depends upon a state of equilibrium existing between internal forces which govern the functioning of body and mind. This equilibrium results when man lives in harmony with his external environment.

The ancient Greeks also levied a special tax that guaranteed an annual salary to doctors. This was to supplement the money they obtained through their fees. The tax aided communities that were seeking doctors.

Greece was the intellectual center of the western world and continued to enlighten those people who attempted to enslave her.

The first of these conquerors was Philip II of Macedonia, the father of *Alexander the Great*. At Philip's death in 336 B.C., Alexander started his career of conquest, subduing Thebes (335 B.C.) and thus gaining ascendancy over all of Greece. The period from 336 to 133 B.C. is often referred to as the *Hellenistic Age*, since the conquered lands under Alexander the Great became Greek in culture and language; Greece herself, however, suffered an intellectual decline.

Alexander, who desired to rule the world, conquered Greece, Asia Minor, Egypt and Persia as far east as northern India. *Alexandria*, on the Nile delta in Egypt, became the new capital of his empire, and replaced Athens as the center of learning and culture. At Alexandria were located a thriving seaport with docks, lighthouses, rich palaces, a celebrated museum and an outstanding library from which shone a beacon of intellectual light, beckoning scholars from all over the world. In reality this was a university where the ancient manuscripts were studied and research was carried out in the arts, literature, physics, mathematics, astronomy and medicine. Medicine remained in the hands of the Greeks, and many outstanding leaders received an education there.

After Alexander's death, one of his generals, Ptolemy, succeeded him as ruler of Egypt, and thus began the Ptolemaic dynasty (323–30 B.C.). The glory of the Alexandrian Empire was short-lived. Octavian's victory over the Egyptian fleet in the battle of Actium in 31 B.C. unified the Roman world and ended Egypt's proud sovereignty.

THE ROMANS

Rome has been a kingdom, a republic, an empire and a city. About 753 B.C. Rome comprised a small section of land in the center of which was a hill with a few crude shelters. Four hundred and eighty years later it contained all of the peninsula we call Italy. By the second century A.D. Rome encompassed the territory we know as England, Spain, France, Switzerland, Austria, Hungary, Italy, Greece, Turkey, Sicily, North Africa and other smaller states and islands. At the present time it is the principal city and capital of Italy.

The Romans borrowed much of their culture from Greece and other conquered countries. They worshiped a similar pantheon of gods and goddesses and built temples in their honor. Ancestor worship was practiced and gradually the Romans inaugurated the custom of worshiping the emperors.

The Babylonian practice of examining the entrails of animals to foretell future events was adopted by the Romans, and the soothsayer was consulted freely. It was said that Alexander the Great would not embark on one of his exploits without the counsel of the soothsayer who used this same technique of *divination*.

In the midst of the practicality and agricultural achievement, there arose the beginnings of a growing leadership ability and organizational acumen on the part of a few. As the transition from kingdom to republic was accomplished, the desire for conquest of land, possessions and people took precedence.

A division in the populace of Rome was apparent with the wealthy becoming wealthier and the poor abysmally poorer. A summary of events at this time would include the exorbitant loss of lives through conquests, a decline in morals because of war, for the few the replacement of simple living by luxurious living, the infusion of Greek culture, the introduction of gladiatorial games, construction of luxurious baths, a decay in political circles, widespread unemployment and wholesale slavery.

The ascension of Julius Caesar to undisputed power following the defeat of his archrival Pompey in 48 B.C. marked the greatest single turning point in the affairs of Rome. Following the assassination of Julius Caesar in 44 B.C., his adopted son Octavian gained control of Italy and in 27 B.C. was proclaimed Augustus, first emperor of Rome. During his reign peace was restored, industry flourished, roads were constructed, and a census of the whole empire was taken.

Emperors good and bad succeeded Octavian. Several of them must have been mentally ill, and one notes the encouragement of paid spies, poisoning political enemies, wholesale murder, infanticide, persecution by burning and by being devoured by wild animals and finally a dictatorial government with a total absence of liberty.

The family as a unit was not a stable one. Marriages by civil contract were made and dissolved easily, and divorce became a general practice.

In the area of entertainment, the famous Olympic games were replaced by the gladiatorial contests. These were games in which two slaves, frequently war prisoners, fought for their lives for the amusement of spectators. The sadistic Roman society soon lost interest in this sport and to add zest to it, wild animals such as lions and tigers were introduced. The events became more and more inhuman.

Finally, Nero introduced the persecutions of Christians. This mistreatment was started to avert the accusations of many who believed that Nero had caused a raging fire that wiped out a slum area. By ruse, the emperor caused suspicion to fall on the Christians and immediately condemned hundreds of them to die in the arena. The program of bread and circuses has been a well publicized one. It is remembered that as the bread dwindled the circuses expanded in intensity and violence.

The value of the individual had fallen very low, and it is no wonder that the only *hospitals* of note were built for the *military*. Nursing homes, *valetudinaria*, were established for sick slaves because slaves were considered valuable. Nursing was done by the slaves, and the practice of medicine was under the aegis of captured Greek physicians who were granted citizenship.

Asklepiades was one of the early Greek physicians to practice in Rome. He had an interesting theory that health was the balance between tension and relaxation.

Galen (Fig. 3–24) was the most renowned of the Greek physicians during this period and for many centuries to come. Born about 130 A.D. in the famous city of Pergamum in Asia Minor, which had been colonized by Greek settlers, Galen had an excellent general and medical education for this period. His major contributions included the restoration of the famous works of Hippocrates for use in medical thinking and study; the selection, use, and method of compounding drugs, many of which are referred to as

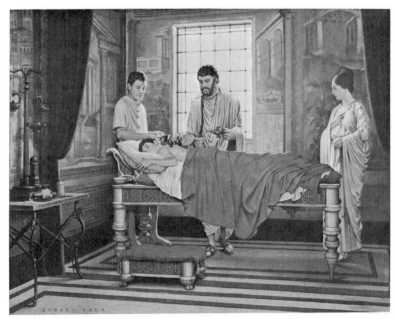

Figure 3–24.   Galen: Influence for forty-five generations. (© 1958 by Parke, Davis & Co.)

"galenicals"; and voluminous works used for the teaching of medical science for many centuries after his death in 201 A.D.

Galen stated that in the process of digestion the liver extracted *natural spirits;* the blood, enriched with natural spirits, passed from the right side of the heart through tiny openings in the septum of the heart into the left side where it was energized by the air from the lungs. The heart synthesized the air and the blood containing natural spirits into the *vital spirits,* which were carried by the arteries. In the brain there was a further transformation into *animal spirits;* the brain stimulated these spirits to travel by way of nerves to the muscles where they caused an extension or contraction of the muscles.

Galen also noted that occupation played a role in illness. He reported certain diseases due to inhalation and a pallor associated with employment in the mines.

Aulus Cornelius Celsus, who lived during the reign of Tiberius Caesar (first century A.D.), is the one to whom we are most indebted for leaving an accurate account of the importance of Greek physicians in Roman medicine. In 1478 his well-known work *De Re Medicina* was one of the few medical books to be printed. The *De Re Medicina* was a compilation of eight books that gave a comprehensive picture of the practice of medicine of Celsus' time.

Celsus wrote the first organized medical history, which has become one of the great Latin classics. He translated works from Greek into Latin, and described the four cardinal symptoms of inflammation—redness, swelling, heat and pain—as *rubor et tumor, cum calore et dolore.*

His writings included the dietary aspects as well as pharmaceutical, medical, surgical, and psychiatric. Forms of therapy that he recommended were sea voyages, changes of scene in the form of trips, moderate exercise, light, massage and warm baths.

Pedanius Dioscorides, a Greek physician of the first century A.D., was a famous leader in the field of pharmacy and author of *De Materia Medica,* which remained for 1500 years the definitive text in botanic medicine. His keen powers of observation helped broaden the knowledge of plants that were usable for drugs. He accompanied the Roman armies, observing, recording and collecting drugs.

The beneficial contributions of the Rom-

ans were in the fields of engineering, public health, sanitation and law. *Aqueducts* were built to supply the city with water from mountain springs many miles away. This water was carried in pipes through the tunnels and across lowlands. Rosen points out that, in addition to the fantastic system of aqueducts, the sophisticated city planning included a water commissioner.[10] The first accounts of the duties of an administrative public health official appeared in *De Aquis Urbis Romae.*

Rosen states that at the height of the Roman Empire, with a population of one million people, about 40 gallons of water per person were consumed per day.[11] In addition, the Romans were desirous of improving the quality of the water and they encouraged the use of settling basins where slaves removed the sediment. Reservoirs, properly enclosed and protected, helped maintain a pure water supply.

Marshes were drained, a sewage system was established and plumbing was introduced into the houses. Records show warnings against the use of polluted water. More precise knowledge of pollution in swampy areas has been revealed in a remarkable Roman note of caution, which stated that ". . . there are bred certain minute creatures which cannot be seen by the eyes, which float in the air and enter the body through the mouth and nose and there cause serious diseases." Malaria, typhoid fever, dysentery as well as diphtheria and tuberculosis plagued the Romans. An epidemic of bubonic plague of historic significance occurred during the reign of Emperor Justinian (483–565 A.D.). The crowded slum areas acted as breeding places for physical and social diseases.

The new public baths became quite fashionable. The Baths of Caracalla (186–217 A.D.) in Rome were expansive, palatial and costly. The baths were named for Caracalla, the emperor who was purported to have ordered the mass murder of 20,000 people. Covering acres of land, they accommodated thousands of persons in the most grandiose manner. The spacious interior had high arched ceilings and was beautifully ornamented with marble and exquisite inlaid mosaics. There were auditoria, gymnasia, reading rooms, patios with cool fountains,

---

[10] *Op. cit.,* p. 39.
[11] *Op. cit.,* p. 40.

soft music and swimming pools to delight the patrons and provide diversional therapy.

For the therapeutic tour of the baths, a person undressed in the apodyterium and received a massage; the warm refreshing waters of the tepidarium were next; increasingly warmer water was provided in the sudadorium, followed by the hot bathing in the calidarium; the final scene occurred in the cold waters of the frigidarium.

The heat of the baths was controlled in the basement beneath the floor where open hearth furnaces manned by slaves sent the heat through a flue system and pipes to the pools above. The pipes were made of soft flexible lead and this may have caused lead poisoning, which, in turn, may have contributed to the physical decline of the Romans. (Another possibility for lead poisoning occurred in the process for preserving and sweetening wine. The wine stood for long periods of time during the so-called sweetening process). In the frigidarium the clear, cold water came from the well-established aqueduct system.

The sun was so important in the Greek and Roman philosophy of living that Apollo and Helios were revered as sun gods. Heliotherapy (sun bathing) was used in classical times and Caelius Aurelianus, a Roman physician during the fifth century A.D., advocated its use for the treatment of rickets, for diseases of bones and joints and skin ailments.

A large swampy section of land was drained by a great arched sewer called the Cloaca Maxima, which emptied into the Tiber River. The land became the basis for the foundation of the famous Roman Forum, the public market place. It was so well constructed that it has withstood the ravages of time and is used today.

THE IRISH CELTS

Ireland was a site of civilized activity as early as 1000 B.C. The story of its early beginnings is embellished with interesting legends and sagas. Ireland has been called Hibernia by the Romans, Ireland by the Norsemen and Erin by countrymen.

The Gaelic-speaking Celts migrated from Europe to Ireland during the middle fourth century B.C. The aboriginal Picts were reduced to vassalage by the socially advanced settlers. It is interesting to note that centuries later when the Irish discontinued the use of the native language and adopted English, they used the mode of English pronunciation of the Elizabethan and Jacobean period, which has been exemplified in Shakespeare's writings.

It is a matter of record that when the Roman spirit was decaying and the light of civilization was waning, the Irish preserved it and contributed to it, inspiring works of literature and poetry, melodious music and gorgeous examples of art. The Irish maintained a real interest in Latin and Greek, and were intrigued by Greek philosophy as well as Greek literature.

In pagan Ireland there were three learned orders: the *druids*, the *brehons* and the *bards*. The druids studied physical and theological science and possessed knowledge of divination and magic. The brehons were lawyers and the bards were poets who preserved much of the fascinating history and traditions of the country.

The Irish were tender-hearted people and, because of the clan system under which they lived, provided dutifully for the needs of the less fortunate. In 300 B.C. in Ireland Princess Macha built a hospital called Broin Bearg or the House of Sorrow.

The Irish were advanced in medical treatments and in the establishment of laws regulating the practice of medicine. In the area of clinical treatments, they recognized the benefit of *moist heat*. Hot compresses, hot water baths, medicated baths and "sweating houses" are mentioned frequently; this is understandable in a damp climate in which "rheumatism" is said to have been prevalent.

Many modern aspects of patient care have been noted in early Irish history. For example, they emphasized the importance of peace of mind for the benefit of patients. This was achieved by careful scrutiny of the patient; persons and things that did not contribute to the welfare of the patient were excluded from the sick room.

Trepanning operations, as observed in the story of an Irish prince, were performed. Because of a severe blow on the head, the prince had lost his memory and physicians resorted to a trepanning operation. Not only was a portion of the skull removed, however, but some of the cerebral material as well. The prince was said to have lost his "organ of forgetting" as a result of the operation, and his memory was restored.

In a twelfth century Celtic *materia medica*, reference is made to the use of mandrake, which was to be used before operations to prevent pain. By this it is seen that the ancient Irish were acquainted with anesthesia for surgical purposes.

The early *obstetrical* practices of the Irish are fascinating and significant in the light of current trends in this field. It was an Irish practice to encourage a mother to deliver her baby while in a kneeling position. A feather mattress (burned after delivery to prevent the spread of infection) was rolled up and the mother knelt on this and leaned against the portion of a chair in front of her, helping herself by exercising as she grasped and pushed during the process of labor. The mother's muscles had been kept in good condition by housework and work in the fields. The birth process was not considered a pathological event but rather a normal physiological experience.

A physician was not in attendance during childbirth, but rather a "wise-woman" or the mother of the one who was having the baby. The Irish mother was out of bed by the third day and back to her chores by the fifth. She took care of her baby in a hammock arrangement on her bed that permitted her to meet the needs of the newborn. These people practiced a forerunner of a "rooming-in" method of baby care.

The practice of medicine was regulated by well-constructed *brehon laws*. One of these laws required that every physician in Ireland keep one door of his house open at all times. The physician's house was to be an open house into which injured and sick might be brought for treatment.

Every physician was expected to permit four medical students to reside in his home. The physician's duties included teaching these young men as he demonstrated the medical care of patients. It is imagined that this prompted doctors to put forth their best efforts as an example to the students. Medical fees were regulated according to the service given to the patient and his ability to pay.

The laws against impostors or people not properly prepared to practice medicine were very strict ones. The Irish felt that those who were ill could be easily deceived, and anyone who took advantage of this "susceptible" state of mind was punished severely:

If an unlawful physician treat a joint or sinew without obtaining an indemnity against liability to damages and with a notice to the patient that he is not a regular physician he is subject to a penalty with compensation to the patient.

Every doctor was held responsible for the treatment of his patients. The brehon laws required that the physician refund fees if he had failed to heal a patient. The patient could use the money to try and find someone who could cure him.

Finally, the law of "sick maintenance" required that provision be made for all who needed curative treatment, nourishing food and a place of care. The persons who were responsible for carrying out these needs were defined clearly and carefully.

The status of woman in Ireland was high. She had legal rights to property, and Irish literature refers to the reverence with which she was treated. One of the outstanding pioneers in the education for women was St. Brigid of Kildare, to be discussed in the section on monasticism.

In pausing to review the achievements and contributions of the ancient cultures, we note that the Sumerians, Babylonians and Egyptians practiced medicine governed by a code imbued with magic principles and did not pursue a scientific quest for the cause of disease; the Hebrews bequeathed to us a good foundation in hygiene, sanitation and preventive medicine; the Chinese laid a firm basis upon which to build the science of pharmacology and therapeutics; the Hindus gave inspiring leadership in the field of surgery; and to the Greeks we owe medical leadership in the theory and practice of clinical medicine and clinical instruction. We notice also, however, how much artistic skill and material wealth accompanied primitive superstition with its lack of medical progress, ruthless brutality and total indifference to the value and equality of the individual.

The Greek spirit of inquiry sparked the use of the scientific approach to problems; this was the beginning of theoretical science, which included medicine. The need for the use of pure reason was extolled. It is tragic that this scientific medical milieu did not spark or act as a catalytic agent for the evolution of nursing!

REFERENCE READINGS

Adams, Francis: *The Genuine Words of Hippocrates.* Baltimore, Williams & Wilkins Co., 1939.

Buck, Pearl: *The Good Earth.* New York, Pocket Books, 1931.

Bulwer-Lytton, Edward: *The Last Days of Pompeii.* New York, Dodd, Mead, & Co., 1834.

Dechanet, J. M.: *Christian Yoga.* New York, Harper & Brothers, 1960.

Gibbon, Edward: *The Decline and Fall of the Roman Empire.* New York, Viking Press.

Hamilton, Edith: *The Greek Way.* New York, Mentor Books, New American Library of World Literature, 1948.

Hume, E. H.: *The Chinese Way in Medicine.* Baltimore, Johns Hopkins Press, 1940.

Lao Tzu: *The Way of Life.* Trans. R. B. Blakney. New York, The New American Library, 1955.

Lin Yutang: *Famous Chinese Short Stories.* New York, Pocket Books, 1952.

Lin Yutang: *The Wisdom of China and India.* New York, Random House, 1942.

MacManus, Seymas: *The Story of the Irish Race.* New York, The Devin-Adair Co., 1907.

Pochin Mould, D. D. C.: *Ireland of the Saints.* London, B. T. Batsford, 1953.

Prabhavananda, S., and Isherwood, C.: *The Song of God: Bhagavad-Gita.* New York, Harper & Brothers, 1954.

Prabhavananda, S., and Manchester, F.: *The Upanishads.* Hollywood, Calif., Vedanta Press, 1948.

Renault, Mary: *The Last of the Wine.* New York, Pantheon Books, 1954.

Stirling, Matthew, et al.: *Indians of the Americas.* Washington, National Geographic Society, 1955.

Stobart, John C.: *The Glory That Was Greece.* Rev. ed. Boston, Beacon Press, 1934.

Tantaquidgeon, Gladys: *A Study of Delaware Indian Medicine Practice and Folk Beliefs.* Harrisburg, Pennsylvania Historical Commission, 1942.

Von Hagen, Victor W.: *Realm of the Incas.* New York, Mentor Books, New American Library of World Literature, 1957.

Walsh, James J.: *The World's Debt to the Irish.* Boston, The Stratford Co., 1926.

Wong, K. C., and Wu, Lieu-Teh: *History of Chinese Medicine.* Shanghai, National Quarantine Service, 1936.

CHAPTER 4

Effects of Spiritual Leadership on the Development of Nursing

Even after nineteen hundred years it is difficult to fully comprehend the impact of the birth of *Jesus Christ* and His teaching on society and the care of the sick. This teaching stressed the need of loving God and one's neighbor; it was a simple philosophy of living a life of love in a world of selfishness and hatred. He was expected; His birth had been announced by prophecy. His coming resulted in the cleavage of time between those events that preceded His birth and those that have followed. He came at a time when much of the world was enslaved. Fear, terror and torture abounded.

It was shortly after Christ began His public life that He preached His Sermon on the Mount, the key to His entire message. Christ saw in every man, even in the poorest and most miserable, a human being whose privilege it was to become a member of the Kingdom of God. There was a recognition of every man's human dignity—a new concept of human worth. His miracles testified to His love, and His attitude toward the sick was a good example in human relations. Instead of "saying the word" and healing the sick, Christ gave individual attention to the needs of all by touching, anointing and taking by the hand (Fig. 4–1). The least gesture of human kindness is noted by Him, even a cup of cold water given in His name does not pass unrewarded. Each act of kindness and charity is of value since each is done for Christ in the person of the distressed. The parable of the Good Samaritan (Fig. 4–2) emphasized the urgency of caring for anyone in need. It

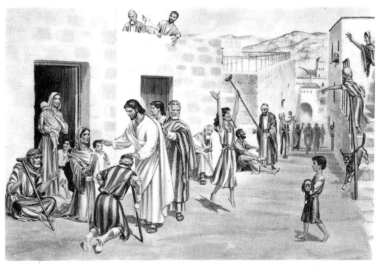

Figure 4–1. Christ, the Healer. (Courtesy of Maryknoll.)

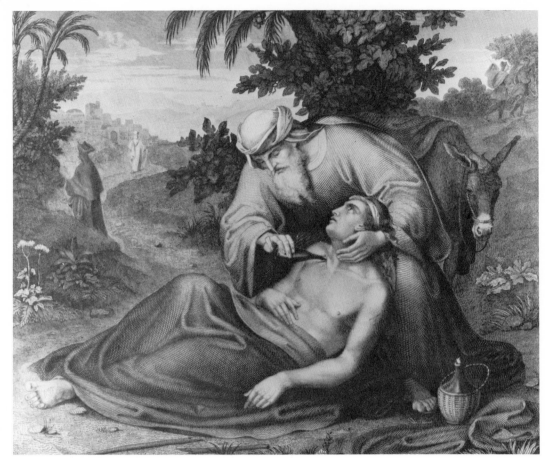

Figure 4–2. The Good Samaritan. This engraving was ordered by Pastor Fliedner for the Order of Deaconesses of Kaiserswerth in 1854. (Author's collection.)

conveyed His message, "upon my return I will reward you." Christ counseled, "Amen, amen I say to you, as long as you did it to one of these my least brethren, you did it unto me." His followers ministered to those in need and envisioned Christ in the recipient.

At the Last Supper Christ gave to His disciples His final instructions, including this commandment: "A new commandment I give you, that you love one another: That as *I have loved you,* you also love one another."[1] This commandment of love was called *new,* for the world before Christ's coming was a world without love. The object of His coming was that of love since He explained, "the Son of man came not to be ministered unto, but to minister, and to give His life as a ransom for many"; and before His death,

He said, "Greater love than this no man hath that he lay down his life for his friends." His command was "Come follow me."

Many historians have recorded stories of the social and spiritual leadership of the Christians as they began to follow in Christ's footsteps. The Carthaginian theologian Tertullian (160?–230? A.D.) wrote:

It is our care of the helpless, our practice of loving kindness that brands us in the eyes of many of our opponents. "Only look," they say, "how they love one another! Look how they are prepared to die for one another."

Eusebius of Caesarea ("the father of ecclesiastical history," 260?–340? A.D.) described a plague in the time of Maximinus Daza:

. . . the Christians were the only people who amid such terrible ills, showed their fellow-feeling and humanity by their actions. Day by

---

[1]John 13:34–35 and 15:12–13.

day some would busy themselves by attending to the dead and burying them; others gathered in one spot all who were afflicted by hunger throughout the whole city and gave them bread.

INCEPTION OF NURSING

This charity—love in action—was apparent in the inception of nursing, which took root, flourished and expanded into the well established field we know today. For nursing was nurtured in the early Christian period, and there were individuals who will be recorded for all time for their example in comforting the afflicted. Solicitously, Veronica wiped the agonized face of Christ, and Mary Magdalene and St. John gave genuine consolation to His Mother.

DEACONESSES

The earliest "bearers of the lamp" (Fig. 4–3) were called visiting nurses. The forerunner of the community health nursing movement of today had its beginning in the first century of the Christian Church. Human suffering had elicited a warm response from individuals down through the years, but the first organized visiting of the sick began with the establishment of the order of *Deaconesses.* They endeavored to practice the *Corporal Works of Mercy.*

Note the basic human needs that were incorporated into the Corporal Works of Mercy:

To feed the hungry.
To give water to the thirsty.
To clothe the naked.
To visit the imprisoned.
To shelter the homeless.
To care for the sick.
To bury the dead.

Consider the implications of those works of mercy for the earliest nurses down to the present. In addition to the obvious need to provide for those who were underprivileged and culturally deprived, the nurse recognized the need for food by those who were malnourished physically, intellectually and spiritually, as well as those who could not serve themselves. In addition to quenching the thirst for water, they realized the tremendous thirst for human compassion. They realized the necessity for clothing a person with the warmth of understanding and love, as well

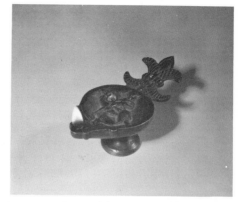

Figure 4–3. Lamp of the type carried by early Christian nurses. (Author's collection.)

as physically. They also perceived the importance of visiting the imprisoned persons of all ages, in all kinds of institutions, especially those confined for long periods, who were neglected or forgotten and who needed to know that people still cared about them.

These nurses incorporated in their care the act of sheltering the homeless who needed to feel warmth and hospitality in a new or strange environment. Care of the sick merited special attention in the Corporal Works of Mercy. Nursing had been the forced occupation of slaves and, therefore, those who worked in the field may not have had the dedication or the broader dimension required to meet the needs of the patients.

The opportunity to give spiritual meaning to both the care given to patients and the suffering borne by patients has been stressed by Christ in the following: "As long as you did it to one of these . . . you did it to me."— and "Pick up your cross and follow me." These nurses were following the command of their Master and imitating Him who spent His life ministering to those in need.

There must have been a pattern of organization based on a district plan. The objectives of their service were the provision of care for the sick in their homes as well as the distribution of aid to the needy.

The early Christians sold what they possessed and gave it to the poor. In their thinking "charity" was synonymous with "love." The Church became the central charity organization because there were no other organized charities from which to obtain clothing, food and other necessities. The deaconess, in distributing the food and medicines that she carried in a basket (the visiting nurse's bag of that period), was the forerunner of the social worker and the public health nurse. She detected needs and brought the thinking and material resources of her group to the patient who needed this care.

The care given by the deaconess probably consisted of bathing patients, especially those who had communicable diseases and were feverish; dressing wounds, including the applications of dressings to burnt areas; giving foods and forcing fluids; and bringing physical and spiritual comfort to all patients, especially to the dying. In this era, greater emphasis was placed upon relieving suffering than on curing or preventing illness. The benefits of scientific progress were lacking, but there was an overflowing of love, charity and tenderness. Home remedies, such as herbs, minerals, diet, bathing and, where possible, fresh air, were relied upon.

The marvels of structure and beauty of wealthy Rome have been portrayed all too well, but the deaconesses and the Christian Roman matrons carried out their duties in the slum sections of the empire. The abysmal poverty of the citizenry has been mentioned and it was in this setting that Christians labored to bring relief to the suffering and depressed. These patients had little of the necessities and were crowded into small tenement areas where little fresh air was available, and much sickness, sorrow, want, misery and distress were present.

Phoebe, a friend of St. Paul, was the first deaconess and thus the first visiting nurse. From the Bible we have learned that she was entrusted with the letters of St. Paul,[2] and he said of her nursing care: "For she also assisted many and myself also."

The date of the Epistle to the Romans in which there is reference to Phoebe is about 58 A.D. Note has been made of her wealth and important social status and the realization that she had business that necessitated travel to the capital of the Empire. Phoebe was clearly an educated woman, as well.

The writings of St. John Chrysostom (d. 404 A.D.), the Bishop of Constantinople (known as "The Golden Mouth" in recognition of his remarkable eloquence), described the activities of another deaconess, *St. Olympias*. The daughter of a count of the Roman Empire, Olympias inherited an immense fortune when her parents died during her childhood. She married and held a position of social prestige as the wife of the prefect of Constantinople. Left a childless widow at the age of 18, Olympias erected a convent in which a large number of relatives and friends devoted themselves to works of charity and the service of God. Her servants were freed and given the opportunity of joining her convent as sisters.

The Order of Deaconesses attained a position of importance for many years but gradually died out.

MATRONS

A group of noble *Roman matrons* distinguished themselves in the field of nursing. These were women of wealth, intelligence and social leadership who, having been converted to Christianity, founded hospitals and convents and worked for the good of others.

St. Helena (250–330 A.D.), Flavia Helena, was the mother of Constantine the Great, the ruler of the Roman Empire, and the daughter of an innkeeper of Drepanum, in Bithynia (Fig. 4–4). She became the Empress of Rome when she married Constantine Chlorus. She embraced Christianity and dedicated the remainder of her life to the needy. She gave generously to the poor and built shelters and churches for the pilgrims who were determined to visit the "Holy Places." Helena is believed to have found the relics of the True Cross, and has been credited with the establishment of a house for the aged called a *gerokomion*.

Constantine revered his saintly mother and her influence over him was quite pronounced. He rebuilt Drepanum and renamed it Helenopolis in her honor; he also bestowed upon her the supreme title of Augusta.

Empress Flacilla, the wife of Theodosius the Great (346?–395 A.D.) and the daughter of Claudius Antonius, the Prefect of Gaul, went to the hospital daily to attend the sick. There, she washed and dressed the patients, made their beds, prepared food and served them when they were unable to eat. The empress was especially interested in assisting persons with a physical handicap.

St. Marcella converted her luxurious palace on Aventine Hill into a monastery. A scholar, Marcella encouraged other Roman matrons

---

[2]St. Paul to the Romans 16:1–2.

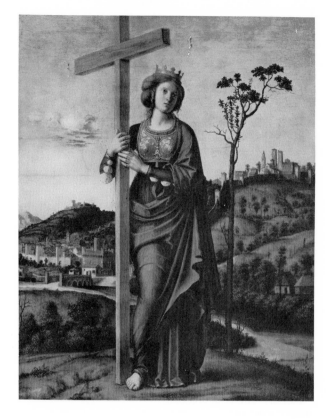

Figure 4–4. St. Helena. Cima Da Conegliano, ca. 1459–1517. (Samuel H. Kress Collection. Courtesy of National Gallery of Art, Washington, D.C.)

of intelligence and spiritual depth to join her in studying Latin and Greek literature, Hebrew and the Scriptures. Of her keenness of mind St. Jerome (340?–420 A.D.) has written, "All that I have learnt with great study and long meditation the blessed Marcella learnt also, but with great facility and without giving up any of her other occupations or neglecting any of her pursuits." Marcella taught the care of the sick to her followers, and her conventual plan encouraged further education for women. Indeed she might be considered the first nurse educator. Marcella was killed by barbarians during the sack of Rome.

St. Fabiola (Fig. 4–5) was one of the most charming, popular and capable members of Marcella's group. She belonged to the patrician family of Fabian and had led a very worldly life, but because of the influence of St. Jerome and Marcella she gave up her earthly pleasures and lavished her immense wealth on the poor and sick. Through her efforts in 390 A.D., the first general public hospital was built in Rome. St. Jerome describes it as a "nosocomium," a place for only the sick. Not content with giving her fortune

to the needy, Fabiola waited on the patients herself, giving special care to those with repulsive sores. She died in the year 399, and her funeral was a manifestation of the gratitude of her patients and of the people of Rome.

St. Jerome summed up the contributions of Fabiola in his famous eulogy after her death:

There she gathered together all the sick from the highways and streets, and herself nursed the unhappy, emaciated victims of hunger and disease. Can I describe here the varied scourges which afflicted human beings?—the mutilated, blinded countenances, the partially destroyed limbs, the livid hands, swollen bodies and wasted extremities? . . . . How often have I seen her carrying in her arms those piteous, dirty, and revolting victims of a frightful malady! How often have I seen her wash wounds whose fetid odour prevented every one else from even looking at them! She fed the sick with her own hands, and revived the dying with small and frequent portions of nourishment. I know that many wealthy persons cannot overcome the repugnance caused by such works of charity; . . . . I do not judge them . . . but, if I had a hundred tongues and a clarion voice I could not enumerate the number of patients for

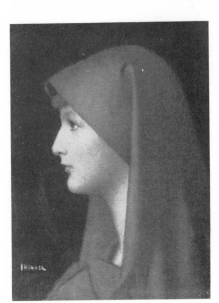

Figure 4–5. Fabiola. (J. J. Henner, 1829–1905, courtesy of Louvre Museum.)

whom Fabiola provided solace and care. The poor who were well envied those who were sick.[3]

There have been indications that Fabiola may have encouraged the construction of a hospice or home for convalescent patients.

St. Paula (347–404 A.D.) was a Roman matron of noble birth, a descendent of the Gracchi and the Scipios, of the line of Agamemnon, and her possessions included the city of Necropolis built by Augustus. This great wealth held no appeal for her, however, and, largely because of the efforts of Marcella, she was converted to Christianity, and entered the monastery on Aventine Hill. Paula was one of the most learned women of this period and a scholar of Hebrew. She assisted St. Jerome (who encouraged each woman to develop her mind through reading and study while increasing her skills in caring for the sick) in his Latin translation of the Scriptures, known as the Vulgate. (See Figure 4–6.) Accompanied by her daughter, Eustochium, Paula sailed for Palestine about 385 and settled in Bethlehem. On the road to Bethlehem she built shelters for pilgrims and hospitals for the sick.

There she founded four monasteries and built a hospital in which it has been said that she and her community of sisters nursed the

sick "with untiring zeal." In St. Jerome's story of the life of St. Paula, he has said:

> She was marvellous, debonair, and pietous to them that were sick, and comforted them, and served them right humbly; and gave them largely to eat such as they asked; but to herself she was hard in her sickness and scarce. . . . She was oft by them that were sick, and she laid the pillows aright and in point; and she rubbed their feet, and boiled water to wash them; and it seemed to her that the less she did to the sick in service, so much the less service did she to God.

St. Jerome provided the inspirational leadership behind the activities and contributions of these Roman matrons. His great spiritual depth was accompanied by a love of learning and an ability to motivate and teach others.

In the selfish, indifferent society of Rome the remarkable contrast of these matrons in caring for the sick and less fortunate was strikingly apparent. It was most unusual for women of high social standing to change from a life of luxury to one of generous service. It was gratifying also to note that high intellectual ability accompanied the practical

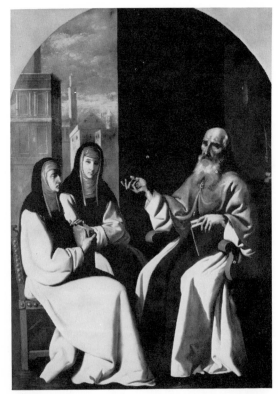

Figure 4–6. St. Jerome with St. Paula and St. Eustochium. (Samuel H. Kress Collection, Zurbaran, 1598–1664. Courtesy of National Gallery of Art, Washington, D.C.)

[3]Letter to Oceanus (LXXVII) in *A Select Library of Nicene and Post-Nicene Fathers of the Christian Church.* Second series, Vol. VI, Letters of St. Jerome. New York, Schaff & Wace, 1893.

skill and loving kindness of these women in nursing. Love was the motivating force for these early Christian women. Fired with the enthusiasm of converts, anxious to lay down their lives for their newly acquired faith, channeling this spiritual growth into the outpouring of love for their neighbor, they showered their attention on the sick and needy so that in ministering to the least of these their brothers they would be ministering unto their Lord.

Members of a brotherhood known as *Parabolani* provided an opportunity for male nurses in the early Church period. This brotherhood was supposedly organized during the great plague in Alexandria, which occurred in the second half of the third century. This group undertook to care for the sick and bury the dead.

Concerning the activities of the *parabolani*, Miss Austin has presented the following account taken from *Hypatia*, a historical novel by Charles Kingsley:

So Philammon went out with the parabolani, a sort of organized guild of district visitors. . . . And in their company he saw that afternoon the dark side of that world whereof the harbor panorama had been the bright one. In squalid misery, filth, profligacy, ignorance, ferocity, discontent, neglected in body, house and soul by the civil authorities, proving their existence only in aimless and sanguinary riots, there they starved and rotted, heap on heap, the masses of the old Greek population, close to the great food-exporting harbor of the world. Among these, fiercely perhaps, and fanatically, but still among them and for them, labored those district visitors night and day. And so Philammon toiled away with them, carrying food and clothing, helping sick to the hospital, and dead to the burial; cleaning out the infected houses—for the fever was all but perennial in those quarters—comforting the dying with the good news of forgiveness from above, till the larger number had to return for evening service. He, however, was kept by his superior watching at a sick bedside, and it was late at night before he got home, and was reported to Peter the Reader as having acquitted himself like "a man of God," as, indeed, without the least thought of doing anything noble or self-sacrificing, he had truly done, being a monk.[4]

St. Sebastian received the ministrations of these early Christian nurses when sorely in need of compassionate, skilled nursing care. During the reign of Emperor Diocletian (284–305 A.D.), Sebastian became company commander in the Praetorian Guards. In 286 A.D. his religious affiliation with the Christian Church and his public declaration of his faith, caused him to be fastened to a stake and shot to death by arrows. That night

---

[4] Austin, Anne L.: *History of Nursing Source Book*. New York, G. P. Putnam's Sons, 1957, p. 62.

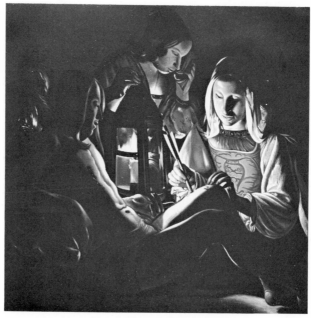

Figure 4–7. St. Sebastian nursed by St. Irene. (Georges de La Tour, French, 1598–1652. Courtesy of Detroit Institute of Arts.)

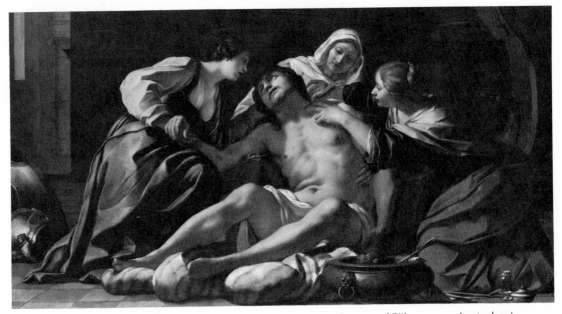

Figure 4–8. St. Sebastian nursed by St. Irene and other nurses. (Courtesy of Rijksmuseum, Amsterdam.)

Irene, the widow of his martyred friend St. Castulus, found that Sebastian was still alive and she and her associates cared for him.

St. Sebastian became one of the most popular subjects in medieval art and many museums around the world possess an artistic portrayal of him. It is of interest to note that many of these paintings highlight the nursing care given by St. Irene and her colleagues (Figs. 4–7 and 4–8).

For many years St. Sebastian was beseeched prayerfully to prevent or cure pestilential diseases which people felt were shot into one's body by invisible arrows.

ACHIEVEMENT OF CHRISTIAN NURSES

These nurses were not just comforters, they were nurturers—observing, listening, assessing, consoling, teaching, giving care as well as caring about the patient and his family. Teaching has been an important duty of Christians since the command "Go and teach all nations." Spiritual, mental and physical health have been involved.

These intellectually and socially skilled leaders identified the basic ingredients of nursing care through careful assessment of need. They realized the dependency of the acutely ill patient upon his nurse for vital life processes.

The nurse role of healer as well as builder of health was achieved where possible by cleaning up the filth and squalor and by rectifying human indignities and degradation. Nurses, in effect, were early social reformers. The site of health delivery occurred where the need existed—in the community, in the hospital, in the home, in the hostel of a pilgrim, in a home for the elderly. The response to human need prompted nurses to care for persons of all ages, all types of illnesses, and physical handicaps. Even the presence of a nurse educator and students of nursing was noted.

When a nursing assessment was determined, intervention was provided by nurses if nursing care was indicated, otherwise the observation was interpreted to the physician if medical care was needed or to the spiritual advisor if spiritual care was warranted. These early Christian nurses emerged from a high social status, shared their learning and techniques with interested recruits, were motivated by a strong spiritual force and were independent practitioners.

PHYSICIANS

Even medicine was infused with human warmth and compassion. One of the best known doctors of this period is *St. Luke*, the Evangelist, who was a native of Antioch and a Greek (Fig. 4–9). Called the "beloved physician" by St. Paul, Luke's writings indicated interest in medical aspects and gave evidence of medical preparation. Several historians suggest that Luke may have studied at the famous school at Tarsus, the rival of Alexandria and Athens, and that he could have met St. Paul there. As a physician Luke traveled extensively and may have been a doctor on board ship. In addition to his literary ability and medical skill, Luke was a noted artist.

St. Cosmas and *St. Damian* (Fig. 4–10) were twin brothers, Arabs by birth and Christians by upbringing, who specialized in the twin professions of medicine and pharmacy. They practiced the art of healing in Asia Minor, attaining an enviable reputation until their careers came to an abrupt end through the persecutions of the Emperor Diocletian. Two other doctors who were martyred during these persecutions were *St. Blaise*, a bishop,

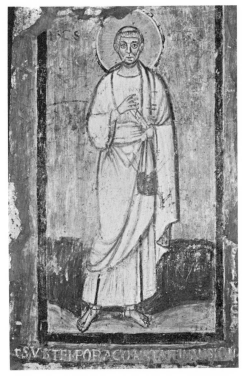

Figure 4–9. St. Luke. Seventh century catacomb wall painting, at the underground Basilica of St. Felix and Adauctus, Rome. (Courtesy of "What's New.")

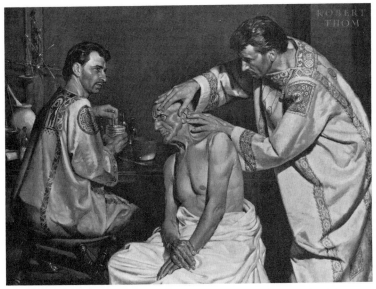

Figure 4–10. Representation of Damian and Cosmas (ca. 300 A.D.). An early example of the team concept in medicine. (© 1952 by Parke, Davis & Co.)

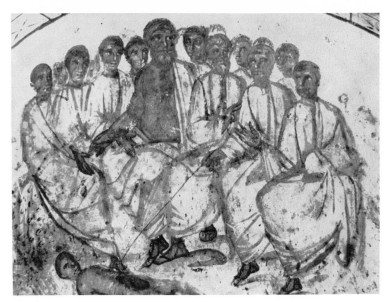

Figure 4–11. Fresco from recently discovered catacombs near the Appian Way. This is a scene of a fourth century medical class. The instructor and students are listening to the discussion of one of the students. (Courtesy of Rev. Antonio Ferrua, S. J., Pontifical Commission of Sacred Archeology.)

and *St. Pantaleon,* the personal physician of Emperor Maximian.

In 312, during the battle of the Milvian Bridge, Emperor Constantine saw a cross in the sky and the words, "In hoc signo vinces" ("In this sign thou shalt conquer"). Winning the battle, Constantine became a Christian, officially recognized the Church and freed it from persecution. Consequently, the Christians no longer had to confine their activities to the catacombs; hospitals, churches and other institutions began to develop.

On the walls in the catacombs muralists painted scenes of significance. One depicts doctors conducting a clinical class for medical students (Fig. 4–11). The master teacher is observed as a student directs a question to him and the quizzical expression on the faces of the students has been captured by the muralist.

HOSPITALS

From the moment the significance of Christ's teaching penetrated the thinking of the early Christians, special places were set aside in their homes for hospitality and the actual care of the sick. These were called *Christrooms,* showing a literal interpretation of the words of Christ, ". . . I was a stranger and you took me in. . . ." These rooms, whether in the home of a bishop, deaconess or other person, were called *diakonia. Xenodochia* was the name given to shelters built for sick and poor pilgrims, and *nosocomia* was the name given to hospitals built by St. Zoticus in Constantinople during the reign of Emperor Constantine.

A hospital planned only for the sick was organized at *Edessa, ca.* 350, to provide care for the victims of a frightful epidemic. With money given to him *St. Ephrem* bought 300 beds and provided care for the critically ill. It is said that he assisted in the care of these sick patients. Later this hospital became the clinical center for a medical school.

One of the most famous hospitals of this period was the *Basilias,* built in Caesarea by *St. Basil* (330?–379? A.D.) and his sister Macrina, both of whom are reputed to have studied medicine. The Basilias was not only a hospital as we know it but was also an institution that cared for the crippled and the poor. There was a separate building for children, another for elderly people, a place of hospitality for strangers and a building for the care of patients with leprosy. St. Basil included a special unit where the physically handicapped could learn a new trade and thus reenter society equipped with the ability to support themselves.

The motive behind the construction of such a hospital is interesting to consider. In the beginning, the plan of religious life was organized on a community basis. One of the first to draw such a group together was St. Basil. When St. Basil gave his monks a scheme for their community life, he established hospitals and schools at the gates of the monasteries. This arrangement was instituted because Basil saw the dangers of the monks being preoccupied with their own salvation and as hermits concerned solely with themselves in their relation to God; his novel plan provided for both the care of the sick and the practice of the monks' religious duties. In this way he proved that the love and service of God must be extended to the love and service of one's neighbor. From that time on, nursing, like education, has been part of the religious life and has been one of the principal ways of practicing the worship of God.

In summary, with the coming of Christ and the subsequent advent of Christianity, the value of the individual was emphasized, and the responsibility for recognizing the needs of each individual became apparent. Many were inflamed with the fire of Christ's love and the virtues of sympathy, generosity and service were practiced. The social position of nursing was elevated, and its spiritual base was laid during this period.

Early Middle Ages

The ancient classical civilization was crumbling rapidly, and an era of restoration and reconstruction was supplanting it. The thousand years that followed the collapse of the Roman Empire, referred to as the medieval period of history, have been subdivided further into the early and later Middle Ages.

As the study of the early Middle Ages commences, a deteriorating world is viewed. Everything was falling into ruins. Population was decreasing both in numbers and strength. Crime waves of an indescribable nature terrified the populace. The burden of increasing taxation and the brutality that accompanied the collection of taxes were insufferable; the already hungry and impoverished people were threatened with torture and imprisonment in the hope of extracting concealed possessions. Whenever an increase in tax rate was announced, agonized murmurs arose from the people who, in desperation, considered the possibilities of fleeing the country, selling loved ones or even attempting suicide. Many relinquished their freedom and offered their services to a landowner in a bondage relationship. In reality, a great many were becoming slaves.

The once-powerful Rome now faced destruction because of extreme moral decay, increasing sterility among the patrician class owing to lead poisoning contracted from the use of lead drinking vessels, abysmal poverty worsened by high taxation, and continuance of wars with concomitant indifference to the plight of the victimized peoples. Disorganized and persecuted communities turned to feudalism, monasticism and, in certain regions, to Islam as possible solutions to the chaos they faced.

FEUDALISM

The castle of the feudal lord was a strong stone fortress usually set high on an inaccessible spot. It was enclosed by massive turreted walls and encircled by a moat. The most important fortification of the castle was called the keep, which was the innermost tower within strongly constructed concentric walls. It was here that protection was secured in times of stress.

The noble's wife had charge of the household, and it was she who took care of the sick and wounded.

The atmosphere of the life of the feudal family seemed to encourage the growth of the spirit of chivalry, which came eventually to mean the institution of knighthood. *Chivalry* reflected the spirit of "noblesse oblige," which required the nobly born to protect and defend the weak.

Although feudalism afforded protection to many, the system had two major disadvantages: a strong central government was not possible and constant warfare prevented progress.

MONASTICISM

Monasticism offered an opportunity for men and women to live a good Christian life while pursuing an occupational career of their own choosing. This monastic idea is not found in Christianity alone; it has been found in connection with many other religious groups. Monasticism was noted after the death of Christ when small groups banded together in independent units on a conventual plan, such as Marcella had organized.

A well-established form of monasticism still flourishing today is the order of Benedictines founded by *St. Benedict* (*ca.* 480–543) (Fig. 4–12). Benedict of Nursia was born of noble parents. He was sent to Rome for his basic schooling and while there was repelled by the moral corruption around him. In disgust he fled to the woods of Subiaco to meditate and pray. Later he complied with the invitations of other monks to organize a monastic family. He became their abbas, or father, from which the title abbot is derived. About the year 528 he composed his Rule and undertook the foundation of the Monastery of Subiaco in the Sabine Hills near Rome.

His most famous monastery was *Monte Cassino* (Fig. 4–13), built on a rugged mountain top between Rome and Naples, probably in the year 529. This monastery, built on a

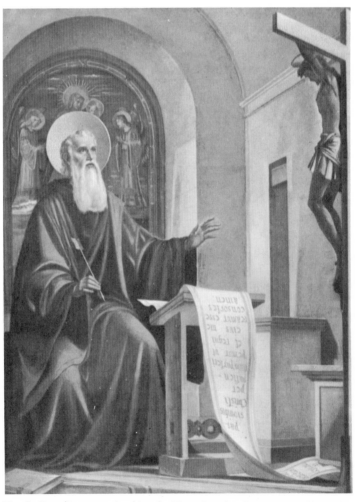

Figure 4–12. St. Benedict composing his rule. (Dom Agostino Saccomanno, Monte Cassino Abbey.)

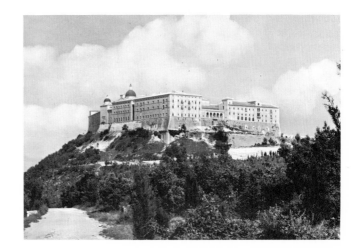

Figure 4–13. Monte Cassino Abbey. (Dom Agostino Saccomanno, Monte Cassino Abbey.)

former stronghold of paganism—one of the temples of Apollo—received great publicity when it was seized by the Nazis as a stronghold and bombed by the Allied forces during World War II.

Other famous Benedictine monasteries include the one at Fulda in Germany, which became world famous under the direction of Abbot Maurus (776–856). This erudite abbot had studied under Alcuin (the teacher of Charlemagne) at the Benedictine Abbey at Tours in France. Abbot Maurus compiled a medical encyclopedia *Physica,* which had a German-Latin glossary of anatomical terms.

The Benedictine monastery of St. Gall in Switzerland (*ca.* 720) became a school of medicine. A ground plan dating back to 820 indicates the presence of a pharmaceutical garden and a pharmacy. A wing contained six beds for the sick.

The rule of St. Benedict brought a stability and a scheme of organization to an age in which chaos and panic reigned. In this period when men fled to the wilderness in large numbers to practice severe forms of penance, Benedict stressed the need of moderation, fruitful labor and discipline. His well known precept, *Ora et labora* (to labor is to pray), has been a guidepost for many Christians through the centuries. He loved the spirit of work, using hands, head and heart. Peace and charity were so important to the Benedictines that they used as their watchword *Pax.* In this atmosphere of peace, love and productive activity, the family spirit was cultivated, for the needs of the community were to be furnished within the monastery walls. Career opportunities were

fostered to meet the growing demands of the community. As workshops of all sorts were erected, the need for teachers was apparent and the monasteries became centers of learning. Not only did the monks engage in practical skills, but they cultivated gardens and prepared medicinal drugs, studied music and languages, copied and illuminated precious manuscripts, and wrote poetry and drama. Actually the monks were scholars, thinkers, librarians and teachers, as well as artisans and farmers. It was the duty of the monk to do for others and share with others, and these centers of activity offered hospitality and shelter to the homeless, care to the sick and refuge to the persecuted. In addition, the monasteries equipped each person with the knowledge and skills necessary to provide him with a livelihood.

The *care of the sick* was an important part of the community life, and one of the rules of St. Benedict stressed that the abbot, who was in charge of the monastery, should arrange for an infirmary. The rule states:

> The care of the sick is to be placed above and before every other duty, as if indeed Christ were being directly served by waiting upon them. It must be the peculiar care of the abbot (or abbess) to see that they suffer from no negligence. The Infirmarian must be thoroughly reliable, known for his piety, diligence and solicitude for his charge.

Shakespeare's portrayal of the monk and his knowledge of medicine is not a figment of his imagination but a true portrayal of the monk in history. Friar Lawrence in *Romeo and Juliet* represents a survival of the fact that from the monastery gardens were derived the sources of plants, herbs and minerals used for healing. We are aware that the monks used a combination of mandrake, hyoscyamus, opium and wild lettuce to induce a state of narcosis in which the patient was insensible to pain. Friar Lawrence suggested that Juliet be placed in such a state "which shall appear like death."

The monasteries fostered an opportunity for women to pursue a career in which they could satisfy their intellectual and spiritual aspirations and develop nursing skills. Many of the women who desired conventual life were gifted with qualities of leadership; the abbesses were skilled executives.

FAMOUS MONASTIC NURSES

St. Brigid (452–523 A.D.), was the daughter of a chieftain of Ulster and became a famous abbess in Ireland and a distinguished scholar, counselor, educator and leader in the healing arts (Fig. 4–14). Under her guidance the monastery at Kildare became well known for its culture as well as for its spirituality and was, in fact, an institution of higher learning for women. Brigid founded schools for children and taught in them herself. In fifth century Ireland, when leprosy was an incurable scourge and lepers were free to roam, they came in droves to Kildare to be bathed

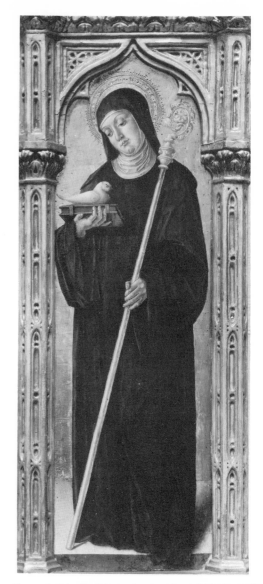

Figure 4–15. St. Scholastica by Vivarini (1450–1499). (Courtesy of Museum of Fine Arts, Boston.)

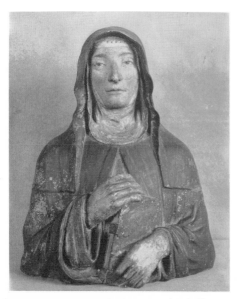

Figure 4–14. St. Brigid. (Courtesy of Isabella Stewart. Gardner Museum, Boston.)

and treated by Brigid. She tended the sick and gave alms to the poor.

Brigid established within her monastery a school of art in which exquisitely illuminated manuscripts were produced as well as gold and silver work of high artistic quality.

Manuscripts have been preserved, copied and illuminated in these monasteries. One of the best examples of these is the world famous Book of Kells, which can be seen in the library of Trinity College in Dublin.

St. Scholastica (Fig. 4–15), the twin sister of St. Benedict, founded an order for women based on his Rule. This Benedictine community for women was started near Monte Cassino, and Scholastica held the office of abbess. Many other famous women of the Benedictine family have contributed in the field of nursing.

St. Radegonde, (*ca.* 519–587), a German princess and the daughter of a Thuringian king, and a grand-niece of the great Gothic king, Theodoric, was a deeply religious, cultured and beautiful girl who had deep sorrow in her life. In her infancy her father was murdered by her uncle; as a young girl she was carried off by Clotaire, the Frankish king of Neustria, when he subjugated her country. She was forced to marry Clotaire, become his queen and was eventually one of his six wives (Fig. 4–16). The king murdered one of these wives with her son and daughter as well as Radegonde's brother. In revulsion she fled from him and sought asylum at a monastery.

Radegonde was a scholar and had marked qualities of leadership. After becoming a nun, she founded the Holy Cross Monastery at Poitiers, a religious settlement of 200 nuns. The care of the sick was the chief activity; study ranked next in importance and two hours every day were devoted to reading literature. The members of her community copied manuscripts and performed dramatic compositions. One wonders if the latter were performed as diversional therapy for the patients. In the hospital she had built, Radegonde bathed the patients herself, giving special care to the lepers. To this group of social outcasts, who were deprived of the necessities of life and love and affection, Radegonde, a queen and nun, bestowed an embrace of welcome and a "leper's kiss." Queen Radegonde's example encouraged many ladies of noble birth to care for the sick, and her influence also extended to the establishment of hospitals.

St. Hilda (614–680 A.D.), the abbess of Streonshalh (now Whitby) in England, was born of noble parents and was a cultured, scholarly woman and a gifted administrator, teacher and counselor. Because of her guidance and inspiration, her community did more than translate, transcribe and illuminate manuscripts; creative writing was encouraged and Caedmon, the first English poet, received his encouragement and guidance here (Fig. 4–17).

Associated with each Benedictine Monastery were the associate members called *oblates.* These members could live within the

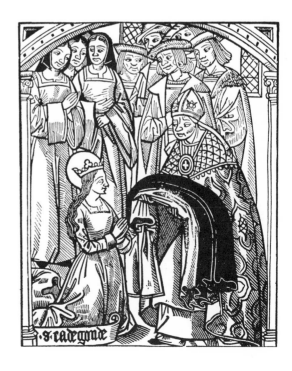

Figure 4–16. St. Radegonde, wife of King Clotaire, receiving religious robes from St. Medard. (From an old woodcut.)

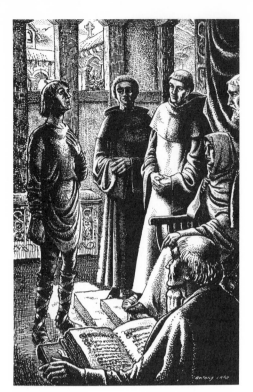

Figure 4–17. Caedmon appearing before Abbess Hilda who encouraged him to tell his tale in his own words. (Roche, *Christians Courageous.* Burns & Oates, Ltd.)

monastery or in their own homes but gave their services to the monastery and in turn received the benefits of such a relationship. This type of monastic affiliation is still in existence.

The capable women in the monasteries were not only the abbesses, but also the many gifted sisters and oblates who contributed to the monastery in a remarkable way. Such a person was the sister, *Hrotswitha* (935–1001), of the Benedictine Abbey at Gandersheim. Hrotswitha entered the monastery at the age of 23 and was tutored by the Mistress of Novices and the Abbess, studying Virgil, Plautus, Horace, Terence and Aristotle. She had great writing ability, and her dramas were given to the literary world in a French translation in 1845. These works glorified Christian feminism and showed how it could conquer the brutality of man. Hrotswitha was one of the great literary personalities of history, and it is said that her plays were enacted by nuns to an audience of nuns.

It is important to realize the part the

monasteries played in the preservation of culture and learning. They stood as an oasis in a desert of insecurity, persecution and suffering. These monasteries offered refuge for the persecuted; encouraged manual labor, formerly the duty of slaves; fostered healthy, purposeful lives devoted to personal piety and promotion of human welfare; developed agricultural experimental stations; motivated artists and skilled craftsmen in architecture, music, painting and in arts and crafts; provided nurses and doctors to care for the sick; cultivated medicinal gardens; advocated personal and professional growth by studying; preserved manuscripts and built the foundation for universities by sending copies of manuscripts from monastery to monastery. Lastly, they were the school teachers of this period. Not only did the monasteries give new creative expression but they preserved the ancient cultural treasures, for when the empire fell, the ancient learning of the classical period would have been lost and forgotten were it not for the monks of the West.

Nursing attracted many of the women of this period and its recruits numbered several queens. *St. Clothilde* (*ca.* 474–544) was a Burgundian princess who married Clovis I, King of the Franks. Widowed, she spent the rest of her life near the Monastery of St. Martin at Tours where she cared for the sick.

Queen Theodolinde, wife of Agilulf, King of the Lombards, worked conscientiously for the sick among the poor and especially for lepers. *St. Bathilde* (*ca.* 634–680), wife of Clovis II, King of the Franks, was kidnapped in childhood and became first a slave, then a queen-consort and finally queen-regent. The foundress of the monasteries at Chelles and Corbie, she retired as a widow to her Abbey at Chelles and ministered to the sick poor.

St. Margaret (1045–1093) married King Malcolm[5] of Scotland. Learned, beautiful and deeply religious, she washed the feet of beggars, gave money to the poor, visited hospitals and ministered to the sick. Margaret helped families in distress, especially displaced persons and ransomed captives of every nation, and founded hospitals, churches and monasteries. Her uncle, St. Edward the Confessor, King of England, is

---

[5] His father was that "gracious Duncan" whose sad fate has been immortalized by Shakespeare. Macbeth usurped his kingdom.

believed to have built the Benedictine monastery in London now called Westminster Abbey.

SPECIAL CARE OF MENTALLY ILL

The first organized plan for the care of mentally ill and mentally retarded children (other than that at St. Basil's in Caesarea) was founded at Gheel in Belgium.

Tradition has its beginnings toward the end of the sixth century in the legend of St. Dymphna, an Irish princess who fled the incestuous demands of her demented father, a king of Ireland. He pursued and murdered her in the forests around present-day Gheel.

The fame of the saintly young girl spread as reports of miraculous cures, especially to those who were mentally ill and emotionally disturbed, occurred at her tomb. People brought their relatives in the hope of a cure. First, a shrine was built and then a church was constructed and dedicated to *St. Dymphna* (Fig. 4–18). The alcoves of these edifices could not contain the number of patients who arrived in Gheel on pilgrimages. A building adjoining St. Dymphna's church housed the pilgrims. This structure, called *Sieckenkamer* or *Chambre des malades,* frequently could not accommodate the large number of mentally ill and mentally retarded guests, and the housewives of Gheel accepted these patients as boarders and as foster members of their families. The populace of Gheel has developed great skill in caring for these foster members and has bestowed love and affection upon them.

Judicious regulations, enacted as early as the fifteenth century by the Municipal Board of Gheel, prevented abuses that might have occurred. When France annexed the Belgian provinces, the institution came under local government. In 1852, it was reorganized by the Belgian government and given the name of "colony."

Today, when a person arrives at Gheel, he is received for observation at the "Infirmary" or central hospital. While there, a plan of care is instituted, including the newest techniques of psychiatry, before he is admitted into the home of the foster family. A home care plan has been developed whereby the psychiatrists and psychiatric nurses at regular intervals visit and check on the patients in their new environment.

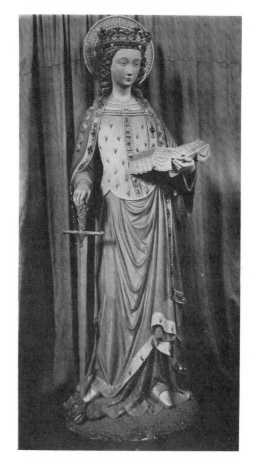

Figure 4–18. St. Dymphna.

The patients entrusted to the Colony of Gheel enjoy, in spite of their misfortune, all the advantages of freedom and of family life, permanent contact with normal persons, voluntary work fitted to their aptitudes and their preferences as well as forms of entertainment.

Gheel has a population of more than 22,000 and contains 5850 families of which approximately 2000 accept patients. From 1926 to 1950, 8358 patients were admitted to the colony. Of this number 2197, or more than 26 per cent, returned to their families cured or improved.[6]

Gheel is now an institutional town under government control and receives children from all countries and situations, placing them under the care of St. Dymphna and her

[6]Gushee, L.: Unpublished translation of brochure obtained by Mrs. Mary Gushee on a visit to Gheel, June 1957.

modern counterparts who are anxious to give loving care to these individuals.

Thus, charity in action is carried out by a community of health professionals and kind-hearted people toward a needy group of individuals which results in supervised family care.

Goldin[7] quotes Dr. Harry Shapiro of the American Museum of Natural History who is involved in a study of Gheel today: "Psychiatrists in this country point out that the treatment is nothing new—but treatment is not the question. What is at issue is the *care* of these people."

The nursing care and supervision was under the direction of the Soeur Hospitalière—hospital sisters under the rule of the Augustinian order—called Augustinian Sisters. This is the oldest order of nursing sisters in existence.

SCHOOL OF SALERNO

In the transition from monastic to lay medicine the *School of Salerno* played an important part. Although the school's beginnings are not well known, it may have been an outgrowth of the Benedictine Abbey of Monte Cassino; the library of Monte Cassino still contains many valuable medical manuscripts, and copies of these may have been sent to the new school. Benedictine monks joined Salerno's faculty, which also consisted of lay men and women. This famous school produced many leaders in the field of medicine and surgery.

Students were given lectures in the classroom and at the bedside of patients, and discussions were encouraged. Methods of treating the patients included drugs, bloodletting, diet and psychotherapy in the form of soothing words and restful music. It is interesting to realize that the importance of psychotherapy in the process of healing was recognized. Anthimus, a physician of Theodoric, wrote a book called *Dietetica* on the importance of nutrition, food selection and preparation. In addition to providing an appropriate diet, the book stressed the theory that the food should be served attractively to encourage the patient to eat.

The importance of a good bedside manner was realized, and a doctor of Salerno was

encouraged to question the messenger who summoned him to the bedside of the patient so that he could consider the patient's condition before seeing him. It is assumed that it was the nursing assessment that was sent to the physician. The doctor was advised to sit and chat pleasantly with the patient so that when he took the pulse it would be a true reading and not an elevated one caused by excitement.

Because of the wise influence of the medical leadership at the School of Salerno, medical legislation was enacted. As early as 1140, a law was passed forbidding anyone to practice medicine without being examined carefully. The essential education required to receive a degree from the School of Salerno and thence to become eligible for the examination for licensure was: three years of premedical study in logic, philosophy and literature, five years of study in medicine and surgery, and one year as an assistant to an experienced practitioner.

It is a well-known fact that very early in its history women studied at Salerno. All branches of learning, including medicine, were opened to women, and copies of many medical licenses granted to women can be seen in the Archives of Naples. A famous woman doctor, Trotula by name, is supposed to have written a book on obstetrics and gynecology and to have been head of the department of diseases of women.

MEDIEVAL HOSPITALS

There were three famous medieval hospitals built outside monastery walls and they are extant today: the Hôtel Dieu in Lyons, the Hôtel Dieu in Paris and the Hospital of the Holy Spirit or the Santo Spirito in Rome.

The *Hôtel Dieu* in Lyons, established in 542, was organized on the pattern of an almshouse and was administered under lay management. The nursing was carried out mainly by repentant women and by widows called sisters (though not a religious group) and by male nurses called brothers. This hospital has achieved an interesting record of accomplishment.

The *Hôtel Dieu* in Paris was founded around 650; it was conducted under lay administration and built on the almshouse pattern. The nursing staff was composed of Augustinian Sisters.

The *Santo Spirito Hospital* in Rome was founded by order of the Pope in 717 and was

[7]Goldin, Grace: "A Painting in Gheel," *Journal of the History of Medicine and Allied Sciences*, Volume XXVI, Number 4, October, 1971, pp. 400–412.

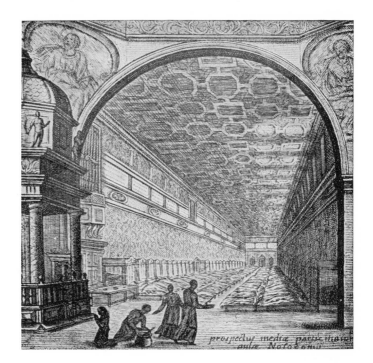

Figure 4–19. A ward in the Santo Spirito Hospital of Rome. (Castiglioni, Arturo: *A History of Medicine.* Alfred A. Knopf, New York.)

built primarily to receive only the sick. This hospital exists today and has inspired the establishment of many others like it (Fig. 4–19).

ISLAM AND ARABIC MEDICINE

A new monotheistic religion called *Islam* arose among the predominantly nomadic peoples of the Arabian peninsula.

Mohammed, the founder of Islam, was born at Mecca in the year 570. In 610 he announced that he had been called by Allah to preach a new religion.

Mohammed commenced his work by striving to sway his fellow men from idolatry to the worship of Allah. Gradually his enthusiastic converts extended this invitation by means of the sword. Each convert was called a "Moslem" or "one who submits."

By the time Mohammed died in 632, Islam had spread by the military genius of Mohammed, and his followers controlled the territories of Egypt, Palestine, Syria and India. Later Roman Africa, Spain and even Constantinople were captured. Twenty-one years after the death of Mohammed, the rule of Islam extended over a territory as great as the Roman Empire.

Two forces ended these sweeping military successes and prevented Islam from spreading over the civilized world. In the East, the eastern part of the Roman Empire—the Byzantine State—was saved by the military skill of the soldiers of Emperor Leo III; in the West, a powerful Frankish duke, Charles Martel, defeated the Arab forces.

The Arabs had learned much in their conquests and they eagerly assimilated the effects of this cultural exchange with other groups. One of these groups that had considerable influence on the field of medicine was that of the Nestorians. They were the followers of a heretical monk, Nestorius, who, after he and some of his followers were expelled from the Byzantine State, settled in Syria and thence migrated to Persia, China and India. The Moslems secured copies of the Greek medical texts of Hippocrates, Galen and Dioscorides from the Nestorians, who assisted in the translation of these manuscripts into Arabic.

The great contributions of the "Golden Age of Arabic Medicine" were concentrated in the areas of compounding drugs; in the advancement of medical knowledge through diagnosis, description and treatment of disease; in requiring licensure after careful examination of physicians and pharmacists; in providing medical leaders and in the construction and administration of exceedingly modern hospitals.

The Arabs were unable to develop a full understanding of anatomy and physiology because dissection was forbidden. Surgery was frowned upon, cautery being more popular than the knife.

Three of the famous physicians of this period were Rhazes (860–932), Avicenna (980–1037) and Maimonides (1135–1204).

Rhazes was a Persian scholar who added to the medical contributions of Hippocrates and Galen by his medical work entitled *The Compendium.* He described the diseases of smallpox and measles in one of his monographs and was a skilled clinician.

Avicenna, a Persian, was one of the great scholars of the Arabic world (Fig. 4–20). Called the "Prince of Physicians," his writings, especially his *Canon of Medicine,* have been considered some of the most important textbooks in the field of medical education; the *Canon of Medicine* was studied in the medical schools of Europe from the twelfth to the seventeenth centuries.

Moses ben Maimon (*Maimonides*) (Fig. 4–21), the third member of the Arabic medical triumvirate, was born in Moslem-controlled Cordova, Spain, of a Jewish family descended from King David. He was an excellent clinician and as his fame spread he became the court physician to the Sultan Saladin. It has been said that during the Crusades Richard the Lion-Hearted, learning of Maimonides' great skill, asked him to return to England with him as his personal physician. The greatest rabbinic scholar of his age,

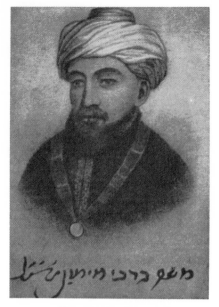

Figure 4–21. Maimonides.

Maimonides is remembered for codifying the Talmud and for composing the beautiful prayer that reads,

And now I turn unto my calling;
Oh, stand by me, my God, in this truly important
  task!
Grant me success! For—
Without Thy loving counsel and support
Man can avail but naught.

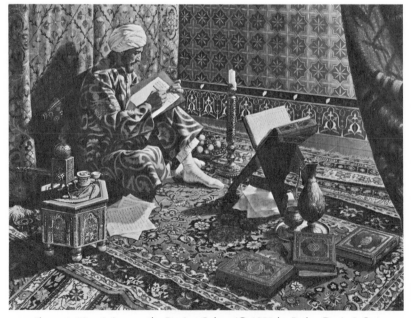

Figure 4–20. Avicenna: the Persian Galen. (© 1953 by Parke, Davis & Co.)

Inspire me with true love for this my art
And for thy creatures.
Oh, grant—
That neither greed nor gain, nor thirst for fame,
nor vain ambition,
May interfere with my activity.
For these, I know, are enemies of Truth and
Love of men,
And might beguile one in profession,
From furthering the welfare of Thy creatures.
Oh, strengthen me!
Grant energy unto both body and the soul,
That I may e'er unhindered ready be
To mitigate the woes,
Sustain and help,
The rich and poor, the good and bad, the enemy
and friend.
Oh, let me e'er behold in the afflicted and the
suffering
Only the human being!

Medical centers at this time were located in Cairo, Alexandria, Damascus and Baghdad. *Hospitals* were part of these centers and were famous for having beautiful architecture, being well equipped, employing unusual ideas of social service,[8] encouraging study

---

[8]For example, on discharge a patient was given money to permit him to convalesce properly before returning to work.

by including lecture rooms and libraries and employing readers and storytellers for the patients.

Alchemy and pharmacology were specialties and the Arabic scientists, highly skilled in compounding medicines, were interested in finding an "elixir of life." Pharmacists were independent practitioners and apothecary shops were common in the Moslem countries.

Moslem women were notably absent in the care of the sick, largely because they were kept in seclusion and shrouded in heavy veils. Polygamy was practiced by Moslem males, and it is said that Islam improved the status of woman only in the sense that it forbade the killing of girl babies, which was permissible in pre-Islamic times.

As the early Middle Ages end, amid distress, poverty and political chaos, it is observed that the Church had grown; Christianity had spread; missionaries carried not only the religious message but civilization as well; benevolent institutions had arisen; and monks and nuns had replaced the deaconesses and matrons in the care of the sick. *Nursing at last had developed roots, purpose, direction and leadership.*

REFERENCE READINGS

Austin, Anne L.: *History of Nursing Source Book.* New York, G. P. Putnam's Sons, 1957.

Blacam, Hugh de: *The Saints of Ireland—the Life Stories of Saints Brigid and Columcille.* Milwaukee, Bruce Publishing Co., 1942.

Caldwell, Taylor: *Dear and Glorious Physician.* New York, Doubleday & Co., 1959.

Curtayne, Alice: *St. Brigid of Ireland.* New York, Sheed & Ward, 1954.

Eckenstein, Lena: *Women under Monasticism.* Cambridge, The University Press, 1896.

Harnack, Adolph: *Luke, the Physician.* New York, G. P. Putnam's Sons, 1909.

Kavanagh, Julia: *Women of Christianity.* New York, D. Appleton Co., 1852.

Kingsley, Charles: *Hypatia.* New York, Lovell, Coryell & Co.

Luce, Clare B.: *Saints for Now.* New York, Sheed & Ward, 1952.

Maynard, Theodore: *St. Benedict and His Monks.* London, Staples Press, 1956.

Merton, Thomas: *The Seven Storey Mountain.* New York, Harcourt, Brace & Co., 1948.

Oursler, Fulton: *The Greatest Story Ever Told.* New York, Doubleday & Co., 1949.

Pond, Marian B.: *Heaven in a Wildflower.* New York, Vantage Press, 1954.

Power, Eileen: *Medieval People.* New York, Barnes & Noble, 1924.

Riesman, David: *The Story of Medicine in the Middle Ages.* New York, Harper & Brothers, 1936.

Roche, Aloysius: *Christians Courageous.* London, Burns & Oates, Ltd.

Sienkiewicz, Henryk: *Quo Vadis?* Boston, Little, Brown & Co., 1896.

Slaughter, Frank G.: *The Road to Bithynia.* New York, Doubleday & Co., 1951.

Smith, C. Raimer: *The Physician Examines the Bible.* New York, Philosophical Library, 1950.

Uhlhorn, Gerhard: *Christian Charity in the Ancient Church.* New York, Charles Scribner, 1883.

Walsh, James J.: *Old Time Makers of Medicine.* New York, Fordham University Press, 1911.

Waugh, Evelyn: *Helena.* Boston, Little, Brown & Co., 1950.

Wheeler, Henry: *Deaconesses, Ancient and Modern.* New York, Hunt & Eaton, 1889.

Wiseman, Cardinal: *Fabiola, or the Church of the Catacombs.* New York, P. J. Kenedy & Sons.

CHAPTER 5

Social and Spiritual Forces in the Expansion of Nursing (1000–1500)

THE CRUSADES

Toward the close of the eleventh century the Seljuk Turks who had embraced Islam became the most warlike segment of the Moslem world. During their tour of conquest they captured Palestine, among other places, and erected mosques in the Holy City of Jerusalem. Cruel persecutions were meted out to the Christians who had been making pilgrimages since the death of Christ. The capture of the Holy Places and the harsh treatment of the pilgrims impelled the European Christians to unite and stop the actions of the "infidel" Turks. Armed intervention seemed the best solution. Thus were initiated the military expeditions of the religious movement known as the *Crusades,* which lasted for nearly two hundred years (1096–1291).

In evaluating the results of the Crusades, there are both favorable and unfavorable aspects to be considered in these two hundred years that served as an avenue of interchange in ideas, customs and disease between the East and West.

It is difficult for us to envision the ordinary difficulties that beset the Crusaders on their journey. Travel was slow and laborious; adequate and nutritious food was hard to procure and harder to preserve; prevention of disease was impossible, and immunity to newly encountered diseases was low in most cases or nonexistent.

Hospitals and shelters had been built for the pilgrims by such persons as St. Helena and St. Paula, but the ones available did not meet the needs of the Crusaders. Fatigue, malnutrition, digestive disturbances from food poisoning, poor sanitary conditions and contact with communicable diseases all contributed to an acute demand for hospitals and providers of health care.

Military Nursing Orders

This brought about one of the major results of the Crusades, the formation of *military nursing orders* that drew large numbers of men into the field of nursing. The membership in these orders consisted of knights, monks, and serving brothers. Careful selection of members was employed because the recognized accolade of knighthood had to be achieved before membership in one of the military nursing orders was established. The monks were spiritual advisors and the serving brothers were highly motivated persons who became assistants to the military nursing knights and the priests.

The *Knights Hospitallers of St. John* were organized originally to staff one of two hospitals that had been built by rich merchants of Amalfi in 1050 A.D. in Jerusalem. The hospital for male patients was placed under the protection of St. John (probably St. John the Baptist) and a monk, Peter Gerhard, took charge (Fig. 5–1). The second hospital, for female patients, was dedicated to St. Mary Magdalene and was staffed by nuns under the direction of a capable Roman lady named Agnes. The purpose of these orders was to care for pilgrims who became ill on their journey to the Holy Land. Their care extended to Moslems and Jews as well as

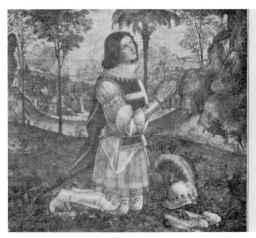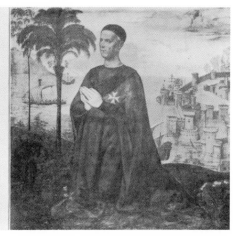

Figure 5–1. A Knight of St. John in armor (at left) and in the black mantle of a military nurse. (From frescoes by Pinturicchio in the Cathedral in Siena.)

Christians. The hospitals in Jerusalem were well equipped. Each patient was provided with a cloak of sheepskin and boots, the forerunner of bathrobes and slippers.

The knights were mainly a nursing order, but assumed a military role when it was essential to defend the hospital and its inmates. Their habit, worn over their suit of armor, was a black mantle with a white *Maltese cross.* (See Figure 5–2.)

Gradually, the knights built additional hospitals, hostels and hospices at strategic points in the mountain passes and at river crossings. When the Knights Hospitallers went to Rhodes, they built extensive fortifications. They set up a Health Commission that prevented an outbreak of the plague by strict enforcement of a 40 day isolation period for all those who had come in contact with plague victims. This is the origin of the term *"quarantine."*

The order settled on the island of Malta in 1530, and the hospital they constructed there is a famous one with many interesting features. As early as 1617, a board was placed at the head of each bed upon which doctor's orders were written. The physicians and surgeons were accompanied on their rounds by a secretary who took down the prescriptions as the doctors dictated them. Nurses remained with the patient.

A method of protection had to be devised to prevent the spread of communicable diseases when ships docked in the harbor. Some measures taken to prevent and control disease in addition to quarantine and isolation were the use of a pure water supply brought by an aqueduct system, drainage canals for the overflow of water, collection and disposal of garbage and burial of the dead outside the city walls.

After the knights had settled on the island of Malta, they reestablished the Sisters of the Knights Hospitallers of St. John who had been forced to flee Jerusalem when that city fell. They had escaped to Europe but came

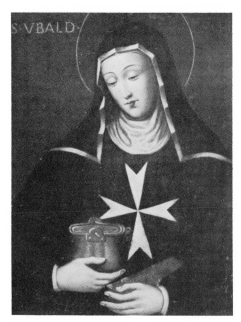

Figure 5–2. Saint Ubaldesca in the military nursing habit of the Hospitallers of St. John.

to Malta and remained there after the Knights had departed from this area in 1798. This order of sisters, wearing the habit of the Hospitallers, still remains to care for the sick of Malta. It has been said that at first the habit of the order was red with the white Maltese cross, but later the red was changed to black.

The Knights Hospitallers of St. John have been known as the Knights of Malta for many years. They have been considered a sovereign power with representatives of ambassadorial rank, and the diplomatic sovereignty is recognized universally. Under the Geneva convention their insignia, the Maltese cross, was awarded the same recognition of immunity by belligerents in war as the Red Cross. As Knights Hospitallers of St. John and later as Knights of Malta, they have given outstanding service in international nursing.

The *Teutonic Knights* came into existence in 1190 during the siege of Acre. This order was comprised of German knights who banded together and converted their tents into emergency hospitals, and who alternately nursed and fought. They, too, took vows to care for the sick, erect hospitals and defend the faith. The Teutonic Knights were distinguished from the Knights of St. John by the white tunic with a black Maltese cross outlined in gold over their coat of mail.

The *Knights of St. Lazarus* were devoted especially to the care of lepers; the name Lazarus was derived from the parable of the leper in the Bible. Many historians seem to indicate that this is the oldest of all knightly orders. It has been associated with the special hospital for lepers that was part of the Basilias built by St. Basil. Though these knights set a valiant example and gave excellent care, the order ceased to exist by 1830.

The Order of the Most Holy Trinity, more popularly known as the *Order of Trinitarians*, was founded in the year 1197. Not only did they render first aid on the battlefield and in plague-infested villages, but they also received the victims into the monastery hospital. They also ransomed the Christians taken prisoner by the Moslems. This group wore a white habit with a red and blue cross on the breast (Fig. 5–3).

The Crusades afforded a glorious opportunity for cultural interchange, especially for contact with *Arabic medicine*. This interchange was particularly valuable in broadening the scope of patient care and hospital planning, and in the development of medical education.

GROWTH OF CITIES

The feudal system declined in importance, and the groups that had previously lived around the feudal castles for protection began to build towns and develop a new social structure.

There were disadvantages to this new way

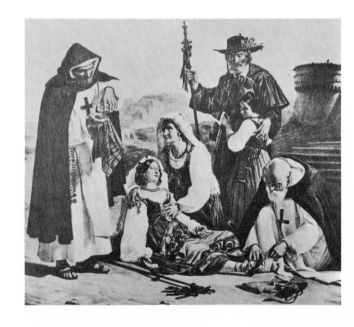

Figure 5–3. Trinitarian Fathers giving first aid.

of life. Living conditions were overcrowded; houses were ill-ventilated and poorly heated; animals shared the family quarters; there was improper sewage and garbage disposal; water supply and resources for preservation of food were inadequate. Continuance of these conditions produced serious consequences.

Frequently food poisoning resulted when food remaining from the previous day was seasoned highly, then served. One historian mentioned a covered casserole that was called "coffin."

Refuse from houses was thrown into the streets. Indeed, it has been said somewhat facetiously that the use of stilts became obligatory in many places. As a result, town edicts were posted requiring the citizenry to stop throwing refuse into the streets. The next injunction reprimanded the throwing of refuse in front of a neighbor's house. In some cities this refuse was removed every four days; in others, every eight days! Where could this garbage and debris be placed? The moat seemed to be a likely place, and so it was used.

This surrounding moat had provided the town with its water supply, but with its "added burden," it was no longer suitable. Fountains and wells became necessities, and a drinking cup was hung on the side.

Public bathhouses were constructed. It was not until the fifteenth century, however, that the sexes were segregated in these baths (Fig. 5–4).

The citizens were concerned at the increase in the disease rate yet were ignorant of the elementary principles of hygiene. They worried about inhaling the foul-smelling air and about the increase in the numbers of rats and vermin. As the disease rate continued to mount, the populace wondered about the possibility of transferring infection by the drinking fountain cup.

With what seemed a solution, all lepers were told to carry their own cups.

The problem of air pollution bothered medieval people because a hygienic precept stressed that "the air in which you live must be light, free from poison and should not stink."

MEDIEVAL TREATMENTS

The importance of the four bodily humors in keeping a person healthy remained the

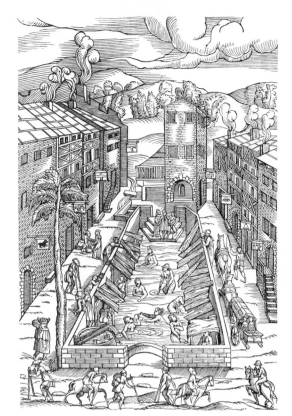

Figure 5–4. A public bathing facility in a European town during the sixteenth century. (Martin: *Deutsches Badewesen in vergangenen Tagen.*)

prime health concept at this time. To prevent or cure disease it was essential to withdraw the corrupt humors from the body. This was done by *purging, cupping, bloodletting* and *leeching.*

A powerful purgative was frequently given followed by the withdrawal of a small amount of blood. This procedure, called bloodletting, was one of the functions of the barber.[1] Leeches were also used for this purpose. These treatments were repeated as frequently as it seemed necessary.

Often, cups were applied to the skin and adhered to it by means of suction, the air having been quickly withdrawn from the cup. These applications acted as counterirritants.

At the height of ancient Greek and Roman medicine, metal cups were used. The ancient American Shamans used sucking tubes for cupping; these were hollow deer bones. Glass cups eventually replaced the metal ones.

The oldest printed blood-letting chart was drawn in 1493. The "Zodiac Man" (Fig. 5–5)

[1]The red and white barber poles are symbolic reminders of this early practice.

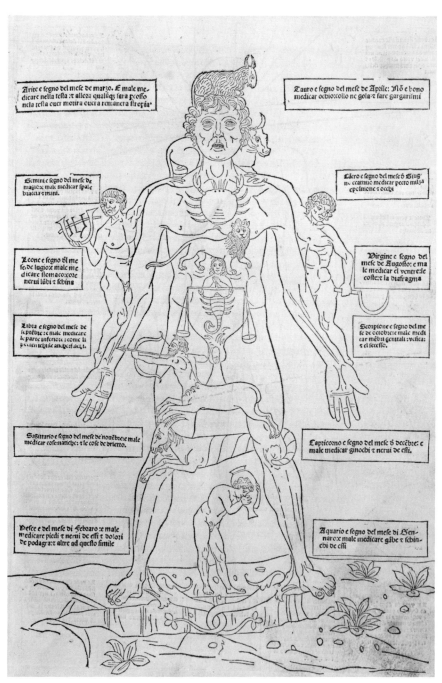

Figure 5–5. The Zodiac Man. Venetian woodcut, ca. 1493. (Courtesy of the Metropolitan Museum of Art, Harris Brisbane Dick Fund, 1938.)

portrays the astrological signs for blood-letting including suggestions for method and time of treatment, related to the humoral pathology of Galen as follows:

Aries, Leo, Sagittarius: warm-dry: yellow bile: choleric temperament
Gemini, Libra, Aquarius: warm-wet: blood: sanguine temperament
Taurus, Virgo, Capricorn: cold-dry: black bile: melancholy temperament.
Cancer, Scorpio, Pisces: cold-wet: phlegm: phlegmatic temperament

Many extraordinary medicines came into vogue at this time, such as one called the *horn of the unicorn*. An animal's horn that was supposed to have the properties of an antidote was hollowed out and used as a cup. The portion of the horn that was removed was powdered and taken as medicine. This was one of the miracle drugs of the Middle Ages and was considered a panacea.

Another medication in which people had implicit faith was the powder scratched from the stone covers of the coffins of saints. This powder was suspended in water and was drunk. Some of the coffin covers had to be replaced three and four times because of the amount of stone scratched away. Herbs were deposited near or on the coffin and a concoction of these herbs was made for the sick person. Often linen was laid on the tomb and then placed on the bed or person of the patient.

The chief diagnostic aid was called water casting or *uroscopy*, which consisted of the examination of urine. Pictures of this technique abound in the artistic contributions of medicine in this period. Indeed, the urine flask became the symbol of medicine.

LEPROSY

The prevalence of the disease called *leprosy*, the genuine fear of it and the attempts to isolate this disease have been historical facts from earliest times. That these people have been treated with much cruelty, little understanding and little kindness is also a known fact. Certain persons, however, gave "over and beyond the call of duty" to welcome, befriend and assist these patients. (See Figure 5–6.)

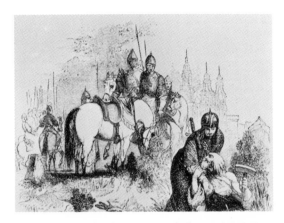

Figure 5–6. The famous Spanish hero, El Cid Campeador, is remembered for many expressions of concern and compassion. He is here portrayed in the act of saving the loor leper from sinking in the swamp.

In medieval communities it was noted that diseases were increasing, especially the disease of leprosy. Due to an inability to diagnose this disease accurately, many diseases of the skin were grouped under the heading "leprosy." All persons suffering from this disease were treated in the same way; they were expelled from the community to protect the healthy. We have mentioned that leper houses, lazarettos and finally leprosaria were built to house these patients when they were critically ill. The number of such establishments is reputed to have been 19,000 in Europe during the thirteenth century.

Special laws, which demanded that lepers announce their approach by shaking a wooden rattle or blowing a horn, were enacted in the Middle Ages. Lepers were permitted to beg for the necessities of life (Fig. 5–7).

The pathetic plight of the leper has been portrayed in art and literature. It has been emphasized that he was a social outcast. Ceremonies for the dead were recited and he was dispossessed of his fortune, title, money and personal possessions. To the rest of the world, the leper was literally dead, permitted to have only the horn, rattle or bell and his own drinking cup. In the past a white cross was the distinctive mark indicating the home or dwelling of a leper.

Norway has doors on churches that open to permit lepers to observe the ceremony, but not mingle with the parishioners.

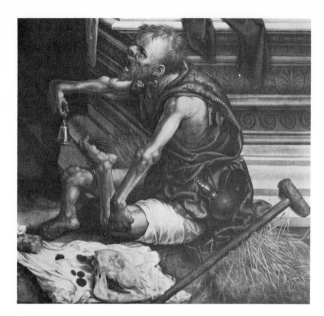

Figure 5–7. A person with advanced lepromatous leprosy. Note the bell and the crutch of the period. From a triptych by Barend Van Orley, ca. 1492–1542. (Courtesy of Royal Museum of Fine Arts, Antwerp.)

BUBONIC PLAGUE

In the fourteenth century a catastrophic outbreak of the *bubonic plague*, known as the Black Death, brought fear and devastation to much of Europe and the rest of the world. Records of this disease had appeared in the Bible, and mention has been made of the epidemics that occurred in the ancient civilized world. The outbreak of bubonic plague in the fourteenth century was one of the most devastating crises in human history and was a period of intense psychological trauma.

In 1345, ships returning from a long voyage to China and India reached the ports of the Black Sea and the Mediterranean. The cargo, when landed, included some of the rats from the ships. With the stage set by the unsanitary conditions described previously, an outbreak of bubonic plague resulted.

A presentation of the clinical picture may help in understanding this historic tragedy. Plague is an acute infectious disease caused by a bacillus called *Yersinia pestis*. Primarily a disease of rodents, particularly rats, the plague is readily transmissible to humans by such parasites as fleas feeding on a diseased rodent. The disease is transmitted also by direct contact with an infected person. After a brief incubation period of about two days, the following clinical picture is observed: chills, fever (101°–105°), severe headache, extreme prostration, vertigo, abscesses

called buboes in the lymph glands and hemorrhage of the superficial blood vessels that gives a bluish-black color (responsible for the popular name "Black Death"). Finally death results. There are three different types of the plague: the bubonic, the septicemic and the pneumonic.

The suddenness of the onset of disease and the brevity of its duration were responsible for the hysteria and panic that accompanied such an epidemic.

The chief means of defense from the disease in the medieval mind was to flee from the infected persons and from the location of the outbreak. Thus families fled from their loved ones, leaving them to die unattended.

The disease reached pandemic (worldwide) proportions eventually and when the plague ended, India was reputed to have been depopulated; China lost thirteen million persons; Cairo was supposed to have lost daily from ten to fifteen thousand lives and altogether at least a quarter of the population of the then-known world had perished.

THE GREAT POX–SYPHILIS

The other great scourge of the Middle Ages was *syphilis*. Its origin remains a mystery.

Syphilis was known before this time but under different names. Medieval syphilis was known first as *mal franzoso, morbus gallicus* or *mala napoletana.* After it became epidemic, it was called the "pocks." By the end of the fourteenth century, physicians were already prescribing mercurial ointments, but these were used for many skin afflictions other than syphilis.

On March 25, 1493, the town crier of Paris was directed to order from the city all afflicted with "the greater pox" (*la grosse vérole*) under pain of being thrown into the Seine River.

Another problem, less dramatic and spectacular but nonetheless real, was that of the frequent feuds. The high incidence of family feuds necessitated nursing care because of the wounds inflicted during these battles. This aspect of life in Italy in the fourteenth century was presented by Shakespeare in *Romeo and Juliet.* The tragic street scenes of fighting and stabbing were not the result of Shakespeare's facile pen and creative mind but were based on factual evidence.

RISE OF MENDICANT ORDERS — EXPANSION OF NURSING

With the rapid spread of misery and sickness and the fright of the plague, religious fervor mounted. A different type of religious ministration was required from that of the period when communities lived around a monastery. The answer to this demand came when St. Francis and St. Dominic each founded three religious orders: the first order was for friars; the second order was for nuns; the third order was for the laity, men and women who continued to lead secular lives.

St. Francis of Assisi (1182–1226) (Fig. 5–8) is undoubtedly one of the best-loved figures in world history. Francis was a worldly, pleasure-loving youth with extraordinary qualities of leadership. After a serious illness in his early twenties, Francis changed his manner of living, becoming concerned about others, and patterned his life after that of his Redeemer.

Disinherited by his merchant father for giving profuse alms to the poor, Francis donned a rough brown tunic, bound it around his waist with a heavy white rope, and went barefooted around the countryside ministering to the poor and outcast.

His first real spiritual challenge may have been his encounter with leprosy. St. Francis, having a marked aversion to leprosy, beheld a

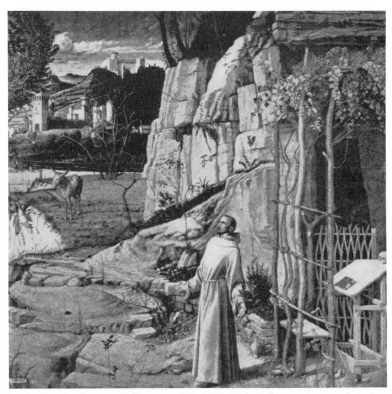

Figure 5–8. St. Francis of Assisi. (Bellini, ca. 1430–1516. Frick Collection, New York. University Prints.)

leper approaching him and begging for alms. After a brief pause, St. Francis embraced the unfortunate man and gave him what money he had. Becoming the champion of lepers, St. Francis and his companions lived next to the leper hospital and ministered to the patients. He made the public acutely aware of the plight of the leper and the problem of leprosy.

Many followers were attracted to this happy, kind and courageous man and in 1209 the Order of Friars Minor, or "little brothers," was formed. The rule of the Franciscans emphasized poverty and humility; they were mendicants and begged for themselves and for the poor. This obligation of mendicancy forced the friars to receive their daily bread as the fruit of their apostolic labors.

In studying the life of St. Francis, a medical practice of this period was noted. It became apparent that Francis' vision was failing and that he would soon become blind. The medical treatment selected was to cauterize his eyes with a red-hot iron without even the benefit of a soothing drug.

The spirit that guided St. Francis of Assisi has been summed up in his prayer:

Lord, make me an instrument of your peace.
  Where there is hatred, let me sow love.
  Where there is injury, pardon.
  Where there is doubt, faith.
  Where there is despair, hope.
  Where there is darkness, light.
  Where there is sadness, joy.
O Divine Master, grant that I may not so much seek
  To be consoled as to console,
  To be understood as to understand,
  To be loved as to love,
  For it is in giving that we receive,
  It is in pardoning that we are pardoned,
  It is in dying that we are born to eternal life.

Before his death in 1226, St. Francis' followers numbered in the thousands. One of his well known followers was the learned *St. Anthony of Padua* (1195–1231) who had been a teacher at the Universities of Paris, Bologna and Padua. Anthony was an eloquent preacher, a benevolent almsgiver and a prison reformer.

St. Clare, the beautiful daughter of a rich and noble family of Assisi, heard St. Francis preach and was motivated to follow his simple life of charity, humility and fervent devotion. Against strong parental opposition, Clare, garbed in her jewels and finery, changed happily into a brown sackcloth habit. Then Clare entered a nearby Benedictine abbey; in a short time a special convent was established for her and other young women who wanted to share this life of poverty and simplicity. Her sister Agnes joined the group and a short time after her father's death her mother joined them also. This second order of St. Francis became known as the order of *Poor Clares* (Fig. 5–9).

The rule of the Poor Clares was essentially the same as that of the Order of Friars. In times of epidemics, the Poor Clares took care of the sick and opened their convent as a hospital.

St. Clare died in 1253, but her order continues and has been described in *A Right to Be Merry.*[2]

While St. Francis was achieving success in Italy, *St. Dominic* was establishing an Order of Preachers, more frequently called the Dominicans. Many eminent scholars arose from these two groups at this time: the Dominican Albertus Magnus (1206–1280) and the Franciscan Roger Bacon (1214–1294) contributed to the beginnings of experimental science by emphasizing the value of observation, experimentation and the use of inductive reasoning. Known as the Prince of Scholastics, the Dominican St. Thomas Aquinas (1225?–1274) studied under the Benedictines at Monte Cassino and, sometime after 1265, began his greatest work, *Summa Theologica.*

The *Third Orders* of St. Francis and St. Dominic were established for many of the distinguished persons whose occupations and obligations could not permit them to live a conventual life, but who felt a need for this spiritual bond and wanted an opportunity to share in the accomplishments of the Order. Into the Third Order of St. Francis came such well known persons as St. Louis IX, the King of France; St. Elizabeth of the royal house of Hungary; Dante, the famous poet; and three great scientists in the field of electricity, Volta, Galvani and Ampère.

St. Elizabeth of Hungary (1207–1231) (Fig. 5–10), the daughter of King Andreas II and

---

[2]Sister Mary Francis, P. C.: *A Right to Be Merry.* New York, Sheed & Ward, 1956.

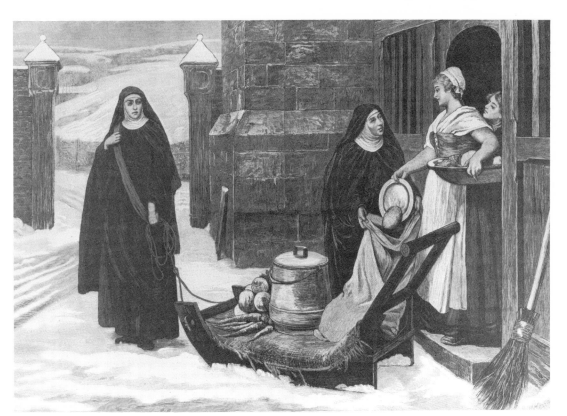

Figure 5–9. Mendicants begging "For The Poor," from a painting by W. F. Yeames (1875). (Author's collection.)

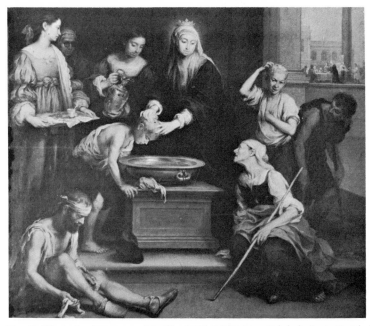

Figure 5–10. St. Elizabeth of Hungary. (Murillo, 1618–1682; Hospital de la Santa Caridad, Seville.)

Queen Gertrude of Hungary, was betrothed at four years of age to Ludwig, son of the Landgrave of Thuringia. They were married at an early age (1221) and were a devoted couple. Elizabeth was cheerful and fun-loving and exemplary for her goodness, generosity and sympathy. After her marriage, Elizabeth had a turnstile built into one of the castle gates, and she herself distributed alms daily to the poor and needy. During the famine of 1226, Elizabeth organized a distribution of food, depleting the castle granaries for the purpose. She would take the hour's walk from the castle to the nearby town to visit the sick in their homes, attending personally those who were ill and staying with the dying.

Elizabeth joined the Third Order of St. Francis and devoted her entire time, strength and energy to the needs of the sick poor. She built hospitals and directed her services especially to the lepers. Prisoners received her attention also and she bathed the wounds inflicted by their chains.

Before his death during one of the Crusades, Ludwig had cooperated with Elizabeth in her projects, partly because he had been permitted to witness several instances of her unusual sanctity. After his death, however, Elizabeth was expelled from her husband's castle, the Wartburg, and those to whom she had given so generously refused to assist her. Elizabeth settled at Marburg where she spent the remaining years of her short life (she died in 1231 at the age of 24) nursing the sick in the Marburg hospital that she had founded.

St. Louis IX (1214–1270) was especially interested in the three great needs of humanity — education, justice and charity — and he devoted his life to achieving these for his subjects (Fig. 5–11).

Louis' endeavors in the field of education resulted in the building of the Saint-Chapelle in Paris and in the founding of the Sorbonne College of the University of Paris. Louis stressed the need for properly educated persons to care for the sick and emphasized the necessity of adequate medical education. He himself waited on the sick, bathed them, served them and attended to their needs regardless of their unsightly appearance. Lepers received special care from him. Louis' justice and charity endeared him to his subjects and when he died on one of the Crusades he was mourned by Christians and

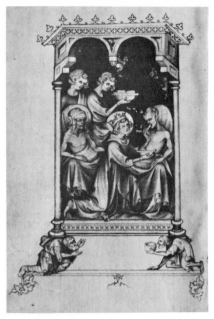

Figure 5–11. St. Louis administers to the sick in a medieval hospital. (Jean Pucelle, ca. 1325.) This is one of many illustrations depicting scenes from the life of St. Louis that appeared in a small book of prayers belonging to his granddaughter, Jeanne D'Evreux, Queen of France and wife of Charles IV.

Moslems alike. Under his reign, France enjoyed prosperity, peace and progress.

Members of the Third Order of St. Dominic were known first in Italy by the name Mantellate. These were lay persons who continued to live at home but bound themselves to a more religious schedule of life. They wore the Dominican religious habit, which consisted of a white tunic girded by a leather belt, a white veil over the head and a black cloak or mantella.

The first young single girl to join the Mantellate was a blind and deformed girl named *Margaret of Metola* (1287–1320), the daughter of wealthy parents who abandoned her because of her physical afflictions. Margaret spent the majority of her 33 years devoting herself to the needs of others. She visited and nursed the sick and gave special attention to prisoners who were kept in underground prison cells without sunlight, fresh air, sanitary facilities or heat. These prisoners suffered from lack of food and clothing, from the stench, from "jail fever" and from the wounds inflicted by their chains. Only the few who could afford to bribe their jailors received the bare necessities of life when these were obtainable. Yet every day, Margaret and her white-robed companions entered the prison armed with bundles of food, clothing, bedding and medicines.

St. Catherine of Siena (1347–1380) (Fig. 5–12) was born Catherine Benincasa, the 25th child of a well-to-do merchant and his wife. Catherine became a forceful, gifted, clear-thinking and diplomatic leader and writer. At the age of 18, joining the Mantellate and receiving the habit of the Third Order of St. Dominic, Catherine began her many works of mercy.

St. Catherine has been noted for the kindness and tenderness that she extended to persons with the most loathsome of diseases. When a poor woman with leprosy was refused admission to a hospital, Catherine begged that the woman be admitted, promising to care for her.

During the epidemic of the bubonic plague, the shadowy figure of Catherine could be seen going around the streets of Siena at night. With a lighted lantern she would look for forsaken victims so that she might comfort them. She ministered to the plague victims who were hospitalized. Mrs. Curtayne depicts Catherine carrying a bottle of cologne and bringing some refreshment into the stench of the hospital rooms. Catherine rallied her friends and they, too, "braced themselves to bend close to the livid, swollen faces, choking down the nausea of that pestilential odour."[3] There was very little to be done for these plague victims; to be willing to stay with them and comfort them was a supreme sacrifice.

Catherine of Siena's influence has been great. The nineteenth century English poet A. C. Swinburne praised her accomplishments in his poem, "The Laud of St. Catherine:"

> Then in her sacred saving hands
> She took the sorrows of the lands,
> With maiden palms she lifted up
> The sick time's blood-imbittered cup,
> And in her virgin garment furled
> The faint limbs of a wounded world,
> Clothed with calm love and clear desire,
> She went forth in her soul's attire,
> A missive fire.[4]

SECULAR NURSING ORDERS

There were other groups of workers who joined together yet were not bound by vows to monastic life. These members could terminate their vocations at any time and either return, settle down to married life or devote themselves to any other occupation. Such groups have been referred to as *secular nursing orders,* and they visited the sick, took care of foundlings and orphans and brought the sick to hospitals.

The *Order of Antonines,* or Hospital Brothers of St. Anthony, was founded about 1095. This group of laymen specialized in the care of patients suffering with a disease called St. Anthony's Fire (Fig. 5–13). Special hospitals were built for the sufferers of this disease, and the Antonines were successful in caring for these tragic victims.

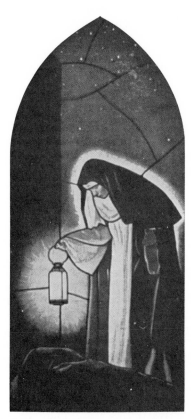

Figure 5–12. St. Catherine of Siena. (Courtesy of Will Ross, Inc.)

---

[3] Curtayne, Alice: *St. Catherine of Siena.* New York, The Macmillan Co., 1929, p. 75.

[4] Brown, E. K.: *Victorian Poetry.* New York, Thomas Nelson & Sons, 1942.

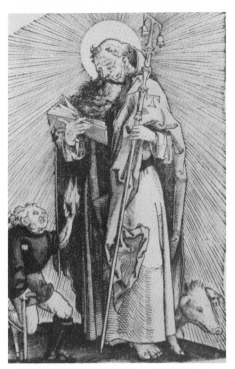

Figure 5–13. The great Egyptian hermit, St. Anthony, is represented with a victim of St. Anthony's Fire, or ergotism. (Woodcut by Johannes Wechtlin, *ca.* 1490–1530.)

In his book *The Day of St. Anthony's Fire*,[5] which presents the 1951 outbreak of this affliction (which occurred in Pont-Saint-Esprit in France), Fuller states:

In 1089, an observer wrote: "We could see many 'ergotists' in the village, bowels devoured by sacred fire, either dying wretchedly or living with gangrened limbs." When the town of La Motte-au-Bois in the province of Dauphiné, some hundred kilometers from Pont-Saint-Esprit, was stricken by ergotism in the Middle Ages, a nobleman and his son, both afflicted with the disease, called on St. Anthony and were cured by what they thought was the presence of St. Anthony's relics in the town. The relics had been captured by the Saracens in 532 and taken to Constantinople, but they had been brought back to Dauphiné by a conscientious pilgrim. The nobleman and his son then set up a lay society to cure the ill who were smitten by the disease. Even then the disease was nothing new. Ergot in rye had been mentioned in the Bible by the prophet Amos; Pliny had mentioned it in his *Natural History*. It was used in the tenth century in Thuringia for its strange power to hasten childbirth; it is still used under controlled modern

medicine for the same thing today. "There is a tingling and burning of the hands and feet," one writer described the symptoms, "and then a frightful heartburn. Fingers and toes are bent nearly doubled and clamped; the mouth is full of foam. Often the tongue is lacerated by the strength of the convulsions. There is a severe secretion of spittle. The sick utter that they are being destroyed by a burning fire. They feel great giddiness, and some of them become blind; the intellectual capacities are polluted, a fog comes over and destroys the mind."

The more sophisticated observations of the nineteenth century recognized that ergot was a parasitic fungus growth on grain, called *Claviceps purpurea*. A dense tissue forms in the ovaries of rye and gradually replaces the entire substance of the grain with a hard, purple, curved body called the sclerotium. This is the commercial source for pharmaceutical ergot, recognized in modern medicine as a very useful but often puzzling drug. It was only in the nineteen-thirties that many of the ergot alkaloids were discovered and defined chemically, but even today many facts are elusive. One thing is certain: All the ergot alkaloids are derivatives of lysergic acid, a chemical that still has much mystery surrounding it.

The hallucinatory manifestations of this disease have been documented in many dramatic references.

The *Beguines* of Flanders, Belgium (1184), were one of the most prominent of these secular nursing orders for women. Lambert le Begue, Bishop of Liege, was impelled by the belief that a person could live a religious life by devoting himself to good works without joining one of the established religious orders of the church. He suggested the founding of this community of women who would live together without taking vows or giving up their property or possessions. They were free to leave the group at any time or to marry.

The Beguines erected communal hermitages known as "Beguinages" on the outskirts of towns. These communities were arranged on a cottage plan, grouped around one large central structure, usually the church. Each cottage accommodated from two to four persons. The Beguinages at Bruges (*ca.* 1184) and at Ghent (*ca.* 1234) are well known (Fig. 5–14).

Each new member received her preparation under a more experienced member on an apprenticeship basis. These women devoted themselves to the needs of widows and orphans of the Crusaders. They pooled resources for they did not accept payment for services to the sick.

[5] Fuller, John G.: *The Day of St. Anthony's Fire.* New York, The Macmillan Co., 1968, pp. 117–118.

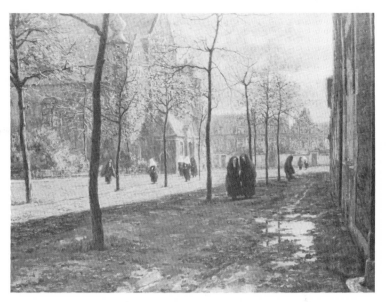

Figure 5–14. Members of the order of the Beguines leaving the Church of St. Elizabeth and heading toward the Beguinage at Ghent in Belgium. Painting by Ferdinand Willaert. (Author's collection.)

The Beguines devoted themselves to the care of the sick and were praised for their ministrations during war, famine and epidemics. They converted their houses into hospitals and worked as volunteer nurses. They distributed food and clothing during such catastrophic occasions as the Napoleonic Wars and the epidemic that followed, during the cholera epidemics and during the famine and industrial crises of the nineteenth century.

The Beguines built a hospital close to the Beguinage and established an order of sisters called the Sisters of Matilda to staff these hospitals. One of the most famous of these hospitals is the Hôtel Dieu at Beaune, which was founded in 1443 (Figs. 5–15 and 5–16). Although the primary work of the sisters was

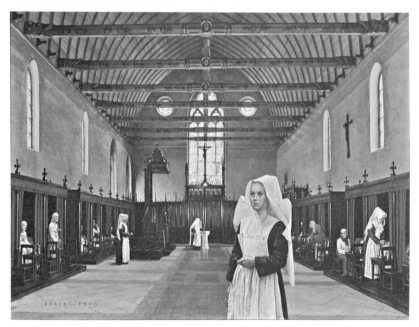

Figure 5–15. Hotel Dieu, Beaune, France. (© 1958 by Parke, Davis & Co.)

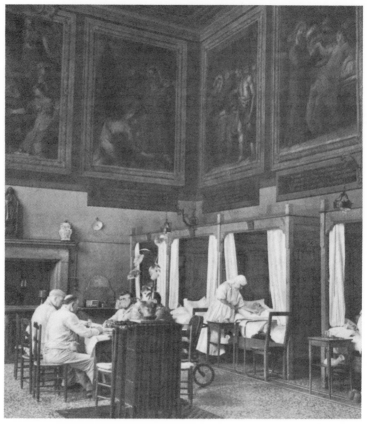

Figure 5–16. A Sister at the Hôtel Dieu in Beaune giving care to a patient in a room compartment. Ambulatory patients enjoy meals at the table in the center. Note the works of art.

nursing in the hospital, they did give care to the sick in their homes, staying with the dying and consoling the families of the bereaved.

The desire of women to join such a philanthropic project is apparent when we realize that by the end of the thirteenth century there was hardly a community that did not have a Beguinage, many of the larger cities having several, and the Beguines numbered about 200,000.

An order of men, the *Brethren of the Common Life*, was founded at this time by Gerhard Groot. At first, these men devoted themselves to the care of the sick poor and visited them in their homes. They were interested chiefly in teaching children who were bedridden. After a time they became the schoolmasters of the period, and such well known persons as Erasmus and Thomas à Kempis became members.

The *Sisters of the Common Life* specialized in the care of the sick, of which instruction of sick children was an integral part. These sisters took no vows, lived together in a conventual plan and could leave the group at any time.

The *Misericordia*, founded in 1244, was another group of religious laymen. Their chief contribution to medieval society was the volunteer ambulance work that they carried on in many Italian cities. The Misericordia are sometimes known as the "Masked Brotherhood" because of the masks that they wore on duty (Fig. 5–17). It is believed that this group felt that their unique contribution would gain spiritual merit if they prevented themselves (the givers) from being recognized by others.

The Italian city of Florence still boasts of the benevolence of the Brothers of Misericordia. In 1961, it was reported that 2500 members devote at least an hour a week for the charitable purposes of caring for the sick and needy. In their headquarters at the Piazza del Duomo assemble men of this

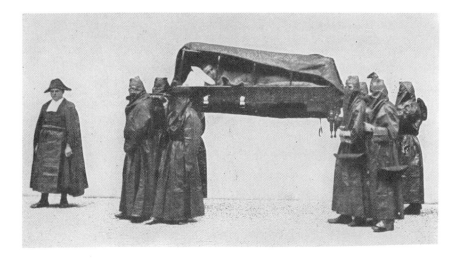

Figure 5–17. The Brothers of the Misericordia taking a patient to the hospital in Florence.

brotherhood who come from all walks of life including doctors, lawyers, students, civil and public servants. These brothers are prepared to assist the afflicted at any hour, for a carefully planned rotational schedule allows for a staff of twenty men on duty at every hour of the day or night.

The black-robed brothers are respected and admired for their great acts of charity. Although they wear the same identifying robe, the hood is no longer pulled down over the face today except during the funeral of one of the members.

Towards the end of the twelfth century, the *Order of the Holy Ghost* was founded in connection with the famous medical school at Montpellier in Southern France. The medical school was granted a charter in 1180, and the Order nursed the poor in homes and hospitals and were in charge of nursing at the Santo Spirito Hospital in Rome.

The Alexian Brothers, formed during the scourge of the bubonic plague in 1348, was a group of laymen united to care for the plague sufferers. They undertook the burial of the dead. In 1469 this group was organized under Augustinian rule and took as their patron saint St. Alexius, a fifth century Roman, who nursed the sick in the hospital built by St. Ephrem at Edessa. This order continues to serve the sick and has an enviable record of accomplishments.

The Alexian Brothers' Hospital School of Nursing in Chicago has been the largest all-male nursing school in the United States.

They maintain and staff several large general hospitals for men and boys as well as a rest home and home for elderly men. Memorial Hospital and Clinic at Boys Town, Nebraska, is also staffed by the Alexian Brothers. Nursing is only one of the many fields in which the brothers serve for the betterment of society.

INDIVIDUAL NURSES

Besides the part that organized groups played in the nursing achievements of this period, there were also certain individuals who were exemplary in their expansion of the field of nursing.

St. Hildegarde (1098?–1179) (Fig. 5–18), one of the most erudite women of the Middle Ages, was born of noble parents and at the age of eight was sent to be educated to the Benedictine cloister at Disibodenberg. At the end of her schooling, Hildegarde entered this monastery and years later became its abbess. She also founded another Benedictine cloister near Bingen on the Rhine.

Hildegarde was a scholar and eagerly absorbed the vast amount of scientific writings that had been accumulated in the monastery. The fruits of her labors appeared in a series of books, some of which were concerned with theological subjects but at least two were related to the field of medicine: *Liber Simplicis Medicinae* and *Liber Compositae Medicinae*. These books were assumed to have been written for the nuns in charge of the infirmaries

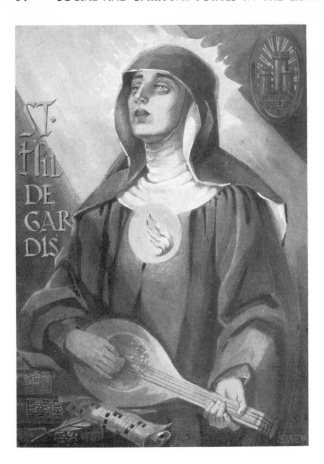

Figure 5–18. St. Hildegarde. (Bosk, J.: *Patrons of Our Names in Word and Picture,* Neuland Verlag.)

in the numerous Benedictine monasteries. There was a need for such references, for these infirmarians were not only responsible for the care of the nuns but cared as well for sick travelers who stayed at the convent guest houses.

In the sixteenth century the first of these books was edited under the title *Physica St. Hildegardis.* It contained nine books. The second volume, consisting of five books, presented the general diseases of the human body and the causes, symptoms and treatment of diseases. It was a compendium of information based on scientific investigation. Hildegarde discussed the vibration and pulsation of the blood in the veins; the regulation of vital activities by the brain, spinal cord and nerves; and the importance of understanding normal and abnormal psychology.

Her accumulated knowledge encompassed medical science, nursing, music, herb gardening and natural science, accompanied by a spiritual and religious philosophy of fantastic scope. Her books indicate her constant educational pursuits as well as her original thinking. Her medical works were written between 1151 and 1159, when she was nearly 60 years old.

She was skilled in understanding the politics of the day and even predicted consequences that would occur, such as the fall of the German Empire, the turbulence of the Papacy and the coming of the Reformation. She corresponded with prelates, princes and other persons of high as well as lower stations of life.

St. Hildegarde, who knew many things that were unknown to the physicians of her day, was both doctor and nurse—but her greatest accomplishments were contributions to the scientific foundation of nursing and medicine.

Hildegarde's works proved not only that the monasteries collected and housed the works of intellectual endeavors, but that their residents were encouraged to peruse these works and add to the accumulation of knowledge.

Abbess Euphemia, who was the director of a Benedictine monastery in Hampshire, England, from 1226 to 1257, was reputed to be a pioneer of modern hospital design. Euphemia designed the plans for an infirmary that contained beneath it a course of water, flowing with such force that all the refuse was carried away. This was a more attractive and sanitary infirmary than was noted in other areas during this period.

Cunegundes, a niece of St. Elizabeth of Hungary, married Boleslaus, the King of Poland. Cunegundes visited the poor and the sick in the hospitals, and she gave special care to lepers. After the death of her husband, Cunegundes entered a monastery of the Poor Clares.

Queen Elizabeth of Portugal (known also as St. Isabel, 1271–1336), a grandniece of Elizabeth of Hungary, devoted her life to charity. She gave food and lodging to the poor, established a house for penitent prostitutes who were given special training so that they might reenter society as useful citizens, instituted a hospital for foundlings and nursed the sick in the hospitals. At the death of her husband, Elizabeth joined the Poor Clares and died in the convent at Coimbra which she had founded.

St. Roch (1295?–1327) was the son of the governor of the city of Montpellier in France. At the death of his parents when he was about eighteen years of age, Roch distributed his large fortune to the poor and set out on a pilgrimage. When he reached Italy, he saw the devastation caused by the bubonic plague and offered his services in nursing the sick. Roch contracted the disease but was miraculously cured, and in the several paintings of him the "bubo" of the disease can be noted on his leg (Fig. 5–19).

Queen Isabella of Castile married Ferdinand, King of Aragon in 1469. Isabella has been credited with having introduced the tent-type hospitals and ambulances for the injured on the battlefields. She visited and cared for the wounded and showed skill in caring for the sick.

Queen Matilda, affectionately called "Good Queen Maud," was the wife of King Henry I of England and the daughter of King Mal-

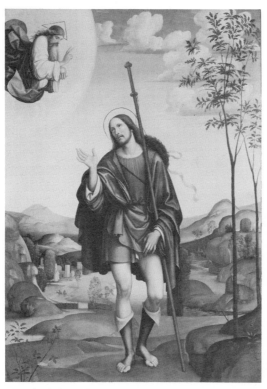

Figure 5–19.   St. Roch pointing to the bubo in his groin. From a painting by Francesco Francia (1450–1517). (Courtesy of The Metropolitan Museum of Art, gift of George R. Hann, 1965.)

colm III of Scotland and Queen Margaret. In addition to founding hospitals, she personally gave care to the sick.

MIDWIFERY

Obstetrics and gynecology were practiced by *midwives*. These women had developed their skill by observation and experience, for they had borne children. The paintings of this period frequently indicate the presence of the midwife and the nursemaid who cared for the baby. Often the nursemaid is shown using either her arm or foot as a thermometer to test the water before bathing the new baby. In difficult labor the midwife asked the advice of the physician, but he did not come to examine the patient or to assume the duties of the midwife. Among primitive peoples delivery has been carried out in a squatting or sitting position (Figs. 5–20 and 5–21), and in early days in Europe the obstetrical chair or v-shaped stool was used. Later, delivery in bed was the accepted method. (See Figure 5–22.)

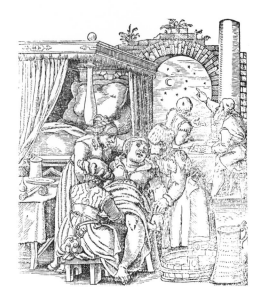

Figure 5–21. A delivery during the Renaissance, by Jakob Ruff, 1500–1558. Belligerent midwives guard the lying-in chamber against medical interference. The physician-astrologer at the window casts a horoscope of the newborn. (Courtesy of National Library of Medicine, Bethesda, Md.)

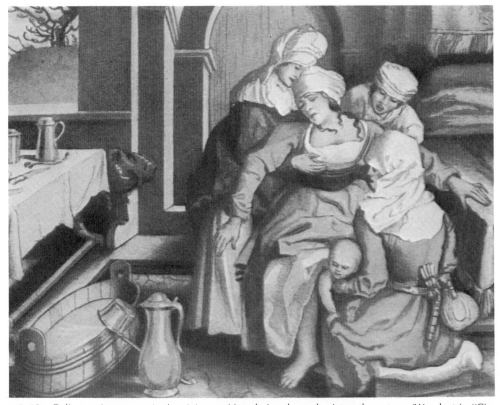

Figure 5–20. Delivery of a woman in the sitting position during the early sixteenth century. (Woodcut in "Cicero de officus," Augsburg, Steyner, 1531.)

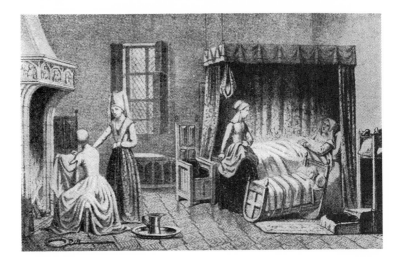

Figure 5–22. Obstetric ward of Dutch hospital in the fifteenth century. Note rooming-in aspect of child care.

ORGANIZATION OF HOSPITALS

We have mentioned that crowded living conditions and an increase in the spread of disease caused a demand for more hospitals, for the existing ones had been organized as almshouses, orphanages and hospices for travelers, as well as accommodations for the sick. *Pope Innocent III* (1161–1216) was a dominant force behind the movement to visit existing hospitals and then construct the necessary ones as efficiently and attractively as possible.

The first hospital in England was established at York and was built by Athelstane about 936. This was also a poorhouse and had a department for lepers. Queen Matilda founded St. Giles' Hospital in 1101 to care for 40 lepers. For many years this leper hospital was the most important of its kind in the British Isles. She also was the motivating spirit behind the building of the Hospital of St. Katherine in London in 1148. The charter of this hospital included the opportunity for nursing the sick poor in their homes. Many centuries later, the Jubilee Institute for District Nursing adopted this charter. Women of noble birth did both the nursing in these hospitals and district work in the homes of the poor.

St. Bartholomew's Hospital (cf. Fig. 5–23) in London was built in 1123 because of the encouragement of Rahere, formerly the king's jester, who became an Augustinian monk. *St. Thomas' Hospital,* also in London, was founded by Richard, the prior of Bermondsey, in

1213. Later this hospital was made famous when it was used by Florence Nightingale as the center for clinical experience for her students. This hospital and St. Bartholomew's

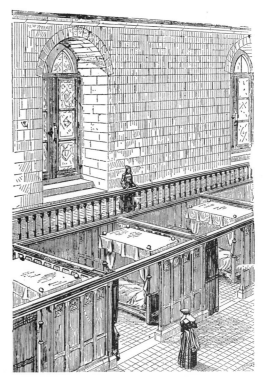

Figure 5–23. Ward in hospital founded in 1293 at Tounerre in France by Marguerite of Bourgogne, sister of St. Louis IX. It was airy, well ventilated and had richly carved woodwork and beautifully colored stained glass windows.

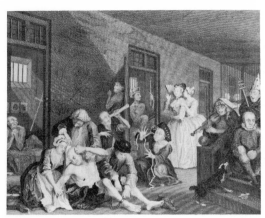

Figure 5–24. Bedlam. Engraving by William Hogarth (1697–1764) from The Rake's Progress, London, 1735.

were the only ones spared during the closing of religious monasteries, convents and hospitals during the Reformation.

Bethlehem Hospital, commonly known as Bedlam, was originally a hospice of St. Mary of Bethlehem. Later, in addition to the general hospital, provisions were made for the care of mentally ill patients. In the fourteenth century Bethlehem was designed exclusively for the mentally ill, and the *Nursing Mirror* states: "In 1377 it became the first *lunatic asylum* in Britain and the second one in Europe." This article mentions that when patients responded to medical treatment they were encouraged to go out into the streets and beg for their living. Wearing a metal armband that indicated their mental condition, these patients were called "Tom o' Bedlams." The article reports that the "violent ones who were interned were kept in chains and cells and treated with considerable inhumanity" because it was believed that these patients "had neither understanding nor feeling."

Patients who were mentally ill were received into wards in general hospitals for the "insane" or in separate buildings called "asylums." The word *asylum* implies security, but these asylums were more for the protection and comfort of the community than for the security of the patients. Centuries ago asylums were in effect prisons; our practice of having a person who is mentally ill committed to a psychiatric hospital by a judge or court is a survival of medieval methods. The care of the patient was custodial in nature and the attendants were chosen for their physical strength.

These mentally ill patients were treated as animals, often being half starved and kept under filthy conditions. For centuries their treatment was based on the idea that they felt neither heat nor cold. People had a fixed idea that they were possessed by devils or that they were being punished for their sins. Iron manacles and chains were used for restraint and there was a time when it was thought that fright and tortures were useful in driving out "madness"; this was the "shock therapy" of the period.

In the eighteenth century, Bedlam was one of the tourist attractions of London. Visitors came to be amused at the antics of the inmates (Fig. 5–24). This was a source of revenue for the hospital.

The *Hospital of Santa Maria della Scala* in Siena is of special interest because it was here that St. Catherine of Siena gave such valiant care to the plague sufferers. Her major efforts were directed to the patients who were in the attached house for lepers. This hospital continues to attract visitors because of its beautiful interior frescoes and artistic paintings.

It was the custom of this period to display paintings in the hospitals to provide diversional therapy for patients. This was done at *St. John's Hospital* at Bruges in Belgium, which was founded in 1118 by Augustinian monks and nuns as a hospice for travelers. The older buildings are preserved as a museum, but six masterpieces of the Flemish painter, Hans Memling, have made this hospital the envy of the world's art galleries (Fig. 5–25). A fascinating account of this hospital and Johannes Beerblock's painting of the great hall have been presented by Mrs. Goldin.[6]

The Hospital of the Innocents in Florence, another famous hospital, was built as a foundling asylum because of the large number of children who were abandoned and either left to die or became the property of the person who found them (Figs. 5–26 and 5–27). The *Ospedale Santa Maria degli Innocenti* was built in 1451 with the financial assistance of the guild of silk merchants. This hospital exemplified beautiful architecture and was adorned with the famous medallions of Della Robbia. A type of foster parent plan whereby new

[6]Goldin, Grace: "A Walk Through a Ward of the Eighteenth Century," *Journal of the History of Medicine and Allied Sciences*, 1967, Volume XXII, Number 2.

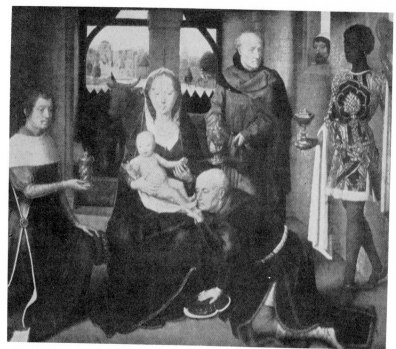

Figure 5–25. One of the famous masterpieces of art at St. John's Hospital at Bruges. (Memling, ca. 1430–1494, St. John's Hospital. University Prints.)

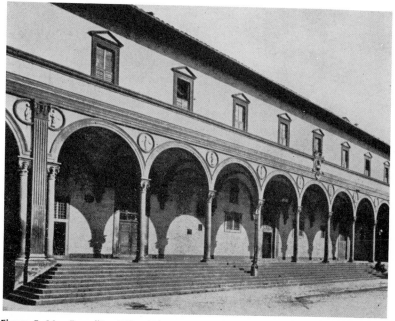

Figure 5–26. Foundlings' Hospital (Innocenti), Florence, ca. 1421. (University Prints.)

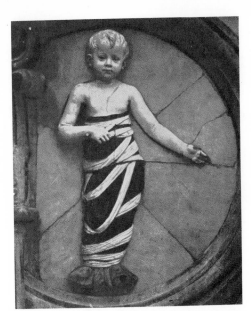

Figure 5–27. Bambino. (Andrea Della Robbia, 1435–1525, Hospital of the Innocents, Florence. University Prints.)

parents had to promise to treat the orphans as their own children was instituted in the Ospedale Santa Maria. Either the hospital or the new families taught the children trades and provided the girls with dowries. This hospital is administered by the Sisters of Charity of St. Vincent de Paul.

GUILDS

The *guilds*, associations for workmen and tradesmen, were important factors in the Middle Ages. Divided into the three categories of apprentice, craftsman and master craftsman, these guilds protected the worker, the product and the public.

The apprenticeship method of learning a skill was stressed and expanded. Higher standards of work were encouraged; prices were set; unethical practices were forbidden; and certain social insurance was provided for the worker and his family.

UNIVERSITIES AND LEARNING

The founding of universities was a cultural achievement of monumental significance. As there were few institutions of learning, stu-

dents traveled great distances, first to the schools connected with the monasteries, then to the cathedral schools[7] and finally to the universities.

Latin was the universal language, used for teaching in all schools. Thus, it was easy for teachers to give and students to accept knowledge, regardless of nationality.

The curriculum in the universities emphasized the seven liberal arts: rhetoric, grammar, logic or dialectics, mathematics (including geometry), astronomy, music and metaphysics. The graduate departments of these universities consisted of philosophy, law, theology and medicine. Upon passing an examination, the student was awarded a bachelor of arts degree, and the master's and doctor's degrees were also conferred.

Learning flourished and an intellectual awakening was occurring. This stimulus was given added impetus by the invention of movable type by *Johann Gutenberg* in 1438. Previous to this, books were copied laboriously, but with the printing press books became more readily available.

A renaissance occurred in the fields of literature and art. Petrarch, Dante, Boccaccio, Cervantes and Chaucer wrote their literary masterpieces; thousands of singing poets, or troubadours, roamed the countryside; and religious plays based on the life of Christ and on the lives of the saints were performed.[8]

Two visual media used for teaching were beautiful tapestries and magnificent stained glass windows; many were picture chronicles that told a story with liveliness and with exquisite color.

MEDICINE

A renaissance did not occur, however, in the field of medicine because doctors had implicit faith in the ancient *humoral theory*, the four humors of the body—blood, phlegm,

[7] These schools were attached to the great cathedrals and were started by Charlemagne and his teacher Alcuin. The most famous of the cathedral schools were those of Chartres, Notre Dame, Lyons, Metz, Tours, Rheims and Orleans.

[8] The famous Oberammergau Passion Play is supposed to have started when the bubonic plague was carried to that city by a visitor. Untold havoc was caused, and the townsfolk promised to produce the play every ten years if the plague ended. See Crawford, R.: *The Plague and Pestilence in Literature and Art.* London, Oxford University Press, 1914.

yellow bile and black bile. If one of these humors diminished or increased in quantity or changed in quality, disease occurred. Not only was the physical makeup of the person influenced by these humors, but also his personality was affected by them.

Many doctors of this period were also firm believers in alchemy and astrology, the latter being based on the belief that the celestial bodies influenced the lives of men. The humors were supposed to be controlled by the planets, and one decided when to take medicine or when to be bled according to the astrological signs (Fig. 5–28).

There were several leaders in the field of medicine. Mondino de Luzzi (*ca.* 1270–1326), called *Mundinus*, was a graduate of the University of Bologna in 1306 and taught in the medical school. He specialized in anatomy, dissected bodies and completed a manual on anatomy in 1316 that was published in 1487. He assigned the actual dissection of bodies to an assistant while he counseled from his chair. A female assistant to Mundinus had remarkable skill in dissecting and injecting the arteries and veins with a different colored liquid that soon hardened.

Mundinus' dissection manual was widely

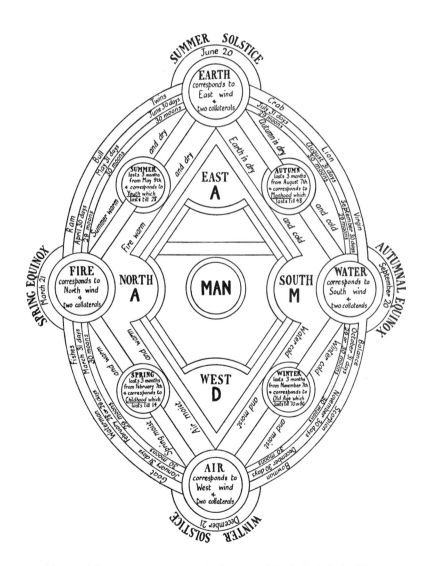

Figure 5–28. A translation of the Macrocosm as conceived in 1011 A.D. by Byrhtferth of Ramsey. (Grattan and Singer: *Anglo-Saxon Magic and Medicine.*)

used after the invention of printing, especially as a guide for medical students and students of art. It is known that the artists of this era dissected bodies in order to paint more accurately.

Guy de Chauliac (1300–1368), considered the greatest surgeon of the Middle Ages, wrote *Chirurgia Magna,* which became a textbook of surgery. De Chauliac recommended surgical intervention for certain conditions of the skull, the chest and the abdomen, and set an excellent example by caring for plague victims while many other doctors fled from the scene.

Cardinal Nicholas of Cusa (1401–1464), known as *Cusanus,* was the son of a wealthy ship owner. He was an able scholar, an expert in canon law and, being a skilled mathematician interested in natural science, suggested an ingenious method of measuring pulse rate. In this period, time was determined by the ancient water-clock method, which measured the intervals of time elapsing during the flow of a specific quantity of water. Cusanus' suggestion was to weigh the amounts of water that flowed during 100 pulse beats of a number of "healthy" individuals of the same age and build. This could be used as a standard, and deviations could be judged by comparison with the normal pulse rate.

Cusanus wrote a provocative book entitled *The Idiot,* which motivated a study of nature and influenced a rebirth of study of science. He employed the Socratic method in Platonic dialogue form, stimulated the thought processes and finally provided a solution through analytical techniques and intuition. He proposed the doctrine of what he called "learned ignorance," which results from an increased awareness of the "more one knows the more there is to know."

His strong mathematical and scientific background was applied to the studies of man. He was aware of the fact that the rate of the pulse and breathing could be measured and would vary according to different illnesses as well as be influenced by physical and social surroundings and even by climate.

Cusanus ends the dialogue in *The Idiot* by announcing, "experimental knowledge requireth large writings for the more they are, so much the more easily may we come from the experiments, to the Art which is drawn

from them." It is interesting to note that Cusanus anticipated Copernicus in his belief in the earth's rotation and revolution around the sun.

The guild system penetrated into the field of medicine. Many surgeons had delegated certain aspects of their work to barbers and midwives, a fact officially recognized by King Charles V of France in the fourteenth century when he granted to barbers the right to do bleeding and minor surgery. The guild regulations on this privilege varied with the times and the localities. For example, Reisman notes that in 1415 in Florence "no one under the age of fifteen should be apprenticed to a doctor of medicine, to a surgeon, barber, midwife or any one else having to do with the sick. Apprentices were required to establish their reputation for honesty, morality, mental and physical fitness, and had to be natives of Florence and of legitimate birth."[9]

In summarizing the progress of the later Middle Ages, we see that the Crusades stimulated the growth of the military nursing orders, unwittingly encouraged the spread of disease and brought Europe into contact with Arabic medicine. The sudden spread of urban developments increased the possibility for cultural growth, but sanitary and hygienic conditions caused the spread of disease. Certain medical treatments, beliefs and practices were retained from earlier periods while new ones were added. Hospitals of historical interest were built; religious orders were formed and contributed many well-known leaders and groups that specialized in the care of the sick. Travel and commerce flourished and acted as a culture medium for the development of new tastes and interests. Educational institutions were organized and learning flourished. Although there were accomplishments in such fields as art, architecture and literature, no striking achievements were noted in medicine.

It has been documented that nurses responded to the needs of society in times of persecution, warfare and pestilential crises. Recruits to nursing continued to be drawn from individuals of high intellectual and social background.

---

[9]*Op. cit.,* p. 229.

REFERENCE READINGS

Bedford, W. K. R., and Holbeche, Richard: *The Order of the Hospital of St. John of Jerusalem.* London, F. E. Robinson & Co., 1902.

Bonniwell, William: *Margaret of Metola.* New York, P. J. Kenedy & Sons, 1952.

Chesteron, Gilbert K.: *St. Francis of Assisi.* New York, Doran Co., 1924. (Available as an Image Book, 1957.)

Clay, Rotha Mary: *Medieval Hospitals of England.* London, Methuen & Co., 1909.

Crawfurd, R.: *The Plague and Pestilence in Literature and Art.* New York, Oxford University Press, 1914.

Curtayne, Alice: *St. Catherine of Siena.* New York, Sheed & Ward, 1935.

Cushing, Richard J.: *St. Catherine of Siena.* Boston, Daughters of St. Paul, 1957.

Fuller, John G.: *The Day of St. Anthony's Fire.* New York, The Macmillan Co., 1968.

The Hours of Jeanne D'Evreux, Queen of France. New York, The Cloisters, Metropolitan Museum of Art, 1957.

Giordani, Igino: *Catherine of Siena.* Milwaukee, Bruce Publishing Co., 1959.

Grattan, J. H. G., and Singer, Charles: *Anglo-Saxon Magic and Medicine.* New York, Oxford University Press, 1952.

Hoff, Hebbel E.: "Nicolaus of Cusa," *Journal of the History of Medicine and Allied Sciences, 19*:101–108, 1964.

Murphy, Dennis G.: *They Did Not Pass By.* London, Catholic Book Club, 1957.

Ogden, Brother Daniel: *Of Valiant Men* — A Chronicle of the Congregation of Alexian Brothers. Wisconsin, The Novitiate Press, 1957.

Robeck, Nesta de: *Saint Elizabeth of Hungary.* Milwaukee, Bruce Publishing Co., 1953.

Schermerhorn, Elizabeth: *On the Trail of the Eight Pointed Cross.* A study of the heritage of the Knights Hospitallers in feudal Europe. New York, G. P. Putnam's Sons, 1940.

Sister Mary Francis, P. C.: *A Right to Be Merry.* New York, Sheed & Ward, 1956.

Thomas Aquinas, St.: *Basic Writings.* New York, Random House.

Walsh, James J.: *The Catholic Church and Healing.* New York, The Macmillan Co., 1927.

Walsh, James J.: *Old Time Makers of Medicine.* New York, Fordham University Press, 1911.

Walsh, James J.: *What Civilization Owes to Italy.* Boston, The Stratford Co., 1923.

Wohl, Louis de: *The Quiet Light.* Philadelphia, J. B. Lippincott Co., 1950.

Wohl, Louis de: *The Last Crusader.* Philadelphia, J. B. Lippincott Co., 1956.

Wohl, Louis de: *The Joyful Beggar.* Philadelphia, J. B. Lippincott Co., 1958.

Wohl, Louis de: *Lay Siege to Heaven.* Philadelphia, J. B. Lippincott Co., 1961.

Ziegler, Phillip: *The Black Death.* New York, John Day Co., 1969.

CHAPTER 6

Emergence of Nursing Leadership During the Renaissance (1500–1700)

The 200 years between 1500 and 1700 witnessed tremendous expansion economically, politically, socially and intellectually. The extension of trade encouraged new techniques involving labor-saving devices with a concomitant rise in the standard of living. Skilled craftsmen broadened the use of textiles, metal and glass. The improvement in magnification and vision, combined with the spirit of inquiry, led to the construction of microscopes and telescopes. An urge to experiment with these instruments, together with the utilization of mathematical procedures, developed a good scientific base for new dimensions in patient care.

Aids for the improvement of vision, in addition to *Gutenberg's* invention of the printing press, opened new avenues of learning. Formerly education was only available to the wealthy. Books had been written laboriously and painstakingly copied; they were almost nonexistent. A renaissance occurred in the centers of learning, with explosion of knowledge and creative thinking blossoming within the university setting. Medical education found its way into the university framework. The preparation for nursing was not established under the aegis of an institution of higher learning but careful selection of candidates and a planned program of nursing education was initiated during this period.

EXPANSION OF NURSING

The sixteenth century also witnessed another movement—the *Reformation,* which started as a reform and ended as a revolt producing a cleavage in Christianity. The "reformers" suppressed the Catholic religious orders under whose charge the hospitals became places of horror and a period of stagnation ensued. Much has been written about the squalor of the hospitals and the inadequacy of their attendants. During the bubonic plague in London in 1665, these attendants were described as "dirty, ugly, unwholesome hags."

When Henry VIII closed the monasteries in 1535, it was the aged, the sick, the orphans and the dispossessed who suffered most. The English government wiped out the organization of monastic relief without planning a replacement.

Many died of starvation; the homeless and destitute resorted to begging. A statute against vagrancy was issued by Edward VI, who succeeded Henry in 1547. If a person was discovered begging, he or she was branded with a red hot iron with a letter B on the chest. If a person reported the vagrant to the authorities, the vagrant became the slave of the informant. The owner was granted the right to beat, chain or force him to labor in whatever manner he desired. Orphaned children could be retained as apprentices to whatever person found the child. These children could be chained if the master so desired.

In 1552, a committee was appointed to study the problem of poverty in London. Records reveal that some people were so poor that mice were one source of food.

In 1557, rules were formulated by which the charitable institutions for the sick poor were to be managed. Under this system, many hospitals became "houses of correction." Any patient able to work was recruited for service and the work day extended from five o'clock in the morning to eight o'clock in the evening.

Queen Elizabeth passed the first English Poor Law prescribing a compulsory poor tax on every parish. The relief of the poor was no longer an individual problem dependent for solution upon voluntary acts of Christian charity but a national duty exacting a compulsory contribution toward its alleviation.

In 1597, the poor laws were revised since the problem of vagrancy continued. In an attempt to rectify this situation, vagrants were whipped until their bodies were bloody.

For a second offense, the vagrant was sent to the galleys to be chained in boats as an oarsman. The philosophy of seeing Christ in the least of these brethren had been forgotten. Even the sick poor in hospitals were referred to as objects of charity.

Warfare, such as the *Thirty Years' War* (1618–1648), famine and plague still ravaged Europe. Devastating outbreaks of typhus and bubonic plague occurred. As a result of the latter, Germany lost from one half to three quarters of her population. It was during this period (in 1665) that the bubonic plague reached England (Figs. 6–1 and 6–2).

When a person contracted the plague, the

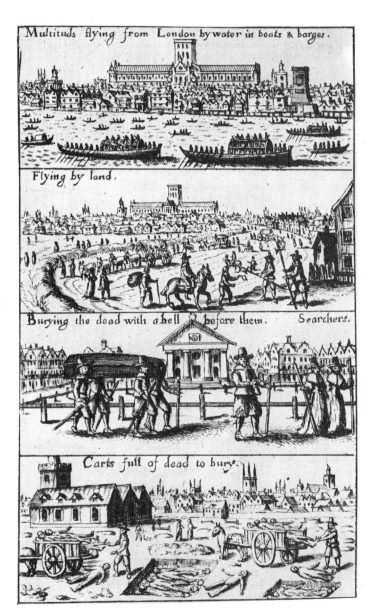

Figure 6–1. Plague scenes in London, 1665. (Caraman, Philip: *Henry Morse, Priest of the Plague.* Farrar, Straus & Cudahy, 1957.)

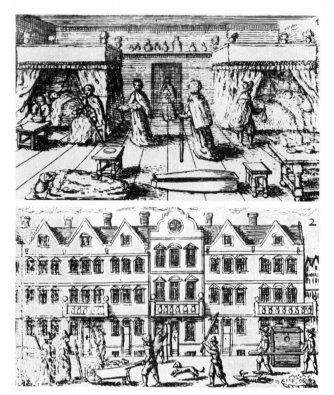

Figure 6–2. Plague scenes. *Above,* a room in a plague-infested house. Several sick patients are in bed, one walks around the room and, in the foreground, a corpse is ready to be placed in the coffin.

Below, a row of London houses boarded up with red crosses on the locked doors. This is an example of enforced quarantine. Two bearers are carrying a sick person to the pest house in a sedan chair. Dog catchers are killing dogs and loading them in wheelbarrows. (Caraman, Philip: *Henry Morse, Priest of the Plague.* Farrar, Straus & Cudahy, 1957.)

house was boarded up with the well members forced to become prisoners with the sick one. Fires were ordered to be kept burning in the streets, one before every sixth house, for three days, continuously, to purify the air.

Plague physicians wore a long red or black leather gown, leather gauntlets and a mask with glass-covered openings for the eyes and a long beak filled with fumigants and antiseptics, and carried pomander containers filled with sweet smelling spices (Fig. 6–3).

Elaborate precautions were taken in the burial of the dead, at night. Dog catchers prowled the streets, killing stray dogs and removing their bodies for burial. The huge mounds of earth are mute testimony to the plight of the English during this scourge. In one of these mounds 50,000 bodies were said to be interred.

Figure 6–4 depicts the costume worn by physicians during the plague of the seventeenth century. Many satirical comments and caricatures described the appearance of the doctor and the costume he wore to protect himself. Indeed, Hecker has commented, "human science and art appear particularly

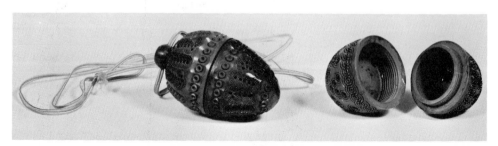

Figure 6–3. Pomander containers held to the nose to scent the air one inhaled. Scented herbs, potpourri, filled the container. (Author's collection.)

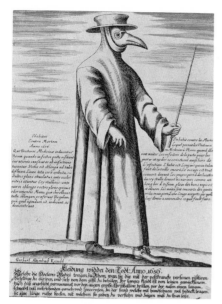

Figure 6–4. The Plague Doctor. An engraving by Gerhart Altzenback, seventeenth century. (Courtesy of Yale Medical Library, Clements C. Fry Collection.)

weak, in great pestilences, because they have to contend with powers of nature, of which they have no knowledge."[1]

The emotional trauma must have been devastating. Loved ones were abandoned. Hospital service was inadequate; many people

---

[1]Hecker, J. F. C.: *The Epidemics of the Middle Ages.* London, 1846, p. 50.

died on the street. There was a need for organized charity. The severe fire in London brought destruction to the breeding place of rats.

In France, no longer could workers carry on their trade in their own homes. The artisan now lived on back streets or slept in the attic of his master, often going to bed hungry. His working day was a long one, sometimes seventeen continuous hours.

In this period of marked intellectual enlightenment and achievement, it is noted that the knowledge of hygiene was poor. (See Figure 6–5.) People bathed infrequently although there were many famous medicinal baths. The value of fresh air was not understood or appreciated. When someone was ill, the doors and windows were closed for fear of cold and draughts. Another unfortunate occurrence was the *window tax*, which fostered the spread of disease because hundreds of hospital windows plus those in homes were blocked up or bricked over to save money. There were those, however, whose standard of living was much higher, whose homes were comfortable and less unsanitary and whose diet was better balanced.

In the sixteenth century, infants were commonly breast-fed, but wet-nursing was available, and baby farming was a notorious evil. The exceedingly high infant mortality rate was due to extremely poor public and personal hygiene. Cities had no drainage; filth and infection were rampant.

The medical treatment given during this

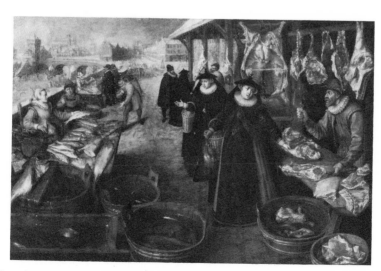

Figure 6–5. Fish and Meat Market, by Lucas van Valckenborgh (1535–1597). (Courtesy of The Montreal Museum of Fine Arts.)

period is revealed in a consideration of the treatment given to King Charles II in 1685:

A pint of blood was removed from his right arm, then eight ounces from his shoulder, and then in succession he was given an emetic, two physics and an enema containing fifteen substances. Then his head was shaved, a blister was raised on the scalp, a sneezing powder was given to purge the brain, then cowslip powder to strengthen it. Meanwhile, more emetics, soothing drinks and still more bleeding was continued, followed by plaster of pitch and pigeon dung applied to the royal feet.

The following substances were taken internally: melon seeds, slippery elm, black cherry water, extract of lily-of-the-valley, peony, lavender, pears dissolved in vinegar, gentian root, nutmeg and finally, forty drops of an extract of the human skull. As a last resort, the bezoar stone was employed, but the king died anyway (cf. Fig. 6–6).

In 1649, during the worst of the famine, the Abbess of Port Royale writes as follows:

This poor country is a horrible sight; it is stripped of everything. The soldiers take possession of the farms and have the corn threshed, but will not give a single grain to the owners, who beg for it as an alms. It is impossible to plow, there are no more horses—all have been carried off. The peasants are reduced to sleeping in the woods and are thankful to have them as a refuge from murderers. And if they only had enough bread to half satisfy their hunger, they would indeed count themselves happy.[2]

Three years later she again writes:

All the armies are equally undisciplined and vie with one another in lawlessness. The author-

ities in Paris are trying to send back the peasants to gather in the corn;[3] but as soon as it is reaped the marauders come to slay and steal and disperse all in a general route.

Of course the class which suffered most under this general misery was the poor, both the peasant in the country and the artisan in the city. The famine bread that they ate was made of barley and oats mixed with straw. The Jesuit Relations of 1651 say that in one parish the poor subsisted on "straw mixed with earth" and that their staple dish was "mice which the inhabitants hunt, so desperate are they from hunger."

There was a need for a social reform; a solution was forthcoming that revolutionized the care of the sick.

St. Francis de Sales (1567–1622) envisioned a group of women forming a voluntary association for friendly visiting of the poor and nursing the sick. The organization that materialized might be considered one of the early visiting nurse associations. St. Francis de Sales first encouraged and motivated influential ladies to give money and time to an organized service for the sick poor. They were to visit the sick daily, bathe, dress and care for them and take home their linen to be

---

[3] The refugees had flocked to Paris and in 1652 there were 100,000 beggars in the capital.

---

[2] Hugon, p. 172.

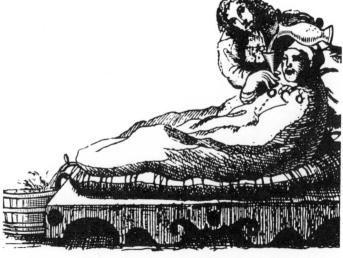

Figure 6–6. A seventeenth century method of reducing the body temperature of a patient with a fever. Patient is placed in a leather sack and cold water is poured into a funnel. The water runs over the body and is collected in a wooden tub at the foot of the couch.

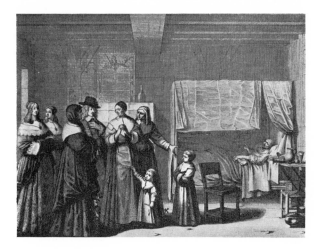

Figure 6–7. Visiting the sick in the seventeenth century. (Brainard, Annie M.: *The Evolution of Public Health Nursing.*)

washed. (Fig. 6–7). It was his desire that this order of women should be without external vows, and they were free to visit the sick in their homes and minister to their needs.

The order was called the *Order of the Visitation of Mary.* The cofoundress and director of this order was a woman, Madame de Chantal, who was experienced in visiting nursing. She was wed to Baron de Chantal, who, after eight years of happy married life, was shot while hunting.

Madame de Chantal and the members of her group visited the sick in their homes, cleaned and dressed their wounds, made their beds, gave them clothes, took home their linen, boiled it to remove impurities, mended and returned it to the patient. She assisted them when they were dying, and when they were dead, she washed and prepared them for burial.

It was *St. Vincent de Paul* (1576–1669) who introduced modern principles of visiting nursing and social service because his conception of charity was a new one for that period. He believed that not only rich and influential persons but also the poor and humble could contribute to the relief of distress by brotherly sympathy and personal service. He taught that indiscriminate giving was harmful and that one must investigate the condition of the poor, find out their needs, ascertain the causes of the poverty and wherever possible remedy them, such as by finding work for the unemployed. He emphasized the concept of "helping people to help themselves." This was an advanced step and extremely modern thinking. He realized the right of the poor to their family life, and

the benefit to be derived from a recognition of the family unit. He urged that the family be kept together, even if rent had to be paid for a period of time. This, too, was certainly a modern idea.

St. Vincent longed to help and comfort his brothers, but he realized the ineffectiveness of his personal service as only one field worker. He felt that if he established large groups of men and women, which would spread out into organized units, they could multiply and encircle the globe.

St. Vincent de Paul founded various charity organizations and directed them as well. He fired others with his enthusiasm.

In 1617, he formed the Society of Missioners, priests trained for special work among the poor; they renewed vows annually.

It was also in 1617 that he first conceived the idea of the Dames de Charité. When he heard of a family's needing assistance, he asked his congregation and got such response that he realized that improperly guided charity could do more harm than good. He suggested to a few ladies the same general plan organized by St. Francis de Sales; these women were called Dames de Charité, their work was mainly visiting nursing. The ladies went from cottage to cottage visiting patients, making sick patients as comfortable as possible, giving food, preparing medicine, and consoling the dying and distressed. This new organization spread throughout France.

Medical as well as nursing care was becoming available for the poor. Doctors gave their services freely and their lives as well in times of epidemics; they were not prepared to protect themselves and others from infections.

Medical charities were directed by Theophrastus Renardot, who had established an association for this purpose in 1612. By 1640, the King recognized the value of his work and gave him free reign to assist the poor.

Soon, several doctors joined him and set aside two days a week to visit sick poor and prescribe remedies. (See Figure 6–8.) Now there were doctors diagnosing cases, ladies giving bedside care and charity associations available to investigate conditions and give material relief.

These groups continued for 10 years, but St. Vincent felt the need for a person who could teach, direct and coordinate the work of the Dames de Charité. Madame Le Gras became the First Supervisor of these visiting nurses. Louise Le Gras (later known as *St. Louise de Marillac*) was a woman of noble birth who was a widow when St. Vincent presented his plan to her, which she accepted.

She would receive directions and counsel from St. Vincent. Then, when she arrived in a village, she would give the Dames de Charité instructions. She accompanied them on their rounds, helping them, advising them, assisting them in their duties and making suggestions about other ways of giving care to their patients. Gradually the enthusiasm of these ladies lessened, for their husbands objected to their absence from home for such lengthy periods.

In 1633, the *Sisters of Charity* were founded and became a secular nursing order of superior character. Young, single girls who were interested in this program were recruited. They were required to be intelligent, refined young women who were sincerely interested in the sick poor. They were called Les Filles de Charité or the Sisters of Charity. A systematic educational program, which consisted of experience in the hospital, visiting in homes and caring for the sick, was established. The program was a combination of social service to the poor and nursing of the sick. The sisters were given a carefully planned program of education before practicing as nurses. Overwork was forbidden by St. Vincent.

St. Louise de Marillac was prepared for

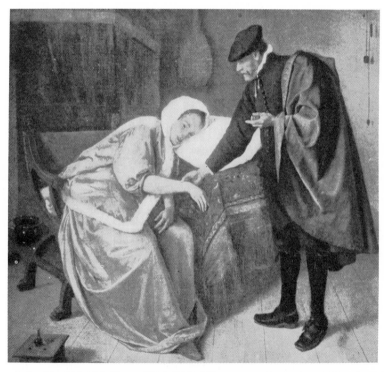

Figure 6–8. The Sick Girl. (Steen, 1626–1679, Rijksmuseum, Amsterdam. University Prints.)

this task. She had an excellent educational background, which was rare for a woman in this time.

Applications came from great distances and St. Louise selected her class with care, as noted by the following letter:

I have no wish to receive any persons except such as are suitable to our life, as regards both health of body and sanity of mind. You know how important this is to a community. I must, therefore, beg you to ascertain whether their desire to come here is prompted by a wish to see Paris, or a desire to make a living for themselves. . . . We do not want those who have no desire to work at their spiritual perfection in the service of God. They should have no motive in coming except the one of serving God and their neighbor.

St. Louise wrote this letter toward the end of 1639. Good health, a sound mind, a respectable background, a desire to serve God in the field of teaching, nursing or social service and labor unceasingly at her own perfection, has been the only dowry required of a girl who wishes to become a Daughter of Charity.[4]

Thus arose the second religious order to be founded by St. Vincent de Paul. St. Vincent taught the Sisters of Charity to find the presence of God in the service of the afflicted. They were to have no grille, no veil, no cell, no cloister. He said, "the streets of the city or the houses of the sick shall be your cells, your chapel the parish church, obedience your solitude, the fear of God your grating, a strict and holy modesty your only veil."

The costume of the Sisters of Charity had been the gray-blue gown and apron of rough woolen cloth worn by the French peasant of the period, with a stiff white collar and a headdress called a cornette (Fig. 6–9).

Into this dark period of nursing came these young, enthusiastic, well prepared nurses called Sisters of Charity. Their zeal became infectious, many recruits joined them and this flourishing order has encircled the globe. They have performed every work of charity: nursing in hospitals and homes, teaching in schools, taking charge of orphanages, giving heroic service during such wars as the Napoleonic Wars, the Crimean War and the Civil War in the United States and, since its inception, they have given courageous care

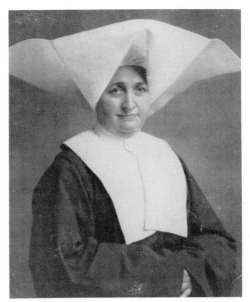

Figure 6–9. A Sister of Charity of St. Vincent de Paul.

to the patients in the National Leprosarium in Carville, Louisiana.

St. Vincent de Paul encouraged the Sisters of Charity to expand their role and develop special skills in caring for abandoned children (Fig. 6–10). In 1640 he founded the Hospital for Foundlings. He had been dismayed that the so-called receiving institution for abandoned children, La Couche, gave the children to anyone who asked for them. Not infrequently professional beggars claimed them and mutilated their bodies in order to arouse pity and collect more money.

The idea of human brotherhood, of love of one's neighbor, of responsibility for the bodily and material needs of one's fellow creature, originating in Christian love, was being revived. (See Figure 6–11.)

St. John of God was born in Portugal in 1495. For some mysterious reason, he disappeared from his home when he was eight years of age and grew up in Spain, spending the greater part of his first 22 years as a shepherd. The next 18 years were filled with the duties of a soldier, which hardened him in both body and soul. The life of a soldier of this period involved revelry, drunkenness, cruelty to the poor and suffering, looting expeditions and the gathering of booty.

At the age of forty, he left the army and

---

[4]*Then — and Now with the Daughters of Charity.* Normandy, Mo., Marillac Seminary, 1946, p. 20.

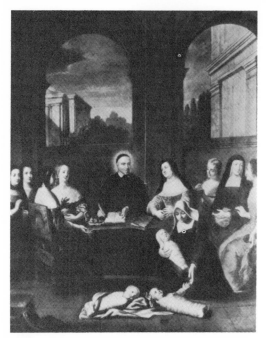

Figure 6–10. St. Vincent de Paul, with St. Louise de Marillac, entreating the Ladies of Charity to continue their efforts on behalf of foundlings. A Sister of Charity is caring for three abandoned infants.

beings who had to beg for a meager subsistence. Returning to Spain, he became a shepherd and reflected on the wasted life he had lived. He made a pilgrimage of repentance.

On the journey to Granada, he encountered a child weary from walking. St. John carried this little one on his shoulder until the end of the journey. When John placed him on the ground, the child said, "John of God, Granada shall be your cross."

He heard a sermon once which stressed the glory of being made a fool for the sake of Christ. John's most unusual reaction to this sermon resulted in his being hustled off to what was then referred to as a lunatic asylum. The picture of the care of the mentally ill of that period was gruesome. The typical treatment was the whip. St. John was stretched out on the floor, hands and feet, and flogged with a double knotted cord. At the termination of this procedure, he was locked in solitary confinement.

When he was released, St. John returned to Granada, gathered all the homeless vagrants and crippled persons into a house that he rented and gave them special care. It was the custom to display one's infirmity in order to beg for charity. When he found those who were too deformed to crawl to his abode, he carried them on his back. (Fig. 6–12). St. John of God begged for alms in order to feed and purchase medicines for these derelicts. Thus was laid the foundation

entered the employ of a gentleman farmer who assigned him the task of caring for his horses. The best of care was lavished upon these animals, in sharp contrast to the desperate plight of the starving human

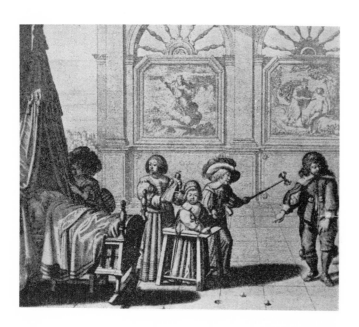

Figure 6–11. Seventeenth century nursery from engraving by A. Bosse (1602–1676). Children learned to walk by means of a walking frame. (Ciba Symposia, August, 1940.)

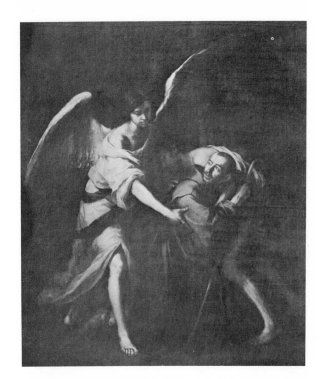

Figure 6–12. St. John of God. (Murillo, 1618–1682, Hospital de la Santa Caridad, Seville.)

for the famous Hospital of St. John of God at Granada.

The Bishop sent for him, insisted that he be known by the name John of God, wear a religious habit, and promised that funds and volunteers would be forthcoming for a better hospital. Benefactors became generous and many begged to assist him in his ministrations. In this new institution, money was allocated from the city treasury to pay for supplies and medical service for the patients. Each patient had a private bed, which was unique in this era when beds contained three, four, or more patients. Patients with contagious diseases were isolated, and an outpatient department was instituted.

St. John had a special interest in abandoned children, admitting them to the hospital until foster or adoptive parents could be found. All patients received superior care, but the ones who were mentally ill were lavished with tender love and understanding. There was an acute need for a kinder and more enlightened type of care of the mentally ill and mentally retarded. The abuse and cruelty meted out to these poor victims has been an appalling fact.

The *Brothers Hospitallers of St. John of God*, the order he founded, grew and thrived. They adopted the Rule of St. Augustine.

They opened hospitals at Madrid, Cordova, Toledo, Naples and Paris (Figs. 6–13 and 6–14). Less than 50 years after the death of their founder, the order had spread to every Christian kingdom in Europe and other continents. Wherever explorer ships happened to go, the Brothers of St. John of God followed to open hospitals for the natives and bring consolation for body as well as soul.

An ambulance unit staffed by the brothers accompanied the forces of King Philip II and Don Juan in their campaign against the Turks. In their daily activities, they sometimes ministered to the needs of those who were fighting. The brothers came to Central and South America as early as 1602, and they often faced severe opposition from the Indian witch doctors of the New World.

In many provinces of the Order of Hospitallers of St. John, the brothers are physicians, surgeons, dentists and pharmacists, although the greater number are registered nurses. They have been the personal infirmarians to the Popes as well as directors of the Vatican Pharmacy. Nursing homes for the aged and also for patients with long-term illnesses have been under the aegis of this order. They have maintained residences for homeless men, utilizing opportunities to assist in rehabilitation and eventual return to

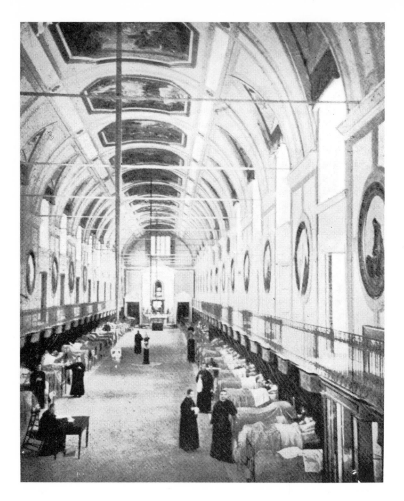

Figure 6–13. First hospital in Italy, "La Pace" at Naples, operated by the Hospitaller Brothers of St. John of God. Note the magnificent paintings on ceiling and walls. (McMahon, Norbert, O.S.J.D.: *The Story of the Hospitallers of St. John of God.* Newman Press.)

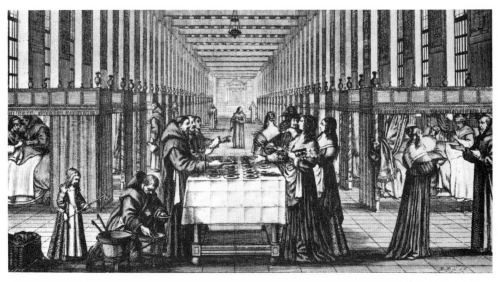

Figure 6–14. The Queen of France and ladies of the court serving the sick at the Brothers' Hospital in Paris. (McMahon, Norbert, O.S.J.D.: *The Story of the Hospitallers of St. John of God.* Newman Press.)

society. Indochina, a fruitful mission field supported by the Canadian Province, has had leper colonies staffed by these brothers. This order of brothers has a long record of devoted service to the needy.

A most enlightening picture of a hospital and the care of patients in Portuguese Goa (an enclave on the western coast of India) in the seventeenth century has been preserved and presented in Blunt's portrayal of the translations of the "Viaggi," the travels of Pietro Della Valle.[5] (Goa was annexed to Portugal in 1510 by Alfonso de Albuquerque. It was a city of wealth in the late sixteenth century and the site of the Church of Bom Jesus, which contains the tomb of St. Francis Xavier.)

Perhaps the most remarkable institution in Goa was the Royal Hospital for men, founded by Albuquerque and subsequently in the charge of the Jesuits, which in many respects seems to have been at least three hundred years ahead of its time. Pyrard, an impartial and accurate observer, spent several weeks as a patient there in 1608. The building, which was surrounded by spacious gardens where convalescents could wander at will, seemed to him more like a palace than a hospital. Everything in the wards was spotlessly clean. The elegant beds were of red lacquer, chequered or gilded, with fine white cotton sheets and silk coverlets that were changed twice a week. Each new patient on his arrival had his head shaved by a barber, and after being thoroughly scrubbed was issued with pajamas, cap and slippers. He was further provided with a fan, a bottle of drinking-water, a little table and a chamber-pot. Lanterns glazed with oyster-shell glowed gently throughout the night. The food was excellent, patients on full diet receiving for supper a whole fowl each, served on a plate of Chinese porcelain, and being encouraged to ask for a second helping. But wine was only allowed when specially prescribed.

The higher officials of the hospital were all Portuguese, the servants native Christians. The doctors, who visited their fifteen hundred patients morning and evening, were accompanied on their rounds by servants bearing baskets of lint and other medicaments or diffusing incense, and by an apothecary and kitchen clerk, notebooks in hand, who jotted down prescriptions and special diet. Male visitors were allowed from 8 to 11 and from 3 to 6 o'clock and might eat with their friends who could apply for extra rations; they were searched at the gate for arms, and to see that they were not bringing unsuitable food or drink to the sick.

---

[5] Blunt, Wilfred: *Pietro's Pilgrimage*. A journey to India and back at the beginning of the seventeenth century. London, James Barrie, 1953, pp. 255–257.

There were two fine churches attached to the establishment—decorated, like the corridors of the hospital itself, with religious frescoes—in which Mass was celebrated daily, and Jesuit priests visited the wards to hear confessions and administer the Sacrament to those who were too ill to leave their beds.

The principal diseases seem to have been enteric fevers, dysentery, cholera, scurvy and syphilis. Patients were carefully isolated; yet in spite of every precaution and every attention, mortality was very high. This was largely due to a general ignorance of the correct treatment of tropical diseases; to the unhealthy climate; and to the fact that the chief physician was always the Viceroy's private doctor, who, like his master, had also to return to Europe after three years' service, just as he was beginning to acquire some knowledge of local conditions.

St. Camillus De Lellis (1550–1614) was born in Naples of a noble family. His father was a soldier adventurer and the son joined him in this occupation. Very early, he acquired an interest in gambling and developed an astonishing skill at this pastime. It has been said of him that before he was 19 he had learned everything a wicked youth could learn and made free use of his knowledge.

During the course of one fighting episode, both he and his father fell ill of a disease from which his father did not recover. This made a profound impression on the son.

Above his ankle, Camillus had a wound that drained constantly and he applied for admission at the hospital of San Giacomo. Because he had no financial resources, he requested the opportunity to be a servant in return for the care to his infected leg. Progress was noted until leisure time prompted him to resort to his old interest in gambling. This terminated his affiliation with this hospital and the medical care he was receiving.

One day, while he was begging, a rich man offered him the chance to become a laborer on a construction project building a monastery. His companions taunted him for accepting such work, so he refused the offer and followed his companions. As he walked with them, he realized that he had rejected what might have been a special opportunity for a change in his way of life. He turned, retraced his steps, and joined the group of laborers at the monastery.

The hard work may have caused the infection in his leg to flare up. He returned to Rome to the San Giacomo hospital and again asked for work in return for treatment for his leg. For four years he remained there, finally receiving an appointment as superintendent of the servants, which, in that period, included nurses—all male. He labored tirelessly and began to love those he served. He realized that good nursing was dependent on love; also, that the duties of a priest were carried out best where love was present. He determined to encourage others, both nurses and priests, to join him. In order to equip himself for this task, St. Camillus studied for the priesthood and was ordained.

He selected a house in the slum area where pestilence was most abundant and gave his service to the sick poor (Fig. 6–15). At first his efforts were directed toward preparing and providing hospital nurses, but he learned that the sick poor outside of the hospital and in the slum areas were desperately in need of care. He achieved remarkable success in tending the dying and from this service his wonderful order, the *Nursing Order of Ministers of the Sick,* evolved. The members of this order wear a red cross on their cassock.

A hospital for alcoholics was opened in Germany by St. Camillus. His love for patients drew him to the prisons where he gave special care to those condemned to die.

The order, popularly called the Camillian

Fathers and Brothers, gave service as army nurses during several wars. Its members served during World War I. Some worked in the hospital trains set up by the Knights of Malta.

St. Charles of Borromeo (1538–1584) was a wealthy, well educated young man who became Archbishop of Milan. When his family died Charles distributed his wealth to the poor. His free time was spent bringing food and clothing to the poor and visiting the sick. During the plague that devastated Milan in 1575, he nursed the sick and ministered to the dying.

Jeanne Biscot (1601–1664), the daughter of a respected citizen of Arras in northern France, performed outstandingly good nursing work in war, famine, emergencies and pestilences. In 1640, when her home town was attacked, many sick and wounded needed medical attention, preferably in a hospital. Jeanne set an example, which others followed, of dressing wounds, feeding, reviving the sick and needy and assisting the dying. These energetic young ladies requested the right to use a building for a hospital and obtained it. They cared for patients as long as care was needed.

One of Jeanne's special talents lay in her

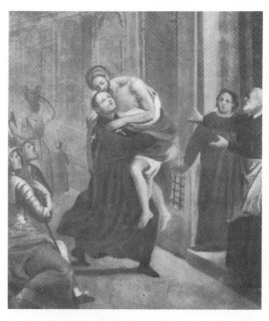

Figure 6–15. In this painting St. Camillus expresses his love and concern for suffering humanity. He carries a beggar into the Hospital of the Holy Ghost and ministers to him.

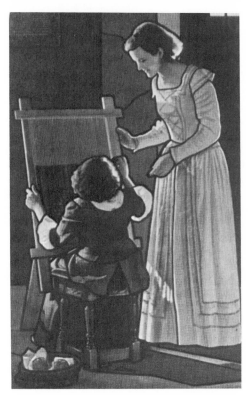

Figure 6–16. Jeanne Biscot. (*They Caught the Torch.* Will Ross, Inc.)

ability to detect and develop the special abilities of her patients (Fig. 6–16). Her hospitals became workshops where community residents of all ages learned to enrich personal skills. To her is given the credit of building a program of occupational therapy.

LIFE IN THE NEW WORLD

The new routes of trade and travel of the period beckoned the Spanish and Portuguese colonists who settled in Mexico and Peru. They brought with them many members of religious orders who were to become the teachers, nurses and doctors in the colonies, and they taught the Spanish language and Christian faith to the Aztec and Inca Indians.

European ideas were carried to the New World, and to the Old World came a wealth of information from the Americas. For example, on Columbus's second expedition, a Dr. Chanca, who was royal physician to King Ferdinand and Queen Isabella, was appointed doctor to the 1500 members of the group. He was a well educated gentleman

who had been professor of medicine at the University of Salamanca. During his sojourn in the Americas he studied the native medicines and many of these remedies, such as balsam of Peru, balsam of Tolu, cascara sagrada, and quinine, were introduced into Europe through his endeavors.

In 1521, Tenochtitlán, the capital of the Aztec civilization, was conquered by Cortés. By 1524, the Hospital of the Immaculate Conception, the *first hospital* on the American continent, was built in the capital, renamed Mexico City, by Cortés (Fig. 6–17). In 1528 Bishop Zumarraga founded the continent's first library with 200 volumes, and by 1534 the first printing press was built. In 1531 another hospital, the Hospital of Santa Fe (Holy Faith), was built in what is now New Mexico. Mission colleges were founded in 1531 at Queretaro and in 1546 at Zacatecas; in 1536 the College of Santa Cruz was established. The Universities of Mexico and Lima, founded in 1551, possessed departments in theology, scripture, canon law, civil law, arts, rhetoric, grammar and medicine. The *first medical school* on the American continent was established at the *University of Mexico* in 1578; the second medical school was affiliated with the University of Lima, in Peru, before 1600.

From the time Jacques Cartier sailed up the Saint Lawrence River in 1535, tales of the fascination of *New France* lured the adventurous. In 1605, the first settlement, the Habitation, was colonized at Port Royal in Nova Scotia. The famous explorer, Samuel de

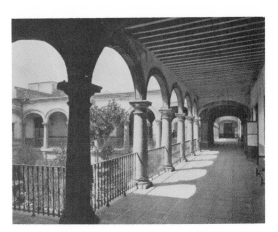

Figure 6–17. Mexico City's Hospital de Jesus, oldest surviving hospital in the Americas, originally named the Hospital of the Immaculate Conception.

Champlain, and the apothecary, Louis Hebert, were two of the members of this pioneer group. Indeed, the first nurse in the French colonies was *Marie Hebert Hubou*, widow of the surgeon-apothecary, Louis Hebert. Marie took care of the sick patients who were recommended to her by Jesuit Fathers.

The reports of life in New France published in the Jesuit bulletin prompted religious nursing sisters to answer the call for help. On August 1, 1639, three sisters of the Order of St. Augustine (Augustinian Sisters) arrived in Quebec and staffed the *Hôtel Dieu* in *Quebec,* built by the Duchess of Aiguillon who was a niece of Cardinal Richelieu (Fig. 6–18). These Augustinian sisters belonged to a cloistered order, and they had been prepared to care for the sick. Their habit consisted of a white woolen dress with a black leather belt and black veil. These sisters gave heroic service during the bleak, cold winters, during the Indian wars and during the epidemics of smallpox and typhus.

Ursuline sisters who were teaching at the mission school were given emergency classes in the care of the sick during the epidemics. Thus instruction in the care of the sick had commenced in the New World.

Jeanne Mance (1606–1673) was born the daughter of well-to-do French parents and was educated at an Ursuline convent. While at the convent school, the stories of heroism from the New World reached France and inspired Jeanne, when her age permitted, to join the courageous band. In 1638, during a severe epidemic, an organization of Ladies of Charity (probably those of St. Vincent de Paul) was formed to care for the sick. Jeanne joined this group and in this way received instruction in nursing care.

On May 17, 1641, Jeanne Mance arrived in Montreal, sponsored financially by the wealthy and philanthropic Madame de Bullion, who asked her to erect a hospital. Jeanne Mance cared for the Iroquois Indians (Fig. 6–19) as well as the colonists, and the Hôtel Dieu in Montreal, founded in 1644, stands as a testimonial to her.

In 1657, Jeanne Mance returned to France

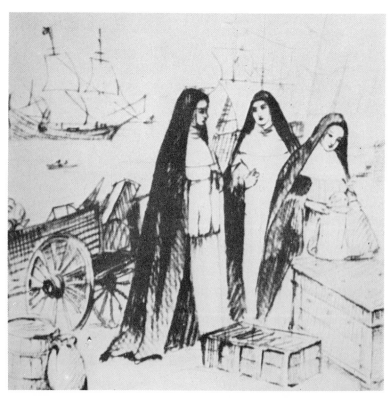

Figure 6–18. Arrival of the first three Augustinian Sisters at Quebec, 1639. (Courtesy of the Hôtel Dieu, Quebec.)

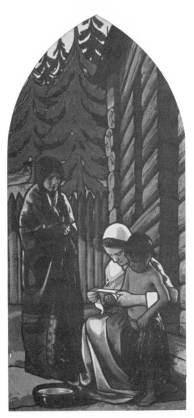

Figure 6–19. Jeanne Mance ministering to a little Indian girl while the mother watches. (*They Caught the Torch.* Will Ross, Inc.)

to recruit personnel. The Hospitallers or *Nursing Sisters of St. Joseph de La Flèche* came over to staff the Hôtel Dieu in Montreal with Jeanne Mance as administrator (Fig. 6–20). From France they sailed on the Saint André, a hospital ship that had terminated its role as such without benefit of fumigation or quarantine. There was an outbreak of pestilence that spread throughout the ship. Jeanne Mance and three of the sisters were infected with the disease but survived.

The care of the sick in colonial America is a fascinating chapter in the history of the English colonists. The settlers were poor and life was difficult in the new land, but the lack of medically prepared persons was a serious problem. Outbreaks of smallpox, scurvy and yellow fever wiped out many of the colonists.

Sir Walter Raleigh sent an expedition to Roanoke Island off the coast of North Carolina. The colony obtained no supplies during the period of warfare with the Spanish

Armada (1588). In 1591, relief ships were sent out only to find that the settlers had disappeared completely. Could the mysterious disappearance be due to starvation or an epidemic? No one knows the answer to this riddle.

The settlers in the Jamestown colony faced a rugged type of existence. During the first three years, all but 60 of the 500 colonists had died from malnutrition or one of the dietary deficiency diseases such as beriberi or scurvy.

In 1620, a type of hospital was constructed that could accommodate 50 persons if at least two patients shared one bed.

The men who practiced medicine in Virginia had great faith in the humoral theory. Medical treatments included withdrawing excessive amounts of humors from the body by using emetics, by purges and by bloodletting.

In the colony at Plymouth, Samuel Fuller, a deacon of the church, acted as physician, using prayer as part of routine treatment. His wife was the first midwife of the colony; Anne Hutchinson and Ann Eliot, wives of prominent men, also practiced midwifery.[6]

---

[6] *Male* midwives were fined!

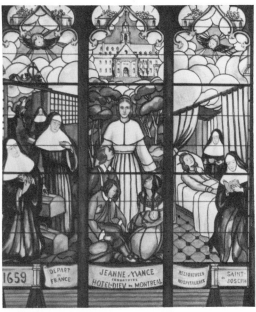

Figure 6–20. In the central panel of a stained glass window in Notre Dame Cathedral in Montreal, Jeanne Mance is surrounded by her patients. On the left are the first three sisters, Hospitallers of St. Joseph, are leaving France in 1659; on the right, they are caring for their patients in Montreal.

Witchcraft was seriously considered a cause of disease or injury. Here and elsewhere it was commonly felt that sickness was punishment for sin. Early colonial records speak of certain persons, both men and women, who were chosen on account of their skill and fitness to care for the sick.

In 1630, the Puritans founded the Massachusetts Bay Company. The influence of the Puritan clergymen was great. In the New England settlements, the clergymen were often the physicians. They were called "preacher doctors."

In the absence of medical schools, the clergy had the best educational preparation to practice medicine. Some laymen performed this task without benefit of education or license. The Rhode Island General Assembly is purported to have granted a degree and a license to practice medicine to a Captain John Cranston for his skill and ability in medical care. It seems an unusual procedure to receive a degree from a group of men not associated in any way with an institution of higher learning, and to receive a license to practice a professional skill without benefit of an examination.

The first governor of the Massachusetts Bay Colony, *John Winthrop* (1587–1649), and his son, John (1616–1676), who became governor of Connecticut, were enlisted as doctors (Fig. 6–21). Their preparation was received largely through correspondence with friends in England and, in like manner, their care of the sick was carried on by letters to patients since they could not visit all of them. These men were two of the many who assumed the duties of apothecary and doctor. Usually they had a chest of medicines and a guide book of suggested remedies for different ailments (Figs. 6–22 and 6–23).

A minister, Reverend Thomas Thacher, "though no Physitian, yet a well-wisher of the sick," felt compelled to write a leaflet for the community to be used during the many and troublesome epidemics of smallpox. The title of this discourse, published in Boston in 1677, was: "A Brief Rule to Guide the Common People of New England how to order themselves and theirs in the Small Pocks, or Measles."

Institutions of higher education were needed in these colonies. In 1636 Harvard College was founded, and in 1693 the College of William and Mary in Williamsburg, Virginia was established. The legislature of the Massachusetts Bay Colony was responsible for the inception of Harvard College because the colony was interested in the promotion of learning and wanted to prepare an educated ministry. For the first fifty years the President of the College did all the teaching;

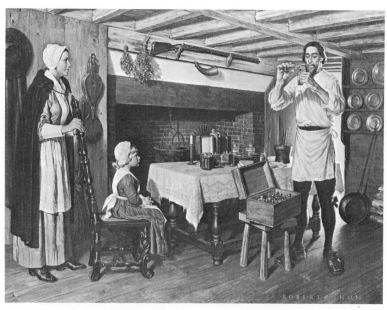

Figure 6–21. Governor who healed the sick. (© 1953 by Parke, Davis & Co.)

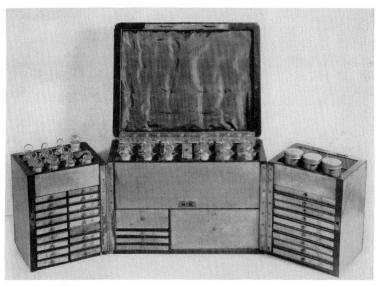

Figure 6–22. A medicine chest of the type used by the colonists and on board ship. Each drawer and section is numbered and described in the accompanying leaflet. (Courtesy of Peabody Museum of Salem, Mass.)

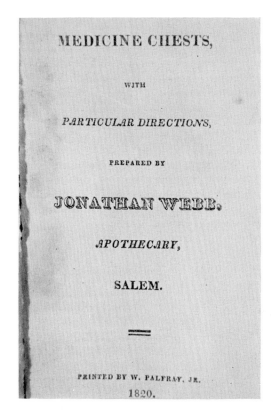

MEDICINE CHESTS,

WITH

PARTICULAR DIRECTIONS,

PREPARED BY

JONATHAN WEBB,

APOTHECARY,

SALEM.

PRINTED BY W. PALFRAY, JR.
1820.

Figure 6–23. The leaflet found in the medicine chest in Figure 6–22. This contains directions for compounding medicines from the ingredients in the medicine chest. (Courtesy of Peabody Museum of Salem, Mass.)

students interested in receiving a medical education went to England or France to receive it.

In 1623 a colony from *Holland* settled in New Netherlands (New York). The *first hospital* in this area was built by the Dutch on Manhattan Island in 1658 with the financial assistance of the West India Company. This was the beginning of New York's Bellevue Hospital, which cared for the sick, the poor and the mentally ill.

Toward the close of the seventeenth century, the *witchcraft* persecutions in Salem, Massachusetts (from January 1692 until May 1693) provided an additional emotional trauma for the colonists.

DEVELOPMENTS IN BIOLOGICAL SCIENCE AND MEDICINE

A renaissance took place in the field of *pharmacy* in the year 1240, when pharmacy secured a legal separation from medicine. By 1498 the first official Pharmacopoeia was published and became the legal guide for all pharmacists. In 1617, King James I granted a charter to the newly formed society of pharmacists known as the "Society of the Art and Mystery of the Apothecaries of the City of London." This extricated pharmacists from the control of the Guild of Grocers; for drugs, spices and herbs, used by apothecaries, were brought from many lands and sold by grocers. This association had placed pharmacists under the influence of the merchant group; after 1617, however, pharmacists emerged as a distinct group of craftsmen.

In the field of *general medicine,* two leaders, Paracelsus and Sydenham, were preeminent.

Phillippus Theophrastus Bombastus von Hohenheim, better known as *Paracelsus,* was one of the most unusual men in medical history. Born in Switzerland in 1493, Paracelsus was a quarrelsome, argumentative person who was credited with igniting the fire of new thinking in the field of medicine. A successful alchemist who was well versed in astrology, Paracelsus formulated many unscientific medical theories as well as many that showed marked ability in guessing, intuition or clear reasoning. He opposed the humoral theory of disease; advocated the use in medicines of many chemicals, such as mercury, sulphur, iron and arsenic; and overthrew the old medical authorities by burning their books publicly and denouncing their authority.[7] In this way, Paracelsus paved the way for the growth of new ideas.

Paracelsus may have had problems because of his strong and often overbearing personality, but he posed a thought-provoking message when he said "Medicine is not only a science, it is also an art . . . it deals with the very processes of life which must be understood before they may be guided."

At the same time, there was an obvious need for knowledge of the human body followed by an intelligent study of its functions.

Another area of expansion was in the development of the fine arts. Christian idealism motivated the arts of sculpture and stained glass, in addition to music. This was one of the greatest periods in the history of art. It was a productive period in medical art because of the drama of human dissection. A very distinguished group of artists laid this foundation and presented accurate knowledge in the field of anatomy and physiology. These artists surpassed their predecessors, the classical sculptors, by not only presenting correct external proportions and appearances but by dissecting bodies to broaden their knowledge. Three of the greatest and most

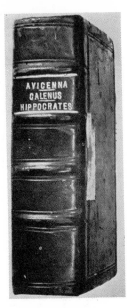

Figure 6–24. Little book, evidently intended to be carried by the medical student or physician, contained the teachings of Hippocrates, Galen and Avicenna. Date of publication is 1649.

innovative artists of the Renaissance were *Dürer, Raphael* and *Michelangelo.* One of the most versatile figures in this period was the Florentine *Leonardo da Vinci* (1452–1519). Many are familiar with his paintings, especially his "Last Supper," "Mona Lisa" and "Virgin of the Rocks." Leonardo, however, was also a sculptor, inventor, mathematician, architect and engineer.

It was small wonder that Leonardo's keen powers of observation were turned to the structure and function of the human body. He dissected the body, and the findings that he recorded in his notebooks were masterpieces of accurate observation that expanded the knowledge of the human body in a remarkable fashion. Leonardo's art was natural and lifelike. He not only portrayed man in a realistic fashion, but he also revealed the person's reaction of fear, pain and frustration as well as happiness and joy.

Andreas Vesalius (Fig. 6–25) (1513–1564), the son of the court apothecary to Emperor Charles V, was born in Brussels. He received his medical education at Louvain and at Padua where he became a member of the faculty. From boyhood, Vesalius had been inordinately fond of dissecting and his first attempts were centered upon animals. In later life, this interest seemed to increase and

---

[7]Medical science and medical teaching continued at this time to be based on the teachings of Hippocrates, Galen and Avicenna. (See Figure 6–24.)

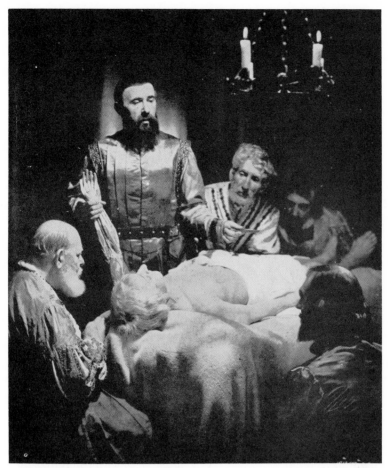

Figure 6–25. Andreas Vesalius (1514–1565). (Courtesy of Davis & Geck Co.)

cemeteries and places of execution yielded him the needed bodies. Although the civil courts permitted the bodies of condemned criminals to be taken by artists, it was not so easy for would-be medical scientists to obtain cadavers; therefore, a close association developed between medical men and grave robbers, or "resurrectionists."

The results of Vesalius' painstaking research were presented in *De humani corporis fabrica libri septem* in 1543. This book was a masterpiece of care and accuracy and presented in clear, readable and visual form the representations of the dissected parts of the human body. Vesalius had established the position of scientific dissection; he had corrected previous inaccuracies, especially those of Galen, but he did not discover the circulation of the blood, which he thought passed through holes in the septum from the right side of the heart into the left side.

The painstaking notes and drawings of Vesalius proved the errors of the past. In his work one notes the confrontation of medieval Galenism with the bases of modern science. It has been recorded that Vesalius sketched in charcoal on the dissection table as he worked. A notebook of a student who was present and watched Vesalius's dissections has been discovered and has provided an excellent primary souce of history.[8]

In the field of *surgery*, the name of *Ambrose Paré* (1510–1590) was a prominent one. Paré started his career as a barber's apprentice, later became an assistant at the Hôtel Dieu and emerged a successful army surgeon. While on duty in the wars, Paré manifested

[8]Ericksson, Ruben, Ed.: *Baldasor Heseler: Andreas Vesalius' first public anatomy at Bologna: 1540. An Eyewitness' Report.* Uppsala and Stockholm (Lychnos Bibliothek 18) 1959.

the gifts that have made him one of the most outstanding surgeons in history.

Gunshot wounds were routinely treated with boiling oil at this time. Paré searched for a substitute and, realizing the injurious effect of this cruel treatment, discontinued its use. He invented many new surgical instruments, made amputation less traumatic by reintroducing the use of ligatures to tie off the blood vessels instead of cauterizing them or sealing the vessels with boiling oil, introduced ingenious artificial limbs and belittled the value and use of powdered mummy and unicorn's horn as medicines. Paré is credited with saying, "I treated him, God cured him."

The first authentically recorded successful blood transfusion on human beings was performed in June, 1667, by *Jean Baptiste Denis,* physician to Louis XIV, in Paris. The patient was a youth 15 or 16 years old who had some obscure fever. The boy made a remarkable recovery following the administration of nine ounces of blood from the carotid artery of a lamb.

An unusual turn of events occurred in legislation when France and England improved the status of barber-surgeons. The climax was reached in 1540 when Henry VIII united the Barber Company with the Guild of Surgeons to form the United Barber-Surgeon Company with Thomas Vicary, the anatomist, as the Master. (See Figure 6–26.)

The surgeons, however, were not so fortunate in obtaining status as the pharmacists were in being separated from the Guild of Grocers.

The first *obstetrical forceps* were devised by a Peter Chamberlen in 1630 in England. For many years, the family told no one of their existence. The secret of the construction of the forceps was ultimately released and they were made for the benefit of all women who needed their use.

Santorio Santorio (1561–1636), a brilliant young man, devised instruments for measuring body weight and temperature (Fig. 6–27). He served for many years as physician to King Maximilian of Poland. Santorio corresponded with his colleague Galileo and applied some of Galileo's ideas to the field of medicine. Santorio has been credited with the invention of three thermometers—one to be placed in the mouth, another with a large bulb to be held in the hand and still another with a funnel into which the patient breathed. He noted also that the excretions of the body were less in volume than the food intake and realized that some of this loss was used in creating energy.

William Harvey (1578–1657) was the major contributor to the field of *physiology.* Harvey grew up in Elizabethan England and, in 1628, he announced his discovery of the *circulation of the blood* with the publication of his *Anatom-*

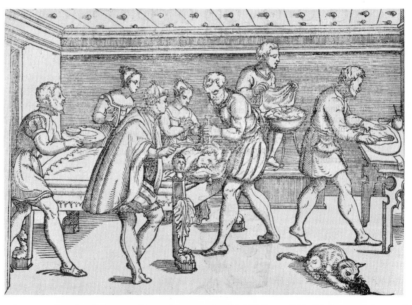

Figure 6–26. A scene showing Johannes Cruce (*ca.* 1573) using the apparatus he designed for trephining. (Courtesy of New York Academy of Medicine.)

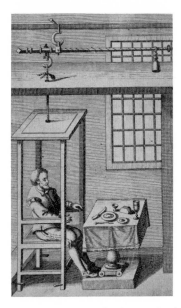

Figure 6–27. Santorio seated in his weight chair, which gauged body weight. His experimentation with aspects influencing body weight was one of the great scientific advances of this period. (Courtesy of New York Academy of Medicine.)

ical Disquisition on the Motion of the Heart and Blood of Animals.

Before Harvey's time, there existed many erroneous notions concerning the blood. Some of these held that the arteries were filled with air, spirits or both, that the veins carried nourishment, that fuliginous vapors were present in the arteries and that the blood did not circulate through the body but rather moved or rocked forward and backward. William Harvey's conclusions can be summarized as follows: the blood moves in a continuous onward direction from the right side of the heart, through the purification system in the lungs, to the left side of the heart whence it is pumped in one direction through the arteries of the body and back to the heart through the veins. The interlacing network of capillaries that formed the connecting link between the arteries and the veins was not described.

Harvey demonstrated excellent research techniques by his careful, painstaking and logical method, and his contribution was of great importance.

Marcello Malpighi (1628–1694), using the newly discovered microscope, reported his observations of the *capillary circulation* in the lungs and mesentery of the frog. This was the important link needed to understand the circulatory system of the body. Another achievement of Malpighi was the discovery of the *red blood corpuscles* in the blood stream (1665).

Scientists were describing nature as accurately as possible in the hope that man would adapt himself to it more effectively. Because Galileo needed instruments to observe natural phenomena, lens grinders devised telescopes. When Sir Isaac Newton described the planets, educated people lost their faith in astrology. Astrology and horoscopes lost their importance in medical care.

The lens grinders also produced *microscopes.* One of the earliest microscopists was Johannes Jansen of Holland who was reputed to have used one about 1590.

Athanasius Kircher (1602–1680), born in Germany, was educated at Fulda and became a Jesuit priest. His interests were many, as seen in his literary achievements, over forty in number, on widely different subjects. One of these works described the wonders of nature revealed to him by means of the microscope. He noted the innumerable "worms" in vinegar and milk, and the countless animalcules in pus and blood that were invisible to the naked eye. Father Kircher was very likely the first scientist to use the microscope in investigating the cause of disease.

Anton van Leeuwenhoek (1632–1723), who was born in Delft, Holland, has been noted for improving the microscope and for identifying certain types of bacteria. Leeuwenhoek had not received a university education or any preparation in medicine. In his leisure he ground lenses, constructed microscopes, studied the objects of nature and drew diagrams of what he observed; in doing this, Leeuwenhoek established the basis for the development of the field of bacteriology. Although animalcules still needed to be identified and classified as bacteria, the "devil spirits" had at last been seen.

Scientists of this era were debating and studying the theory of *spontaneous generation.* An Italian naturalist, *Francesco Redi* (1626–1697), contradicted the idea that living matter such as maggots could spring from non-living matter. He carried out a controlled experiment by placing meat in jars, some uncovered and others covered with parchment and gauze. In a short time maggots appeared in the uncovered jars of meat but not in the covered ones; however, Redi's testimony was not accepted by his contemporaries.

Thomas Sydenham (1624–1689) was a physician who contributed to the field of general medicine. Sydenham was a true follower of Hippocrates, stressing the need for careful observation of the patient, observing symptoms and treating each person's illness on an individual basis. He did not follow the current medical practices completely but used independent thinking. Sydenham advocated fresh air in sickrooms, for windows were not only kept closed at this time, but were concealed by heavy draperies; he encouraged patients with tuberculosis to get fresh air and sunshine by horseback riding; he recommended the simplification of prescriptions (which some-times had filled two and three pages with lists of ingredients), and discarded the useless ones; and he gave a detailed description of prevalent diseases. Sydenham was an eminently able practitioner using the best of the past in his treatments.

In summary, the thread of continuity of leadership in providing nursing care was apparent in this period of the Renaissance. Specially prepared nurses, both women and men, provided nursing care to people of all ages, in varying degrees of health and illness, and in a variety of settings. Nurses expanded their role while continuing to use intellectual skills and judgment in the execution of the physical as well as psychosocial aspects of nursing care.

REFERENCE READINGS

Bertrande, D. C., Sister: *A Woman Named Louise.* Normandy, Mo., Marillac College Press, 1956.

Calvet, Jean: *Saint Vincent de Paul.* Trans. Lancelot C. Sheppard. New York, David McKay Co.

Caraman, Philip: *Henry Morse—Priest of the Plague.* New York, Farrar, Straus & Cudahy, 1957.

Cather, Willa: *Shadows on the Rock.* New York, Alfred A. Knopf, 1946.

Cooper, P.: *The Bellevue Story.* New York, Thomas Y. Crowell, 1948.

Damel-Rops, Henri: *Monsieur Vincent.* New York, Hawthorn Books, 1961.

Defoe, Daniel: *A Journal of the Plague Year* (1721). New York, E. P. Dutton & Co.

Foran, J. K., and Morrissey, Sister Helen: *Jeanne Mance; or, The Angel of the Colony.* Montreal, Sisters of the Hôtel Dieu, 1931.

Gibson, John M., and Mathewson, Mary S.: *Three Centuries of Canadian Nursing.* Toronto, The Macmillan Co., 1947.

Giles, Dorothy: *A Candle in Her Hand.* New York, G. P. Putnam's Sons, 1949.

Heagney, Anne: *God and the General's Daughter.* Milwaukee, Bruce Publishing Co., 1953.

Martindale, Cyril G.: *Life of St. Camillus.* New York, Sheed & Ward, 1946.

McMahon, Norbert: *The Story of the Hospitallers of St. John of God.* Westminster, Md., Newman Press, 1959.

Maynard, Theodore: *Apostle of Charity: The Life of St. Vincent de Paul.* New York, Dial Press, 1939.

Merejkowski, Dmitri: *The Romance of Leonardo da Vinci.* New York, Random House, 1902.

Newcomb, Covelle: *St. John of God.* New York, Dodd, Mead & Co., 1958.

Pachter, Henry: *Paracelsus: Magic into Science.* New York, Collier Books, 1961.

Paget, Stephen: *Ambrose Paré and His Times.* New York, G. P. Putnam's Sons, 1897.

Pepys, Samuel: *Diary (Selections).* New York, Random House.

Repplier, Agnes: *Mère of the Ursulines.* New York, Doubleday, Doran & Co., 1931.

Shellabarger, Samuel: *Captain from Castile.* Boston, Little, Brown & Co., 1945.

Van Loon, Hendrik W.: *R.V.R.: The Life and Times of Rembrandt.* New York, Liveright Publishing Co., 1931.

CHAPTER 7

Nursing and the Pressures of the Eighteenth Century

The accomplishments of the eighteenth century must be viewed against a background of various outbreaks of political strife. Several of these outbreaks ended in armed intervention and revolution in an endeavor to create a more democratic form of government. Three of the revolutions, The Enlightenment, the American Revolution and the French Revolution, sought to spread a doctrine of independence and to emphasize the rights of man. All men were born free and equal and were to be entitled to life, liberty and the pursuit of happiness. The thirteen colonies became the United States of America, "a new nation conceived in liberty and dedicated to the proposition that all men are created equal."

There was need for legislation for improving the sanitary and living conditions for the poor. There had been no attempt at the prevention of disease or at teaching the poor the principles of hygiene and sanitation. Epidemics took a fantastic toll of lives and occasioned severe psychological experiences.

In 1720, when England was threatened with an epidemic of cholera, the Government encouraged Dr. Richard Mead (1673–1754) to publish a book entitled *A Short Discourse Concerning Pestilential Contagion.* This was an attempt to advise and teach prevention of disease. He stressed that, instead of penalizing infected families,[1] a reward should be given to those persons who discovered and reported a case of infectious disease. He stated further that instead of imprisonment of the family, the sick person should be removed, preferably to a place in the country where care could be provided. Dr. Mead did not believe in fumigation, although he felt the acrid smoke of sulphur effectively penetrated a contaminated area. He advocated that all necessary gatherings be cancelled.

During the colonial period in America, the means of communication were limited. People traveled by stagecoach, on horseback, or on foot. There was no regular stagecoach line between New York and Philadelphia until 1766 at which time the trip took three days. Mail was delivered irregularly.

Colonial life in the eighteenth century witnessed distressing outbreaks of disease in epidemic form.

Dr. Caulfield gave a brilliant presentation of one of the catastrophic epidemics that occurred in New England between 1735 and 1740.[2] The epidemic was referred to as "the throat distemper," but was actually three separate epidemics—one of scarlet fever and two of diphtheria. Ultimately, the whole of New England was involved. It was a new disease to that generation and at one point nearly one half of the children died. In the period of five years, five thousand persons died, mostly children and young people.

The best educated man in the New England town was the minister, and often he

---

[1]The former custom, during the times of the plague, required houses in which infected persons resided to be quarantined with a mark of the sign of the cross on the door and the well persons to be shut up with the sick. The imprisonment lasted at least a month after all trace of the disease had disappeared.

[2]Caulfield, Ernest: *A History of the Terrible Epidemic Vulgarly Called The Throat Distemper, Which Occurred in His Majesty's New England Colonies Between 1735–1740.* New Haven, Conn., Yale Journal of Biology and Medicine, 1939.

assumed the role of doctor. Many of the physicians of this period had no medical school background and frequently received their preparation by being apprenticed to some other doctor who also had no formal medical education.

Lacking an understanding of bacterial infection, its cause and method of transfer, they ignored even the most elementary precautions. Ministers and physicians assisted in spreading the disease, carrying the infection on their hands and clothes, to other patients as well as to their own families. Caulfield states that "one of the very noticeable characteristics of the 'throat distemper' epidemic is the frequent occurrence of many deaths in the families of ministers and physicians."[3]

Each family in New England was a self-sustaining unit, and had its own milk supply, water supply, produce, salted pork and poultry. The occasions when the community grouped together were for church meetings, socials, funerals and protection.

One would expect that the spread of infection would be most unlikely. Since the seventeenth century, however, the law decreed that towns with more than fifty families must provide for the education of the children. By 1735, public schools were established throughout New England. The schools were one-room, poorly ventilated buildings, which meant close contact among the children. Another custom contributed to the spread of the infectious disease. When a child died, the neighboring children acted as pallbearers and in addition to coming in contact with the corpse, which in this period was not embalmed,[4] they associated with the dead child's family.

In Kingston, New Hampshire, the "plague of the throat" visited most of the families in town and left them childless. (See Figure 7-1.)

The colonists referred to diphtheria as "canker" and to scarlet fever as "canker rash." Many physicians felt that these diseases were the same except that when a rash was not able to be brought to the surface, the disease was more severe and even fatal. The ingredient in the blood that caused the difference was some "morbifick matter." If an efficacious remedy could be applied that would allow the poisons to reach the skin surface, and evaporate through the pores, a rash would be produced. This "morbifick matter" theory was not new and it is still discussed by older members of this generation when they stress the need for a good sweat to bring out the rash that will assist the poisons of the body to escape.

It was with thanksgiving and deep gratitude that the New England colonists welcomed the end of the "throat distemper."

In 1755, in New York, the first quarantine law was passed. Vessels were quarantined at Bedloe's Island if persons suspected of having contagious diseases were aboard. By legislation in 1784, the State government appointed a health officer to the port to enforce quarantine measures. The first death records were filed in the year 1795 and these reported hundreds of deaths due to the yellow fever epidemic. *Dr. Richard Bayley*, the health officer, attributed this epidemic to the filthy conditions of the city and the crowded living conditions of the poor.

The following year, in 1796, physicians were compelled to report infectious diseases. Ordinances required the disposal of garbage and refuse.

A new threat evolved with the eruption of wars. When the colonies decided to fight in the War of Independence, there was no organized army since the states were not united. Each state had an army that was the spontaneous reaction to patriotism.

During the Battle of Bunker Hill, the need for a medical department for the army was recognized. The Provincial Congress of Massachusetts hired private houses and assembled medical supplies to be used for the sick and wounded. The needs were great. One doctor reported that the distress and plight of the soldiers was indescribable. They lacked shelter, bedding, clothing and adequate food. Infectious diseases were rampant.

Despite the growing pains of a new country as well as the trials and tribulations of older ones, contributions were made in the health fields.

---

[3]*Ibid.*, p. 5.

[4]The body of a person who had died was placed in a coffin and prior to burial, buckets of ice were placed under and around the coffin to assist in preserving the corpse. As the ice melted, the water was thrown out in the yard and could have been a source of infection. The impossibility of burying a body during the cold New England winter months when the ground was frozen presented a source of contagion as well as psychological trauma. When the receiving vaults were unable to accommodate any more coffins, the coffin had to be kept in the coldest place, usually the barn or attic, until the spring thaws.

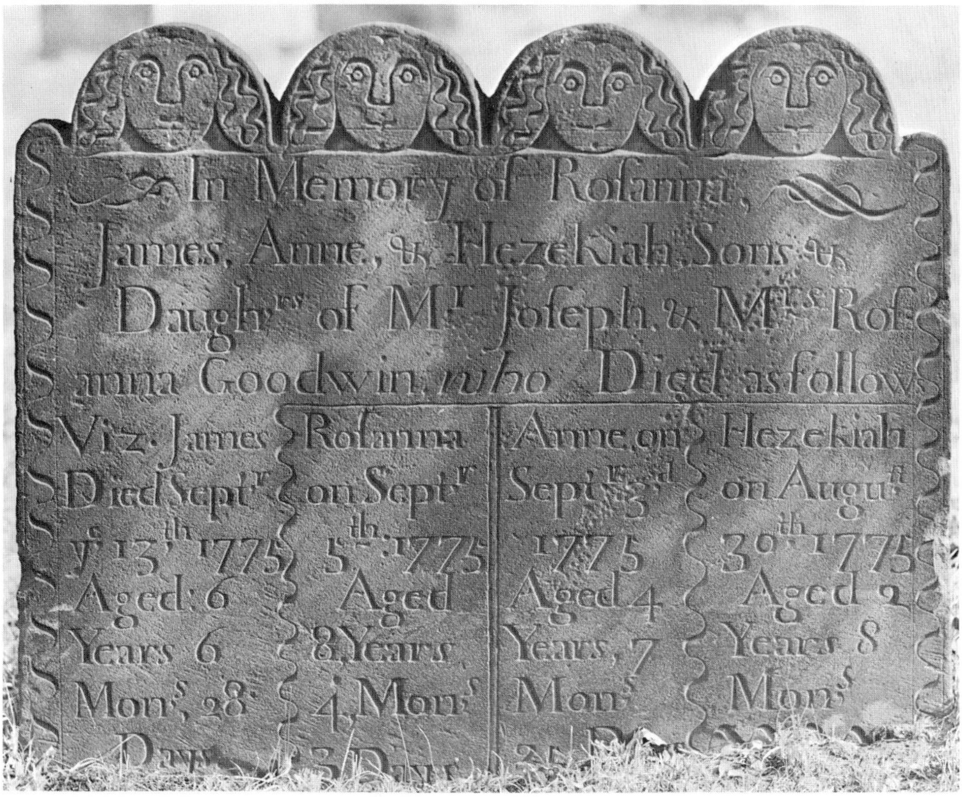

Figure 7-1. A tombstone depicting the tragedy that befell a family in Bloomfield, Connecticut, in an epidemic. (Courtesy of Dr. Wendell C. Hall.)

PROGRESS IN NURSING AND SOCIAL WELFARE

Many social problems as well as physical ills existed at this time. The need for social legislation to relieve the afflictions was apparent.

The person who assumed the role of nurse, keeping people healthy as well as caring for them during illness, was the mother. Her care was as good and patient-centered as her personal qualities, her inventiveness and her applied knowledge could provide. With science striving to become established, in addition to political problems and medical misinformation, her work continued as an independent practitioner. Her skills at providing care and, in many instances, cure have been a tribute to her creativity in planning for comfort and care of her patient.

The ideas for many of the articles, which were designed to help a person feel more comfortable and get well, may have been suggested by the nurses of this period. The number of examples that remain are indicative of the wide acceptance of the comfort measures that were utilized. The importance of nutrition and of keeping a person warm or cool was also recognized.

Women continued to minister to the needs of their families and neighbors. To stay alive in the colonies was a challenge; the women were courageous and heroic. Without central heating, fireplaces were the source of the heat supply. Beds were cold; therefore, long-handled warming pans, usually constructed of brass, were used as bed-warmers. They were filled with live coals and rubbed over the bottom sheet to heat it. When a person was ill, stone jugs filled with hot water, the forerunners of hot water bottles and heating pads, were utilized.

The weight of the soapstones and the stone jugs soon made it apparent that less heavy ones were needed. Many uniquely shaped pottery hot water bottles as well as pewter ones, were designed. The danger of burns, particularly from the pewter ones, does not seem to have been considered.

Mothers used pewter nursing bottles for their "dry-nursing." These were heavy, and the top section unscrewed for the milk to be

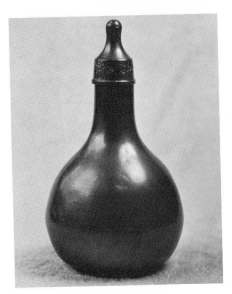

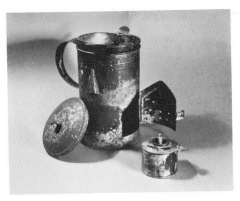

Figure 7–3. Pap warmer. (Author's collection. Photo by DeLores Paul.)

Figure 7–2. Pewter nursing bottle—note the teeth marks. (Courtesy of Miss Kate Hyder.)

poured into the bottom part. The nipple was part of the pewter top section. The dangers of lead poisoning were not recognized, for children used these nursing bottles for several years and their teething marks still remain visible on these bottles (Fig. 7–2).

The eighteenth century combination lamps and food warmers were ingenious devices that provided comfort for the invalid during the long hours of the night (Figs. 7–3 and 7–4). The objective was to keep liquids or nourishing food, principally pap, warm during the night. Pap was a substance made of milk in which oatmeal was cooked and strained. Beaten egg yolks, butter and orange flavor were added. The food was placed in a food pan that fit into a pan of water, much as a double-boiler pan would function. It was a popular food item in the invalid's diet. Beef tea, or the extraction of the juices in

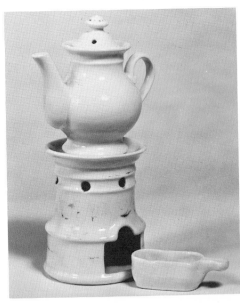

Figure 7–4. A combination night light and broth warmer. A wick was floated on whale oil in the small china dish; the ignited wick furnished light and heat to warm the food. (Author's collection.)

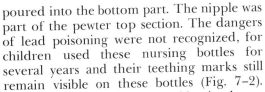

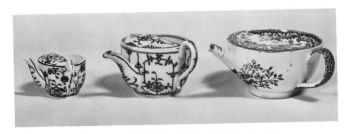

Figure 7–5. Examples of feeding cups. (Author's collection.)

beef made into a broth, was another frequently served dish.

China feeding cups (Fig. 7–5) were designed to permit a patient to serve himself. The sizes of these cups were scaled to meet the personal needs of the patient. Hot water chambered dishes were designed to keep the food as warm as possible as well as to serve as a tray in which to bring the food.

Invalid chairs were devised during this period. Wheel chairs were called "go-chairs" in the eighteenth century. Gout chairs, rocking chairs and fan chairs were produced. The fan chair was invented in an attempt to alleviate the sweltering heat of Philadelphia summers. The chair was designed by a Mr. Cram of Philadelphia and the sponsor of the chair was Dr. Benjamin Rush. The foot moved the fan, which not only cooled a person but also kept the flies from annoying the occupant.

Herbs were used extensively in colonial homes as seasoning in food, as air purifiers, as well as sachet to scent linens and clothes. In addition, mothers concocted many uses for medicinal herbs, which became the bases of medications that are used today. An example of this was the woman in Shropshire, England, who found a remedy that cured dropsy; that herb was foxglove, from which digitalis, a valuable heart medicine, is obtained. Dr. William Withering (1741–1799) discovered that this lady was curing patients with dropsy when it was associated with a heart condition. He extracted from her herb mixture the important ingredient, which was digitalis.

Other than the previously mentioned religious nursing groups, there were no specially prepared nurses.

Nutting[5] states: "The eighteenth century saw a deterioration in nursing and hospital organization, and, naturally, the surroundings of the sick were also changed for the worse. The large airy halls, the cool springs and fountains, and the sweet green gardens of the mediaeval hospitals of France, Spain and the East now gave place to the small dark wards of the city and state institutions of the eighteenth century."

The eighteenth century witnessed the establishment of several important American hospitals.

1731: *Blockley Hospital* (now Philadelphia General Hospital). This hospital received the poor, sick, insane, prisoners and orphans and was connected with a poorhouse. It was an almshouse and workhouse for the aged and infirm of the city. The care of patients was in the hands of servants, criminals and paupers.

1737: *Charity Hospital* of New Orleans. In 1736, in New Orleans, a sailor, Jean Louis, died, leaving a sum of money to be used for the founding of a hospital for the care of the sick. His bequest included funds to purchase necessary equipment. The hospital was constructed in 1737 and served both as a hospital and as an asylum for the poor. After several catastrophes, the hospital was rebuilt in 1832; it had high ceilings, spacious wards and verandas, and was placed under the aegis of the Sisters of Charity in 1834.

1751: *Pennsylvania Hospital* was founded in Philadelphia through the efforts of Dr. Thomas Bond and Benjamin Franklin, both of whom were Quakers. Its purpose was to admit only those who were acutely ill or had received an injury. Strangers as well as the residents of Philadelphia were admitted. It was not an almshouse or poorhouse, but a hospital in the usual sense of the word. The seal of this institution had been that of the Good Samaritan: "Take care of him and I will repay thee."

1770: *Eastern State Hospital*, known as the "Lunatick Hospital," was opened in Williamsburg, Virginia. This was one of the first American state-owned institutions for the mentally ill. In 1770, Governor Fauquier sponsored an act "to make Provision for the support and maintenance of idiots, lunaticks, and other persons of unsound minds."

1771: *New York Hospital* came into existence because of the efforts of public-spirited citizens. In 1771, a royal charter was granted by King George III to "the society of the Hospital in the City of New York in America." It was in the New York Hospital that Dr. Valentine Seaman gave the first series of lectures to nurses in the Colonies.

1786: *The Philadelphia Dispensary* was established through the influence of Quakers.

1796: *The Boston Dispensary* was founded by a group of Boston philanthropists. It had the first dental clinic and the first lung clinic in the nation, as well as the first evening pay clinic for working people. Another unusual aspect was that it had the first food clinic in the world.

[5]Nutting, M. A., and Dock, L.: *A History of Nursing.* New York, G. P. Putnam's Sons, 1935, I, p. 251.

The distressing social conditions existing in the eighteenth century aroused the sympathetic efforts of many persons, including those with political influence. One such person was *John Howard* (1727–1789) who spent years investigating prisons, lazarettos and hospitals in England and on the continent. In a forceful manner he recorded his observations, much to the consternation of the public. As bad as the prison conditions were, including the dungeon horrors, the facilities and care of the mentally ill were worse; the hospitals and nursing conditions were also deplorable. The only praise that he recounted was for the work of the Sisters of Charity and the Beguines.

Filth, poor sanitation and an inadequate and unappetizing diet seemed to be universal. Windows were not opened for fear of drafts nor were patients bathed for fear of getting them chilled.

One of Howard's recommendations was to keep one ward unoccupied so that patients in a ward could be removed to the vacant one while the one to which they had been assigned was cleaned. This was to be done to each ward in rotation.

Hospital nurses of this period were housekeepers, doing the scrubbing and cleaning, when it was done. They were on a low level socially, were unable to read or write and were given to drunkenness and, consequently, to drowsiness. These women were more to be pitied than criticized. They had no desire for their job, nor did they have preparation for it. Fortunately, there were some women serving as nurses who, despite deficient educations, were striving to give devoted service.

Eventually, much progress was noted because of the efforts, courage and endeavors of John Howard.[6]

A prison with a pathetic history of torture was Newgate Prison of East Granby, Connecticut; it was the first Connecticut colonial prison. Prisoners were not segregated according to sex, type of crime or mental condition; the mentally ill and mentally retarded shared quarters with the most vicious criminals. Screams were heard for quite a distance from the dungeons to which all inmates had to descend every night. Physical, emotional and mental disorders were prevalent and infectious diseases terminated many lives.

INFANT WELFARE

In the field of infant welfare much needed to be done. St. Vincent de Paul had championed the cause of the abandoned child in the preceding century. The problem had become a more serious one in the eighteenth century.

Dr. Caulfield has written of the plight of infants in England during this period and of those who tried to alleviate their sufferings.[7]

On the part of the public, there was an attitude of callousness and indifference in a setting of wholesale infanticide. This viewpoint had to be changed before appreciable progress toward reducing infant mortality could be attempted. Records are replete with evidence of neglect, cruelty and sickness as well as infanticide. The exact statistics are not available, but in the early part of the century, the infant mortality rate for children under five years of age was 50 per cent. In London, between 1730 and 1750, 75 per cent of all the babies christened were dead before the age of five. Even Queen Anne, who presumably received the best of care, lost 18 children in early infancy.

The greatest cause of death in infancy was neglect. Wealthy women delegated the care of the children to nursemaids. The infant was nursed either by a wet nurse, which could mean transfer of disease to the child, or by "dry nursing," or bottle-feeding, which meant the possibility of contracting disease from contaminated milk and water. It has been pointed out that the children of the wealthy were neglected because of fashion while those of the poor were abandoned because of poverty.

There was a constant supply of wet nurses available because of the deaths of their own babies. It has been stated that "in some cases the infant mortality was the source of the wet-nurse supply; in other cases, the effect."

The rate of infant mortality was incredibly high in the eighteenth century. The mortality of dry-nursed infants was nearly three times that of the breast-fed ones. The common

---

[6]*Amelia* (1751), by Henry Fielding. This novel expresses the wickedness of the law courts and the evils of the English prisons of the eighteenth century. It presents a picture of confinement in debtor's jail.

[7]Caulfield, Ernest: *The Infant Welfare Movement in the Eighteenth Century.* New York, Paul B. Hoeber, 1931.

entry into the hospital records was "death from want of breast milk." For example, of 10,272 infants admitted to the Dublin Foundling Hospital during 21 years (1775–1796) only 45 survived, a mortality of 99.6 per cent. Many famous foundling hospitals of the period had similar records.

In 1761, *Jean-Jacques Rousseau* published his famous book *Emile*. Book I is a popular treatise on pediatrics and deals with the hygiene and nutrition of infancy. The dangers of mercenary wet-nursing and of tightly swaddling infants are emphasized. It inveighs against women who do not take care of or nurse their own children.

The British painter and engraver *William Hogarth* (1697–1764) used his considerable talent to focus piercing criticism on the social problems of his day. Charles Lamb testifies to Hogarth's dramatic gift when he opines that most "pictures are looked at—his prints

we read."[8] Hogarth's engravings were picture stories of an intense social ferment and of a world craving the pleasures of it (Fig. 7–6).

"Dropping" of infants was a common occurrence. This meant abandoning the infant on the doorstep of wealthy homes[9] or just leaving a child in the street to freeze or starve. Unmarried women occasionally murdered their offspring to earn a livelihood as a wet nurse.

Nurse members of religious orders con-

---

[8] "On the genius and character of Hogarth," *Works of Charles Lamb, Vol. 1*, p. 70, 1818.

[9] *The History of Tom Jones, A Foundling* (1749), by Henry Fielding. One of the great realistic novels, the story of Tom Jones begins with Squire Allworthy's finding him, an infant, crying in his bed. When the baby was discovered, one of Allworthy's comments was, "I suppose she hath only taken this method to provide for her child; and truly I am glad she hath not done worse."

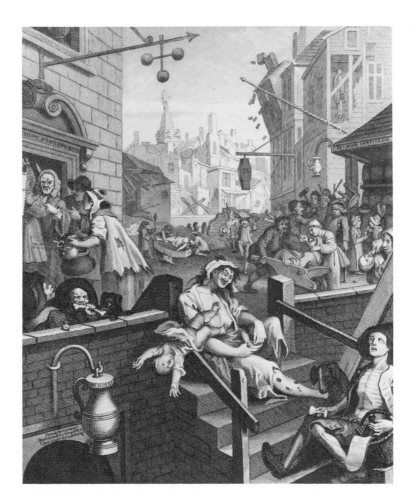

Figure 7–6. Hogarth's famous "Gin Lane" depicts the plight of the child in this period. The frailties of human nature are well displayed in a scene of horrible devastation.

tinued to give nursing care to the well or ill children who were placed in the turnstyles of Foundling Hospitals by mothers who either lacked interest in them or finances to care for them (Fig. 7–7).

Other causes of death as they were reported in this century were: *headmouldshot* or the overriding of the sutures of the cranium, and this included birth injuries to the meninges that resulted in death; *horshoehead* or the separation of the sutures comprising congenital defects of the cranium; *overlaid*, which was due to the practice of nurses' sleeping with infants[10] as well as to the tightness of the stay (Fig. 7–8). The stay consisted of the strings attached to the cap and were tied tightly under the baby's chin; this cap was worn day and night to prevent chilling (Fig. 7–9).

There were some efforts to alleviate this serious situation. *Thomas Coram* (Fig. 7–10) (1668–1751) was instrumental in bringing over and settling in America poor families, known as Oglethorpe's Colony in Georgia.

---

[10]*Pamela* (1740), by Samuel Richardson, was a domestic novel, the first modern novel, a story in a series of letters. The depiction of scenes common to ordinary life was new to English literature. (Nurses were sometimes paid to overlay babies.)

The History of the Adventures of Joseph Andrews and His Friend Mr. Abraham Adams (1742), by Henry Fielding. A satire on Richardson's *Pamela.*

The ARCUTIO.

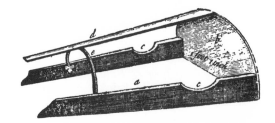

WHEN it is considered how many are charged Over-laid in the Bills of Mortality, it is to be wonder'd that the ARCUTIO's, universally used at *Florence*, are not used here in *England*. The Design above, is drawn in Perspective, with the Dimensions, which are larger than usual ; and is thus described :

a, The Place where the Child lies.
b, The Head-Board.
c, The Hollows for the Nurse's Breasts.
d, A Bar of Wood to lean on, when she suckles the Child.
e, A small Iron Arch to support the said Bar The Length three Feet, two Inches and a half.

Every Nurse in *Florence* is obliged to lay the Child in it, under Pain of Excommunication. The ARCUTIO, with the Child in it, may be safely laid entirely under the Bed-Cloaths in the Winter, without Danger of smothering.

Figure 7–8. An arcutio used to prevent overlaying. (Caulfield, Ernest: *The Infant Welfare Movement in the Eighteenth Century.* Hoeber, Inc.)

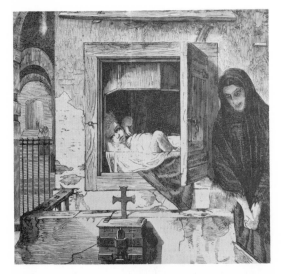

Figure 7–7. A turnstile of the Foundling Hospital in Florence, Italy, where a mother places her baby.

His plan involved erecting huts for deserted infants in which they were to be cared for and nourished properly. He labored for seventeen years on this project, exhausting his funds, then appealed to influential ladies for assistance. Thus, in 1738, the Hospital for Foundlings in London came into being (Fig. 7–11). So many children were brought to this institution that they had to be selected by lot.

William Cadogan (1711–1797), who graduated from Oxford on June 20, 1755 with the Master of Arts degree, and on June 27, 1755 with the degrees of Bachelor of Medicine and Doctor of Medicine, wrote "An Essay upon Nursing and Management of Children." In this, he advocated loose clothing and frequent change of clothing at a time when the body and limbs of a baby were cramped in flannels, swaths and wrappers. Wrapping babies in swaddling clothes had been a custom for ages. Dr. Cadogan also

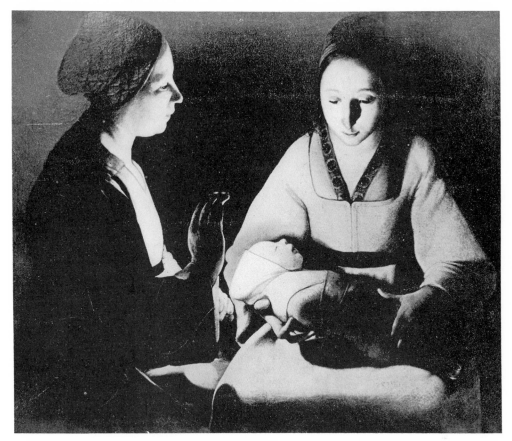

Figure 7–9. Two women with a newborn, tightly swaddled child. Painting by Georges de La Tour, ca. 1600–1652. (Museum in Rennes. Ciba Symposia, 1940.)

stressed the value of daily baths during an era when it was thought that to wash even a baby's head meant subjecting the baby to a cold.

The Foundling Hospital sent printed instructions to all foster mothers for the treatment of minor illnesses.

Jonas Hanway (1712–1786), a philanthropist, was appointed one of the governors of the Foundling Hospital and studied its problems. He became interested in parish workhouses, which were an outgrowth of the English poor laws. The parish workhouse movement, beginning about 1723, was an effort to provide quarters for the poor who were unable to support themselves and their infants. The populace was astonished at the descriptions by Hanway of the conditions that existed. He was successful in persuading Parliament to enact laws for the relief of these infants.

George Armstrong (?–1781) was one of the first English pediatricians. He possessed unusual powers of observation and was an ardent advocate of infant welfare. He was the prime leader behind the dispensary movement. On April 24, 1769, he opened the Dispensary for the Infant Poor. Some important rules he laid down for the parents of patients were: The babies were to be kept neat and clean, and the parents were to preserve order, be thankful for treatment and report on the progress of their children.

He recorded this rich experience at the dispensary in *An Account of the Diseases Most Incident to Children*, which was published in 1771, revised in 1777 and revised again in 1783. This early pediatric textbook presented his diagnostic ability because he wrote about what he saw.

It was Dr. Armstrong who was one of the first to realize that many mothers wanted to nurse their infants but were unable to do so. Dry nursing was recommended. He also

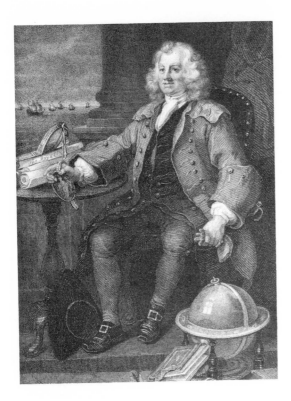

Figure 7–10. Captain Coram, the founder of the Foundling Hospital in London, with the royal charter granted in October, 1739.

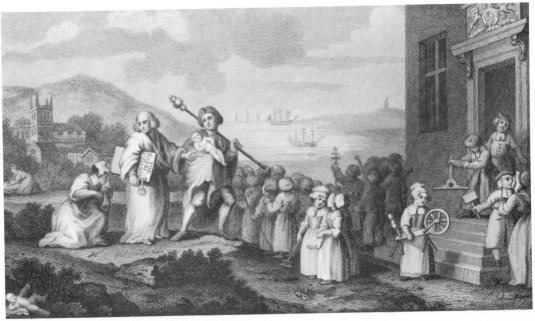

Figure 7–11. The Foundlings. Hogarth's famous scene presents the actions of rescuing the abandoned, helpless infants while providing a Foundling Hospital and an asylum for children, with an industrial training center for youth in a wholesome environment for growth.

suggested that rubbing a baby gently was a soothing remedy, this before the days of psychological experiments.

Infanticide continued to be a public problem into the nineteenth century.

NURSING IN THE REVOLUTIONARY WAR

One writer says, "At the start of the *Revolutionary War* the tale of the medical department was a sorry one. There was practically no organization nor discipline. Surgical instruments were few. Drugs were few and bad; opium and quinine were scarce and ether was then unknown. Trained nurses did not exist. Blundering assistants called 'mates' were the only help the surgeons had." There were only five hospitals in New England, two in New York and two in Philadelphia. In New England after the battle of Bunker Hill, several private houses in Cambridge were made into a hospital with Dr. John Warren in charge. Other hospitals were established near Boston. The nurses were mostly men with no training in nursing. "Improvised hospitals at strategic points were often only halls, churches or hastily constructed sheds. Sometimes an inn was available. Means of transportation were primitive, and long journeys from the battle front left the wounded in grave condition. . . . Despite the exertions of Dr. Benjamin Rush, one of the most distinguished physicians in the Colonies, hospitals were frightfully overcrowded and unsanitary beyond modern conception. Fever and epidemics ran almost unhindered."

In 1777, General Washington ordered that women be engaged to nurse the soldiers; though many were employed, they apparently cooked and served meals but did little nursing. Some women followed their husbands into war and took care of them if they were wounded or ill.

At Valley Forge, in the winter of 1777, small log huts were used as hospitals. Each contained two double and four single bunks made of logs, a table and a fireplace. The operating room was located in a stone schoolhouse, built by William Penn's daughter, Lucy.

An interesting order in Pennsylvania, the German Seventh-Day Baptist, formed a monastic community called the Ephrata Cloister. The habit of the Capuchins or White Friars was adopted by the new monastic community. The brothers wore a long white gown and cowl. The sisters' costume was the same with the addition of a belt with an embroidered rose pattern on it.

After the bloody battle at Brandywine during the American Revolution some 500 wounded soldiers were brought to be nursed by the sisters (Fig. 7–12). The buildings which served as a hospital had to be burned following their occupation to stop the spread of typhus fever. A monument in the monastic cemetery marks the graves of the many soldiers who were buried there.

Nurses had been aboard hospital ships for centuries. An eighteenth century hospital ship in the Mediterranean in 1705 carried five nurses and three laundresses. The duty of these naval nurses was specifically to care for the sick. The work of cleaning and washing was performed by the laundresses while cooks prepared the food.

An interesting assignment for these women nurses was to participate in an early research project.[11] In a pamphlet entitled "An Account of the Experiment made at the desire of the Lords Commissioners of the Admiralty, on board the *Union* Hospital Ship to determine the effect of the Nitrous Acid in destroying Contagion, and the safety with which it may be employed . . .," Dr. James Carmichael Smyth describes the experiment.

The HMS *Union* served many British Naval

---

[11] Singer, Charles. "An Eighteenth Century Naval Ship to Accommodate Women Nurses." *Medical History.* Volume IV. Number 4, October 1960, pp. 283–287.

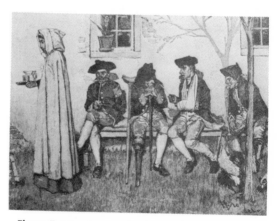

Figure 7–12. A monastic sister at the Ephrata Cloister in Pennsylvania attending the wounded soldiers after the battle at Brandywine.

ships by receiving the sick from them. When a Russian fleet became burdened with typhus fever and endured a very heavy death rate, as many of the Russian sailors as could be accommodated were brought on board the *Union*. They were cared for by the nursing staff consisting of a matron and at least fifteen nurses.

The relationship of lice to typhus fever, frequently called "jail distemper," was unknown. Dr. Smyth and the nurses carried out a regimen that stressed cleanliness, thorough bathing and disinfection of clothes and bedding, and shaving of heads and beards. The patients were placed in newly washed bedding. The sheepskin tunics with the hair turned inward were regarded as sources of infection and were removed in order to carry out the "antiseptic" (this word was used frequently) plan of care. Fresh air and the use of a disinfectant referred to as "antiseptic gas," derived from heating crude nitre (potassium nitrate) with carbon which gave off oxides of nitrogen, killed the lice. Another interesting arrangement on the HMS *Union* was the placement of the sanitary facilities which projected from the side of the ship instead of being inside it.

Dr. Smyth valued good nursing and opposed such things as bleeding and harsh drug therapy.

There were also male nurses assigned to military ships and they wore a special garb. They are familiar from some of the many pictures of Nelson's death at the Battle of Trafalgar in 1815.

NURSING IN THE FRENCH COLONIES DURING THE EIGHTEENTH CENTURY

The most traumatic year in the history of the Hôtel Dieu of Quebec was 1703. In that year, a severe epidemic of smallpox attacked Quebec and eventually the whole of New France. More than 2000 deaths occurred in Quebec. In 1710, a yellow fever epidemic wrought havoc.

The Sisters of the Hôtel Dieu labored tirelessly during both epidemics. Several of the sisters died at their heroic task of caring for the afflicted.

A ship docking in the harbor in 1740 brought 241 plague-stricken patients to the Hôtel Dieu. There was a remarkably low death rate, which indicates skilled nursing care had been given to these patients.

In 1755, another catastrophe confronted the sisters when the Hôtel Dieu was razed by fire. The Bishop of Quebec offered his home and volunteered to be the first orderly.

Two years later the sisters resumed their care of the sick in the newly rebuilt hospital, but they had a new challenge. The year was 1759, and the Augustinian Sisters of the Hôtel Dieu were ordered to go to the General Hospital that was outside of the city. During the French and Indian War, the wounded from the battles of the Plains of Abraham and Sainte-Foye were nursed devotedly by both the Augustinian and the Ursuline Sisters. When Quebec fell to the British, the majority of the sisters returned to their hospital. They received kind treatment from the new regime.

A description of the two hospitals in Quebec as well as the type of women who joined the nursing orders was written in 1769 by Francis Brooke in *The History of Emily Montague*:[12]

The Hotel Dieu is very pleasantly situated with a view of the two rivers and the entrance of the port; the house is cheerful, airy and agreeable; the habit of the nuns extremely becoming, a circumstance a handsome woman ought by no means to overlook; 'tis white with a black gauze veil . . . the nuns of this house are sprightly and have a look of health.

The General Hospital, situated about a mile out of town, is on the borders of the river St. Charles. The order and habit are the same with the Hotel Dieu, except that to the habit is added the cross, generally worn in Europe by canonesses only; a distinction procured for them by their founder St. Vallier, the second bishop of Quebec. The house is, without, a very noble building; and neatness, elegance and propriety reign within. The nuns, who are all of the noblesse, are many of them handsome, and all genteel, lively and well bred; they have an air of the world, their conversation is easy, spirited and polite.

The nursing sisterhoods in Canada came from France to Montreal and Quebec in the seventeenth century. By the eighteenth century, the members of the orders were Canadians.

The *St. Joseph Hospitallers of the Hôtel Dieu of*

---

[12]Gibbon, John M., and Mathewson, Mary S.: *Three Centuries of Canadian Nursing*, Toronto, The Macmillan Co., 1947, p. 53.

Montreal had a rigorous time during the greater part of their first hundred years there. They were beset by problems: lack of money, supplies not arriving from France, fire destroying the hospital, temporarily having to use a portion of a home for the aged, living through the perilous days of the "cold war" while the Indians armed with tomahawks were preparing to attack the English, struggling to care for an extra 500 patients during a smallpox epidemic, surviving the effects of another destruction of their hospital by fire, and coping with a malignant fever epidemic brought by one of the king's ships.

In 1738, *Madame d'Youville*, a widow of means who had been responsible for many philanthropic endeavors, organized a group of women of similar interests. These women became the Soeurs Grises or *Grey Nuns*. Their order was similar to the Order of Visitation founded by St. Francis de Sales. The sisters took care of the sick both in the hospitals and in their homes. They accepted women of all classes of society for membership in this order. The amazingly modern concept of making this a "hospital college" under the aegis of a teaching order was abandoned.

The Grey Nuns differed from the two other nursing orders of sisters in that this new order was not cloistered and included in its program the visitation of the sick in their homes, which was district nursing (visites à domicile). The Community of the Soeurs Grises, under the title of Sisters of Charity of the General Hospital of Montreal, received from Louis XV a charter to operate their hospital. They wore a gray habit with a silver crucifix on the breast (Fig. 7–13).

Mother d'Youville was a capable manager and devised many ways of raising money that was desperately needed for hospital construction, renovation and debts in general.

When English prisoners who had been sick or wounded were convalescing, Mother d'Youville put them to work at their trades and in this way utilized a modern concept of rehabilitation. She sheltered the prisoners in the chapel from the Indians.

When the English captured New France, the various orders of sisters received protection, were not disturbed or prevented from continuing their work and were praised for the care given to all soldiers.

In Canada, a home for abandoned children was established and given the name, *La Crèche d'Youville*. It is still used as a center for

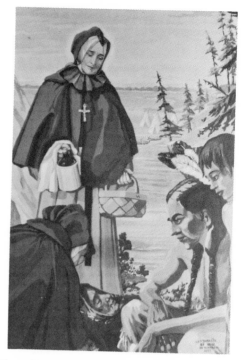

Figure 7–13. In 1755 a smallpox epidemic erupted in Montreal and the surrounding villages. The Grey Nuns nursed the afflicted Indians in their communities.

the placement of abandoned children with foster parents.

In Acadia (Nova Scotia) between 1629–1630 a tiny settlement prospered amid trials and tribulations and came to be known as Port Royal. From its earliest beginnings, it had a type of infirmary for the sick under the supervision of the *Brothers Hospitallers of St. John of God*. Gradually, this developed into a hospital.

Another hospital was constructed at Louisbourg in Cape Breton. Five members of the Brothers Hospitallers of St. John of God were sent to staff this institution; two male nurses, two surgeons, and an apothecary were also assigned.

The British colonized Nova Scotia, and a hospital was constructed for the citizens at Halifax. The matron of this hospital, Sarah Dunlop, has been reported to have worked without pay. This hospital became an almshouse for the poor in 1766.

The English had hospital ships that were described as being utilized when General Howe was moving his army, including sick and convalescing soldiers.

The accomplishments of nursing in eighteenth-century Canada were remarkable. Men and women of nobility who gave superior care in the face of insurmountable odds were recruited.

DEVELOPMENTS IN BIOLOGICAL AND PHYSICAL SCIENCES AND MEDICINE

In the eighteenth century, a basic scientific foundation was continuing to be laid for the eventual blossoming of the health-allied professions.

Daniel Fahrenheit (1686–1736) was born in Danzig and later became a maker of glassware in Amsterdam. He was interested in the measurement of temperatures, and his skill in blowing glass led him into producing thermometers of extraordinary reliability. He made his first thermometer in 1714. Fahrenheit used alcohol at first and then changed to mercury. The gradations reflected the following:

fever heat	112°
human heat	96°
summer heat	76°
temperate	51°
water freezes	32°

Herman Boerhaave (1668–1738), a Dutch physician, was the first to use the mercury thermometer devised by Fahrenheit. It was ten inches in length, required fifteen minutes or more to register and had to be held in place against the person's body. As soon as the thermometer was removed from the body, the mercury fell to room temperature; therefore, it was essential to determine the temperature while the thermometer was in place against the body. Dr. Boerhaave was a clinician of renown and an excellent teacher. He taught his students at the bedside as he made his clinical rounds.

Giovanni Battista Morgagni (1682–1771) was responsible for presenting to the medical world the idea that diseases originated in localized areas of the body, such as in organs or tissues, rather than in an imbalance of humours. In 1761, he published a book entitled *On the Seats and Causes of Disease,* which presented in logical sequence the historical background of each disease, the symptoms, the treatment prescribed and, thence, the pathological findings obtained through autopsies. The data indicated a remarkable amount of knowledge of the previously published literature on the subject.

Stephen Hales (1677–1761), an Anglican clergyman, has been remembered more for his work in biological and physical sciences than for his clerical activities. His special contribution was the research on the circulation of the blood that resulted in a method of determining blood pressure.

He gauged the pressure of the blood by inserting a twelve-foot glass tube into the carotid artery of a horse; the trachea or windpipe of a goose was used for a connective link. Hales noticed that the blood rose and then fell inside the tube in an alternating rise and fall. The height increased during periods of activity on the part of the horse. Thus, he observed the effect of an increased heart rate as a result of effort and strain.

James Lind (1716–1794) discovered the solution to the problem of scurvy, one of the earliest known nutritional deficiencies, which had bedeviled soldiers and sailors from the days of the Crusades. The disease was known to the ancient cultures, but did not become a major catastrophe until long journeys were undertaken with sailors dependent upon rations that had to be stored for many months. Scurvy had taken a greater toll of lives than all naval warfare. Many people developed scurvy when their diet was deficient in fresh fruits and vegetables.

Lind was apprenticed to a physician in Edinburgh, Scotland, and later joined the Royal Navy as a surgeon's mate. During this period, he encountered much scurvy as well as tropical diseases and was concerned about the entire problem of naval hygiene: rat-infested ships, difficulties inherent in obtaining and preserving food and the personal hygiene of the sailors.

In 1747, Lind carried out an experiment with twelve men who had succumbed to scurvy. The most startling response was noted in the men to whom he gave citrus fruits—oranges and lemons (Fig. 7–14).

The results of his careful observations, deliberations and experimentation were reported in his works, *An Essay on the Most Effectual Means of Preserving the Health of Seamen in the Royal Navy,* in 1757, and *An Essay on Diseases Incidental to Europeans in Hot Climates,* in 1768. These writings embodied his suggestions for the care of the patient with scurvy, for upgrading the hygiene and sanitary environment of sailors and for a better comprehension of tropical diseases.

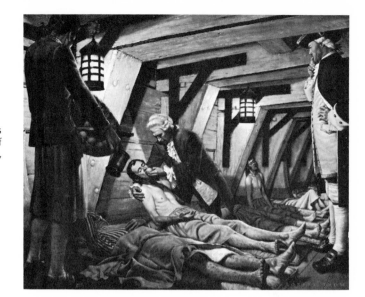

Figure 7–14. Artist's conception of James Lind engaged in his experimental study of sailors with scurvy. (© 1959, by Parke, Davis & Co.)

In addition to the need for citrus fruits in the diet to prevent as well as cure scurvy, his recommendations included: the need for baths and issuance of clean clothing for sailors to curtail the spread of typhus, increase morale and aid in recruitment; an organized program of physical exercise to keep the sailors in good condition; a method of distilling salt water to obtain fresh water; a plan for physical examinations with proper notations on physical record sheets; the use of cinchona bark to prevent malaria; and the inadvisability of going on shore leave in the tropics where malaria was prevalent.

Lind did not live to see his suggestions adopted, but his pioneering efforts in prevention of disease, in the use of an experimental method of gathering data, have been rewarded. Members of the British navy — often referred to as "limeys" — were probably the first group to receive vitamin therapy.

William Hunter (1718–1783) of Scotland was an anatomist, skilled in dissection and a lecturer in anatomy. The anatomical school that he opened in 1746 was a most famous one in London. He eventually became interested in obstetrics, becoming physician-extraordinary to Queen Charlotte, wife of King George III. He published *The Anatomy of the Gravid Uterus* in 1774.

John Hunter (1728–1793), the younger brother of William, joined him in his teaching venture. John had a natural aversion to formal learning for himself, but had rare ability to absorb information and disseminate it in a clear, forceful fashion.

In his school, William Hunter was responsible for providing bodies for dissections. It was John Hunter who joined the so-called *"resurrectionists,"* (men who could be bribed into obtaining corpses from the Potter's Field or various other ways) to obtain bodies.

Surgical technique had been practiced by the barber-surgeons during the past several hundred years. John Hunter's major accomplishments were in practicing surgery and lecturing on anatomy and surgery. His body reposes in Westminster Abbey and the plaque inscription reads: "The Founder of Scientific Surgery."

Leopold Auenbrugger (1722–1809), an Austrian physician, became acutely interested in the processes of disease, especially of the chest. He noticed that when the chest of a healthy person was tapped lightly it sounded like a muffled drum, but in a sick person, the sounds varied especially if the person had an infectious involvement of the chest. In 1761, he published a small brochure entitled *On Percussion of the Chest.*

From time immemorial, *smallpox* had been one of the major scourges of society. The method used by the ancient Chinese has been presented; Rhazes' work in describing the disease has been mentioned; and the wife of the British Ambassador to Turkey, *Lady*

Mary Wortley Montagu (1689–1762) was responsible for introducing to Europe the practice of "engrafting" to prevent smallpox. She described the Turkish method as follows: An old woman would scratch the venom of smallpox into a child's skin. About a week later, the child suffered a higher temperature accompanied by a pustular rash which left scars or pock marks.

After six condemned prisoners of Newgate Prison volunteered for experiments and won their freedom by being inoculated successfully, King George I permitted his two granddaughters to be inoculated. Thereafter, this preventive treatment was warmly received in Britain.

This method was a dubious one because of the dangers of spreading smallpox and keeping the disease condition ever present. The widespread aspect of this disease is shown by the availability of smallpox scabs with which to inoculate. Parents felt the necessity of exposing youngsters because there was a feeling that it was inevitable to contract the disease; thus, to acquire the disease and have it over and done with was more important than prevention.

In 1721, after the infected crew of a vessel from the West Indies landed in the New England colonies, half the population of Boston developed smallpox. About one fourth of these patients died. This was Boston's sixth smallpox epidemic in a century. In 1721, *Cotton Mather* (1663–1728) wrote an "Address to the Physicians of Boston" beseeching them to resort to inoculation.

One of the physicians, *Dr. Zabdiel Boylston*, was willing to try Mather's suggestion. He was successful in his project and at the end of the epidemic, he had inoculated 286 persons, of whom six died (one in 46; the mortality rate for naturally acquired smallpox was one in six).

During the Revolutionary War, the American armies suffered acutely from smallpox. After the Battle of Bunker Hill in 1775, Howe's forces occupied Boston, but his soldiers were incapacitated because of the smallpox epidemic. Washington's meager group of men was stationed in neighboring hills. *General Washington* ordered those men in the army who had not had smallpox to be inoculated.

There were several types of variolation or inoculation such as an arm-to-arm inoculation in which the matter from smallpox pustules was rubbed onto the arm of a healthy person in the hope of conferring immunity. There was always the chance of contracting the disease itself.

Another method consisted of making minute incisions into which some of the variolus pus on cotton was introduced (see Figure 7–15); still another was a thread dipped into the pus and strapped to the arm. Gradually, the methods became more complicated until all were replaced by the newer vaccination described by Jenner in 1798.

Edward Jenner (1749–1823) started his medical career as a student at St. George's Hospital in London and was apprenticed to and studied under John Hunter, living in his home for two years. Hunter's advice to Jenner to be willing to experiment probably motivated the project for which he received international recognition.

In 1796, when cowpox appeared on a farm, Jenner obtained some of the pus from a sore on the hand of one of the dairy maids (Fig. 7–16). He introduced this matter (cowpox virus) by superficial pinprick incisions into the arm of a healthy eight-year-old boy named James Phipps. The vaccinated spot developed a small pustural sore, followed by a scab and a scar. The vaccination proved to be successful when six weeks later Jenner tried to inoculate the boy with smallpox virus. The inoculation failed to take, indicating James's immunity to smallpox. He reported his results in 1798 in a booklet entitled *An Inquiry into the Causes and Effects of the Variolae Vaccinae.*

An important milestone had been reached because someone had been willing and scientifically prepared to experiment with this

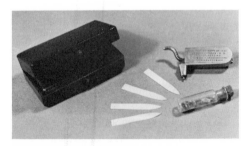

Figure 7–15. The container of necessary ingredients for smallpox inoculation. A bottle of dried smallpox scabs, a metal scarifier to produce the pinprick incisions and the probe-like instruments to introduce the scabs into the superficial pinprick area. (From Mayo Clinic Collection. Photo by DeLores Paul.)

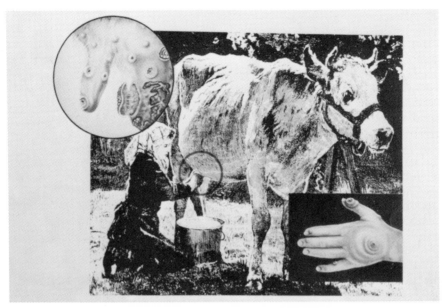

Figure 7–16. Milkmaids contracted cowpox on their hands during the milking process and became immune to smallpox.

method of inoculation to try and prevent infectious diseases.

The physician Carl von Linné (1707–1778), called *Linnaeus*, was a great Swedish botanist who provided a precise classification of plants and animals for natural history. He has been credited with devising the binomial nomenclature, which specified that every natural object was provided a generic or family name and a specific or given name. His orderly classification had a tremendous influence upon the medical theorists of his period.

One of the leaders in medicine who applied the theory of classification to diseases was *Dr. William Cullen* (1710–1790). In 1769 his treatise was translated from Latin into English and was entitled *"Synopsis and Nosology being an Arrangement of Diseases."*

In contrast with the scientific foothold that medical theorists were striving to attain, there were many therapeutic fads and, of course, medical practitioners resorted to the time honored practices of purging, cupping, bleeding and leeching.

An example of a medicinal fad was the use of the *quassia cup.* Quassia was the generic name given by Linnaeus to a small tree of Surinam. The wood has a bitter taste, without odor or aroma, and it was made into "bitter cups." A solution of an alkali, chloroform and water was permitted to stand for a short period of time in the cup and then consumed internally. It was used to reduce fever and as an anthelmintic for threadworm. Quassia cups were officially recognized in the London Pharmacopoeia of 1788.

PSYCHIATRY

Benjamin Rush (1745–1813) was born in Philadelphia of Quaker parents. At the age of 15 in 1760, he received an A.B. degree from the College of New Jersey (now Princeton). The course consisted primarily of Latin, Greek and mathematics; at that time no science was offered. Medicine appealed to him, and he became apprenticed to a Dr. Redman on the staff of the Pennsylvania Hospital for five and a half years. It is interesting to note that Dr. Redman encouraged Benjamin Rush to keep an educational diary called a "commonplace book" into which he inscribed valuable information about patient care.

Rush went to the University of Edinburgh from which he obtained an M.D. in 1768. He became professor of chemistry in the College of Philadelphia, then a professor of medicine when the latter merged with the University of Pennsylvania.

Politics absorbed some of his time and energies, and he was appointed surgeon-general of the army. In 1777, he wrote a directive *To the Officers of the Army of the United States: Directions for Preserving the Health of Soldiers.* Rush was one of four physicians to sign the Declaration of Independence. In 1783 he joined the staff of the Pennsylvania Hospital and while there he introduced clinical instruction.

Among the patients assigned to him were twenty-four "lunatics." These patients were given no treatment medically and were subjected to discomforts and dampness. Benjamin Rush protested against the improper treatment until the legislature appropriated $15,000 for the construction of a ward for the insane. At a time when bathtubs were considered a luxury, he requested and received hot and cold baths for the patients.

He called attention to the need for diversional therapy for psychiatric patients; for suitable companions to listen sympathetically to patients, letting them relieve their subconscious by talking; for a plan for recreation and amusement; for personnel to direct these activities; and, lastly, to separate the mentally ill from those who were convalescing. His requests were granted eventually. In addition to his modern, progressive thinking, he also resorted to bloodletting, violent purging and the use of a special type of chair called a "tranquilizer" (Fig. 7–17).

In 1812, Rush wrote an outstanding monograph on insanity, *Medical Inquiries and Observations upon the Diseases of the Mind.* His treatments were palliative, but the cause of mental illness remained unsolved.

In 1786, Rush founded the Philadelphia dispensary, the first of its kind in this country.

Philippe Pinel (1745–1826) was born in a small village in central France. At a time in the history of France during the days of the French Revolution, the citizenry cried for liberty, equality and fraternity. Yet these were absent in the treatment of the mentally ill. Pinel, normally a timid man of slight, slender build, demanded justice for these patients.

In 1793, a council of three men was responsible for the administration of the Hospital of Paris. Recognizing the worth and ability of Pinel, this council sent for him and informed him that he was the one man in France capable of bringing order out of the chaos

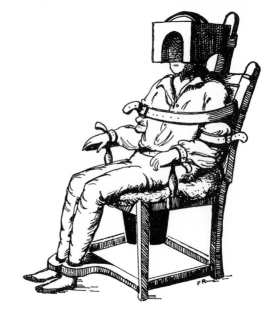

Figure 7–17. A picture of Dr. Rush's tranquilizer chair. (Courtesy of the Pennsylvania Hospital. In: *Some Account of the Pennsylvania Hospital from 1751 to 1938.*)

that was reigning in the insane asylums. He was appointed thereupon to the position of physician-in-chief to the Bicêtre. A description of this institution is impossible, but it was also a prison. The patients who were mentally ill were chained to walls, posts or beds. Violence was the only treatment they received. For a fee, curiosity seekers could obtain amusement by watching these sufferers.

After assuming his new position, he obtained permission from the proper authorities to remove the chains from these patients (Fig. 7–18). A sudden, complete revolution of human intelligence occurred, which demonstrated the efficacy of this new method.

In 1795, he joined the Salpêtrière Hospital founded by Louis XIV to care for poor beggars of Paris. The hospital also provided care for the insane.

Pinel advocated separating the patients who were agitated from those who were calm. To Pinel goes credit for systematizing mental diseases according to symptomatology. This gentle man taught by setting an example of gentleness.

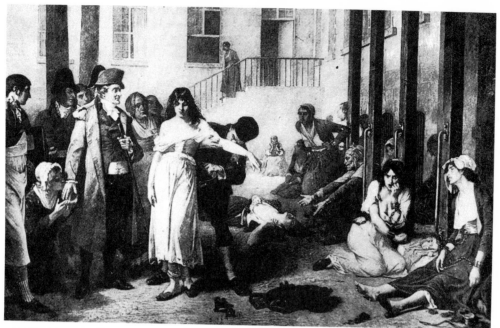

Figure 7–18. The mentally ill at the Salpêtrière are liberated from their chains by Philippe Pinel, 1795. (Ciba Symposia, 1950).

CHEMISTRY, PHYSICS, PHYSIOLOGY

Alchemy was losing prestige, and the science of *chemistry* was just beginning to grow. Several outstanding chemists and apothecaries contributed to a firm foundation in this century.

Henry Cavendish (1731–1810) prepared hydrogen, referred to as inflammable air, by treating iron with acids. He demonstrated that when hydrogen and oxygen were burned, water was obtained.

Joseph Priestley (1733–1804) published in 1767 a *History of Electricity,* which contained a chapter on medical electricity. Another publication discussed his observations on different kinds of air: fixed air (carbon dioxide), inflammable air (hydrogen) and nitrous air (nitrous oxide). His greatest contribution was the discovery of oxygen.

Karl Scheele (1742–1786) was apprenticed for eight years to an apothecary in Sweden who permitted him to experiment in his laboratory. This master not only encouraged Scheele in his thinking and experimenting but also permitted him the use of his extensive library.

Scheele continued his endeavors during the three years of clerkship at a pharmacy.

The world owes a debt of gratitude to the two gentlemen under whom Scheele flourished because rather than assign busy work and menial tasks they permitted him to grow academically.

His discoveries and publications contained information about oxygen, chlorine, fruit acids, tungsten, molybdenum and glycerin.

Antoine Lavoisier (1743–1794) was a wealthy, well educated youth, who owned a laboratory in which he experimented. Priestley and Scheele had isolated oxygen; Lavoisier discovered its uses. It was to him that credit is due for an understanding of the physiology of respiration—how we breathe, how oxygen is utilized and how carbon dioxide is expired during respiration.

Abbé Lazzaro Spallanzani (1729–1799), a well educated gentleman and a priest, taught at several universities. His interest in research led to information on the digestive processes. He discovered the digestive power of saliva, and reaffirmed the solvent property of the gastric juice. He corrected and expanded Lavoisier's theory about oxidation taking place in the lungs and stressed the part the tissues play in respiration, consuming oxygen and giving off carbon dioxide.

Another important contribution helped in

the defeat of the theory of abiogenesis. He believed that if flasks of broth were hermetically sealed and heat applied long enough, no organisms would be found in them. This was a reinforcement of Redi's beliefs.

Benjamin Franklin (1706–1790) has been well known for his contributions to American medicine. He introduced the concept of positive and negative electricity, and it has been stated that he treated paralysis with electrical currents. Included among his achievements to benefit human society are the invention of bifocal lenses, fireplaces and street lamps, acts of statesmanship, including the signing of the Declaration of Independence, and the foundation and successful guidance of the Pennsylvania Hospital. He wrote a history of this hospital, printing it at his own press in 1754.

Luigi Galvani (1737–1798) observed that weak electrical currents caused muscles to contract. He proposed that metals coming in contact with each other generated electricity. Because of his observations and experimentation, he published his famous experiments on electrical stimulations of muscle-nerve preparations in 1792. His discovery laid the foundation for electrophysiology.

Alessandro Volta (1745–1827) invented the epoch-making electric battery. His research showed that a muscle can be placed in a state of continuous contraction or tetany by successive electric stimulations. This led to the use of electric currents in the treatment of disease.

PARAMEDICAL EDUCATION

Frequently the doctor functioned as an apothecary. *Apothecaries* who were not also physicians were in the minority. During the American Revolution, an apothecary, *Andrew Craigie*, was appointed America's first apothecary-general.

The field of *pharmacy* continued to benefit mankind. The Marshall Apothecary was established in Philadelphia in 1729 by *Christopher Marshall* (1709–1797), an immigrant from Dublin, Ireland. His apothecary was the first practical or proprietary school for the training of pharmacists, from which sprang America's first college of pharmacy, Philadelphia College of Pharmacy. His son Charles Marshall became its first president

in 1821. During the Revolutionary War, Christopher Marshall took care of the sick and wounded in the hospitals of Philadelphia. In 1804, Christopher's granddaughter Elizabeth took over the management as *America's first woman pharmacist.*

The *education* of the members of the medical team in this period was sketchy. Many laymen functioned as physicians without an earned degree of doctor of medicine. Apothecaries received little formal educational preparation but had an apprenticeship and much practical training and experience. The M.D. degree was only of relative significance and required various types of preparation including a certain amount of apprenticeship with an apothecary or a surgeon, a semester or two of university classes, a course of study at a dissecting or anatomical school or at one of the hospitals. Any combination of these preparations could suffice, and the gentleman then applied for and received an M.D. degree.

There was no medical school in the English colonies until 1765, and it was very costly to go to Europe for medical preparation.

In North America, the pioneer in medical education was *John Morgan* (1735–1789). Morgan spent several years abroad where he worked with the Hunters, studied with Morgagni and enrolled as a student in Edinburgh from which he graduated in 1763 with the degree of M.D.

He returned to Philadelphia to establish a medical school comparable to those in Europe. It was his firm conviction that a medical school should not be a private venture or proprietary school but rather an integral part of a college or university. He emphasized the need for a good premedical preparation, including Latin, a modern language, mathematics and natural science. His opinions were presented in *A Discourse upon the Institution of Medical Schools in America,* which logically summarized the needs for housing the school for a profession in an institution of higher learning; for proper study of sciences starting with the anatomical structure of the body in order to understand health, illness, and as a *sine qua non* for surgeons. Materia medica, botany, and chemistry were essential to an understanding of diet, medicine and their properties, including a realization of the creation of new substances formed from the change resulting within the body.

It was Dr. Morgan's belief that every practicing physician should have a comparable background of planned instruction; this was impossible with the apprenticeship system. He advocated planned clinical lectures to be given in the clinical setting of the Pennsylvania Hospital.

Another point that his adversaries rebelled against was the separation of the duties of pharmacist from that of medicine and surgery. This practice had arisen in the Colonies out of necessity. In Europe pharmacy and medicine were separate entities. Morgan stressed that prescriptions should be filled by a competent apothecary.

The College of Philadelphia opened in 1765 and Dr. Morgan became the first professor of medicine in the Colonies. Although political strife and warfare disrupted some of its plans and activities, the cornerstone had been laid for medical education in North America.

Finally, a medical school opened in 1765, at the College of Philadelphia (later the University of Pennsylvania).

An educational struggle was brewing between those who learned by training and experience, and those who were well grounded in the theory of scientific investigation. King[13]

presents a letter written by Oliver Goldsmith in 1759 comparing preparation received in Edinburgh (old type) and in Oxford (new type).

The plight of the medical student of the eighteenth century has been well publicized. He became indentured to a practitioner and in return for food, lodging and learning, he helped as a servant, performing many nonmedical functions. His opportunity for education depended not only on the student's resourcefulness, but also on the practitioner's capability and his ability to provide a milieu of inquiry and research. Frequently the student had to join the groups of grave robbers in order to provide the anatomist with the cadavers for dissection and instruction. Figure 7-19, published in 1773, depicts the watchman at the left of the picture holding the resurrectionist who, in turn, is pointing an accusing finger at the scurrying anatomist. The wicker hamper contains the remains of the recently exhumed corpse.

The diary of a medical student of this century has been invaluable for a description of the areas of patient care and medical education.[14]

Medical equipment was costly and scarce. (See Figure 7-20.) The doctor brought his

[13]King, Lester S.: *The Medical World of the Eighteenth Century.* Chicago, University of Chicago Press, 1958, pp. 28-29.

[14]Knyveton, John: *The Diary of a Surgeon in the Year 1751-1752.* Ed. by Ernest Gray, New York, D. Appleton-Century Co., Inc., 1937.

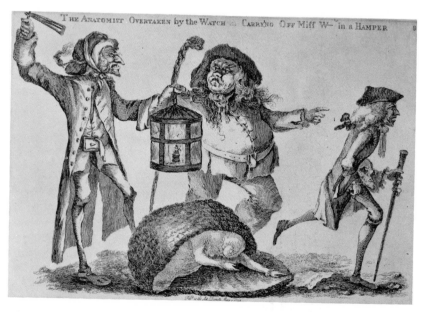

Figure 7-19. The anatomist overtaken by the watch carrying off Miss W— in a hamper. (Engraving by William Austin, 1721-1820. Courtesy of Yale Medical Library, Clements C. Fry Collection.)

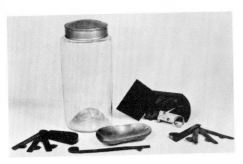

Figure 7–20. Eighteenth century medical equipment—blown glass leech bottle, small leech basin, scarifier and three sets of bleeding knives, the center one being hand-forged. (Author's collection.)

medicines in the medical chest that he carried with him; he also provided the enema equipment for the "clyster" which he administered. A wooden box contained the pewter clyster, which had a nozzle attached to the pewter tubing. The fluid ingredients were poured into the opening beside the plunger; the patient was seated on the nozzle and, when the plunger was released, the fluid was injected with tremendous force (Fig. 7–21).

Another quaint custom of this period was that of the itinerant oculist who traveled throughout the colonies with boxes of glasses to be tried on and selected for assistance in reading.

The sickroom scene of a famous patient is worthy of consideration at this point. In December of 1799, George Washington developed a cold accompanied by a severe sore throat. Soon he had great difficulty in breathing and swallowing. The remedies that were prescribed consisted of mixtures of molasses, vinegar and butter to drink; bleeding done by the overseer of the farm at least three times, removing almost two quarts of blood; rubbing a menthol-type preparation on his throat and then wrapping a piece of flannel saturated with this preparation around his neck; applying a poultice of Spanish flies (made from dried and powdered beetles) to his throat; setting up a vinegar and hot water steam inhalation; and giving calomel as a laxative together with tartar as an emetic. Consultants were summoned and a diagnosis was made by observing the external symptoms. The throat was not inspected, nor the chest listened to. The first diagnosis was quinsy, which was the name given to the condition of a tonsillar abscess. The final diagnosis was "Cynanche trachealis."

It is now believed that diphtheria was the disease, but the bacterial infection coupled with the medical care that he received was the cause of death.

One of the doctors called in on consultation wanted to do a tracheotomy to assist him in breathing and also argued against bleeding because he felt this weakened the patient.

Skilled nursing care is not mentioned as there were no nurses present.

In summary, the eighteenth century witnessed struggles to achieve independence on the part of many peoples, and efforts to conquer pestilential contagion and marked loss of lives and to improve the status of society while laboring under inadequate means of transportation and communication. Achievements were notable in conquering certain diseases, devising diagnostic equipment, developing the beginnings of humane treatment of the mentally ill, and expanding the bases of the sciences of chemistry and physics.

The areas needing strengthening were social legislation for public and industrial health, improvement in medical care and, in the newly formed United States, the recruitment of persons with leadership qualities for nursing and provision of an educational preparation for them.

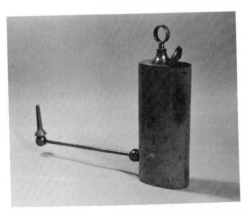

Figure 7–21. A pewter clyster. (From Mayo Clinic Collection. Photo by DeLores Paul.)

REFERENCE READINGS

Andry, Nicholas: *Orthopaedia*. (Facsimile Reproduction of the First Edition in English, London, 1743) Philadelphia, J. B. Lippincott Co., 1961.

Austin, Robert B.: *Early American Medical Imprints 1668–1820*. Washington, D.C., U.S. Department of Health, Education and Welfare, 1961.

Bartlett, Josiah, M.D.: *A Dissertation on the Progress of Medical Science in the Commonwealth of Massachusetts*. Boston, 1810.

Bayley, Richard: *An Account of the Epidemic Fever* which prevailed in the City of New York, during part of the Summer and Fall of 1795. New York, T. and J. Swords, Printers to the Faculty of Physic of Columbia College, 1796.

Caulfield, Ernest: *The Infant Welfare Movement in the Eighteenth Century*. New York, Paul B. Hoeber, 1931.

Caulfield, Ernest: "Some Common Diseases of Colonial Children." *Transactions of the Colonial Society of Massachusetts*, April 1942: 4–65.

Caulfield, Ernest: "The Throat Distemper of 1735–1740." *Yale Journal of Biology and Medicine*, 11:219–272, 277–335, 1939.

Dexter, Elizabeth Anthony: *Career Women of America, 1776–1840*. Francestown, N.H., Marshall Jones Co., 1950.

Dickens, Charles: *A Tale of Two Cities* (1859). New York, E. P. Dutton & Co.

Drinker, C. K.: *Not So Long Ago: A Chronicle of Medicine and Doctors in Colonial Philadelphia*. New York, Oxford University Press, 1937.

Edmunds, Walter: *Drums Along the Mohawk*. Boston, Little, Brown & Co., 1936.

Fielding, Henry: *The History of Tom Jones, a Foundling* (1749). New York, Random House.

Franklin, Benjamin: *Autobiography* (1790). New York, Oxford University Press.

Halsband, Robert: *The Life of Lady Mary Wortley Montagu*. New York, Oxford University Press, 1957.

King, Lester S.: *The Medical World of the Eighteenth Century*. Chicago, University of Chicago Press, 1958.

Kobler, John: *The Reluctant Surgeon: A Biography of John Hunter*. New York, Doubleday & Co., 1960.

Neilson, W., and Neilson, F.: *Verdict for the Doctor—The Case of Benjamin Rush*. New York, Hasting House, 1958.

Packard, Francis R.: *Some Account of the Pennsylvania Hospital*, Philadelphia, The Pennsylvania Hospital, 1938.

Paine, Thomas: *The Rights of Man* (1791). New York, Random House.

Paine, Thomas: *Common Sense* (1776). New York, Random House.

Roddis, Louis H.: *James Lind, Founder of Nautical Medicine*. London, Heinemann, 1951.

Rush, Benjamin: *The Autobiography of Benjamin Rush*. His "Travels Through Life" Together with his "Commonplace Book" for 1789–1813. George W. Corner (ed.). Princeton, N.J., Princeton University Press, 1948.

Van Doren, Carl: *Benjamin Franklin's Autobiographical Writings*. New York, Viking Press, 1945.

Wardrop, James: *On Bloodletting*. London, J. B. Bailliere, 1835.

CHAPTER 8

Response of Nursing to Health Problems of the Early Nineteenth Century

A survey of the nineteenth century reveals a period of expansion politically, geographically, economically, medically, and socially in a century of inventions, discoveries and creativity in every aspect of human endeavor. There were revolts, wars and emotional conflicts even within the newly formed states. It was inevitable that the basic beliefs and principles woven into the fabric of the Constitution would be questioned by the preservation of slavery on democratic soil.

SOCIAL FORCES

There was upheaval in the agricultural and industrial areas because of the application of scientific knowledge to the techniques of production. Power-driven machinery replaced handcraft and human hands; thus, it created mass production, but it also created new problems. The *Industrial Revolution* brought about conditions of poverty, overcrowding, disease and many other social problems.

Under the domestic system of manufacture, a man's work was done at home in a healthy country setting with the family offering assistance. His work might have included carding, spinning, weaving, dyeing or many other skills. The craftsman owned his own tools, purchased whatever raw materials he needed and was in essence a small businessman.

The next step in the evolution of industrial productivity in England and gradually else-where was a system of home industry. Under this system, a businessman with a greater capital outlay could purchase larger quantities of raw materials at lower prices. Skilled workers at home produced the finished product for the businessman who had two concerns: purchasing raw materials and selling the manufactured fabric. The manufacturer was the man who worked in his home, his entire family contributing to his product or service.

In England, toward the end of the eighteenth century, when a series of inventions revolutionized production, machinery replaced handcraft and a factory instead of the home became the work center. The manufacturer became a hired hand; his product was skilled labor. He was now dependent for lodging whereas he once had his own cottage, usually in a rural setting. Factories were noisy and dirty, and the workers had to live close to their work huddled together in poor, sunless homes. Although ultimately the inventions improved society, they caused a change for the worse in living conditions and brought about lack of work for others. This resulted in poverty, that social disease that has been the parent of physical disease.

The whole household worked in England; with low salaries, mothers and even children were forced to work. (Fig. 8–1). Orphans were apprenticed to the overseers of the factories, and these children were treated cruelly. For wages, they were given poor food and lodged in an attic or cellar. The same beds were used by two sets of children, one

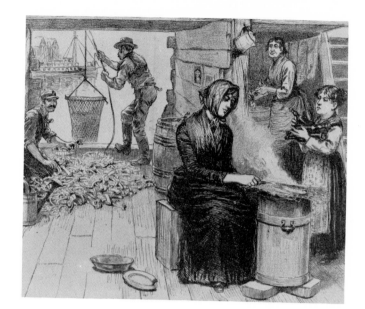

Figure 8–1. Women and children working under most unfavorable conditions. (Courtesy of New York Academy of Medicine and New York City Department of Health.)

during the day and one at night. The working day was a long one, 15 to 16 hours even for little children of five. The indignation against these atrocities to children was expressed by Elizabeth Barrett Browning (1806–1861) in the poem, "The Cry of the Children" (1843).

Alas, alas, the children! They are seeking
   Death in life, as best to have.
They are binding up their hearts away from
   breaking,
   With a cerement from the grave.
Go out, children, from the mine and from
   the city;
   Sing out, children, as the little thrushes do;
Pluck your handfuls of the meadow-cowslips
   pretty;
   Laugh aloud, to feel your fingers let them
   through.
But they answer, "Are your cowslips of the
   meadows
   Like our weeds anear the mine?
Leave us quiet in the dark of the coal-shadows,
   From your pleasures fair and fine.

"For oh!" say the children, "we are weary,
   And we cannot run or leap:
If we cared for any meadows, it were merely
   To drop down in them, and sleep.
Our knees tremble sorely in the stooping;
   We fall upon our faces, trying to go;
And, underneath our heavy eyelids drooping,
   The reddest flower would look as pale as snow;
For all day we drag our burden tiring,
   Through the coal-dark, underground;

Or all day we drive the wheels of iron
   In the factories, round and round."

Within the factories, there was little ventilation and no sunlight; this, in addition to poor housing, constituted a serious health hazard, and many infectious diseases took a heavy toll of life. Trouble was brewing, and riots broke out; unions began to develop.

Philanthropists toiled to achieve the passage of laws to protect the workers and alleviate the situation. In 1819, an act was passed that required that no child under three years of age be employed, that 12 hours a day be the maximum for those under 16 years of age, that time for meals be allowed and that walls and ceilings be white-washed at least twice a year. The law was not enforced.

This was followed in 1833 by the adoption in Parliament of a bill prohibiting night labor to those under 18 years of age, providing that children from nine to 13 were not to work more than 48 hours a week, that those from 13 to 18 were not to work more than 68 hours a week and that children under nine must not be employed. The conscience of the public had been awakened at last. By 1847, a 10 hour workday became a reality for women and young persons, while men continued for 12 hours or more a day.

Other evils, including bad housing, poor sanitation and lack of formal education, were noted. Women and children worked in mines as well as in factories.

PLIGHT OF THE CHILD

In addition to the children who were orphaned and homeless due to epidemics, *foundlings* were being abandoned in many countries, necessitating the construction of institutions to care for them. Public attitude is reflected in the names of existing institutions, such as "Home of the Friendless."

The plight of the child and the shocking treatment they received was highlighted in the infamous Carlock Case in New York City (Fig. 8–2). When a man suspected his servant of theft, he obtained a warrant and went with a warrant officer to search the premises. They found an elderly woman housing three starving almshouse children. The evils of the Almshouse system were exposed, including the health and social problems associated with wet-nursing, the apprenticeship system with its cruel indenture techniques and the mortality of children.

Disease spread in awesome waves through working-class districts. Cholera was the devastating epidemic of the nineteenth century wih major outbreaks in 1832, 1849 and 1866 (Fig. 8–3).

Cholera had existed for centuries in India. The earliest records indicate that Hindus worshipped the goddess of cholera, hoping to placate the goddess so that they would be spared the evils of this dread disease. Other than in India, there was no extensive spread of cholera until the nineteenth century when records indicate pandemic outbreaks. The inception of this disease was associated with abnormal climatic conditions, such as unusual flooding due to heavy rainfall, followed by famine and disease.

In England many reports of diseased cattle indicated an association with Asiatic Cholera. The cattle were slaughtered and because of lack of public health laws, poor people purchased the diseased meat.

Outbreaks of cholera were received in markedly different ways according to the customs and beliefs of people.

Unfortunately, no one knows the real cause of this disease outbreak. The filth of cities and overcrowding of the population, together with impure water supplies, inadequate sewage disposal and unhygienic living conditions, were causative agents. It was because of the disastrous effects of cholera, however, that local boards of health came into being in England, as well as in the United States.

In England, the Board of Health demanded that quarantine regulations be carried out. A special sign, placed on the front of a house, would indicate that this was the dwelling of a person with the disease. Houses had to be "purified" by special methods after the death or recovery of a person suffering from cholera.

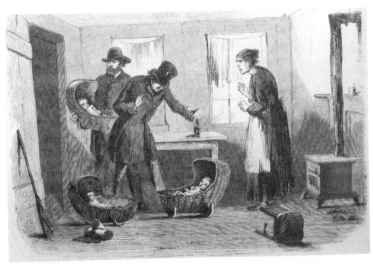

Figure 8–2. Mrs. Carlock and the emaciated and abused infants.

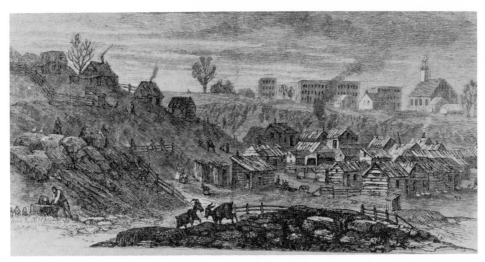

Figure 8–3. The incubators of cholera in New York City. (Courtesy of New York Academy of Medicine and New York City Department of Health.)

Finally, a special cholera house was set up in Exeter, England. It was staffed by two doctors and 24 nurses. The town crier was instructed to obtain additional nurses if this was at all possible.

Fires were lighted in the streets and tar was burned. Clothes were washed in the river, which helped spread the disease to others, although this fact was not comprehended.

Because families were deprived of income, food tickets were distributed during this plight. Soup kitchens were also set up and records reveal the kindness and understanding of the poor to each other.

The disease was devastating and, indeed, the best description of it appears on a monolith inscribed during the days of Alexander the Great: "The lips blue, the face haggard, the eyes hollow, the stomach sunk in, the limbs contracted and crumpled as if by fire. . . ."

At the time of the first cholera outbreak in the United States in 1832, it was considered to be the plight of the sinful. The disease seemed to be attracted to large cities, allied to poverty and slum dwelling and associated with the large numbers of immigrants. The disease even spread across the country with the adventuresome forty-niners.

In 1866, when the Metropolitan Board of Health of the City of New York was instituted, it was recognized by clergy, doctors and municipal workers that cholera outbreaks were preventable (Fig 8–4). Rosenberg's book *The Cholera Years*[1] gives a dramatic and factual account of the panic and terror of this disease in the United States and points up the need for public health workers, including well prepared community nursing workers.

Reading about the lack of understanding of the disease and the panic that ensued emphasizes the need for a new science—the study of the life processes.

There was a growing awareness that health was the responsibility of the public and that the state had a definite duty to protect the public by wise legislation.

Another unusual affliction, a seasonal one, was *milk sickness*, which occurred most severely in drought years. The cause of this dreaded affliction was not ascertained until 1928. A pretty flowering weed with the faint aroma of lilacs, called the white snakeroot because the Indians treated snake bites with its root, was the causative agent. Cows that ate the weed secreted its deadly poison, tremetol, into their milk and both humans and calves consuming the milk succumbed to the lethal effects. Nancy Hanks Lincoln died from this dreaded disease in 1818.

---

[1]Rosenberg, Charles. *The Cholera Years,* Chicago: The University of Chicago Press, 1962.

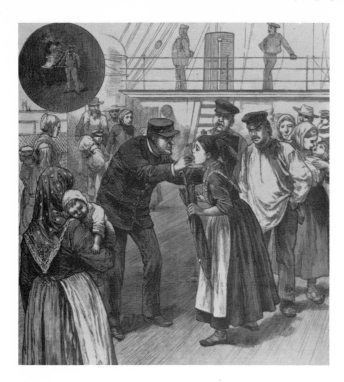

Figure 8–4. An attempt to inspect and quarantine those who might have a contagious disease. (Courtesy of New York Academy of Medicine and New York City Department of Health.)

PROGRESS IN NURSING

With the dawn of the nineteenth century, the actual care of the sick was the responsibility of mothers. Tender, loving care was given to friends as well as family. Every bride purchased or received a cookbook that, in addition to rules and recipes to develop culinary skills, always had a section on first aid and the care of the sick. Perusal of one gives a picture of the rules for prevention of illness in the Connecticut Valley in 1805.[2]

1. Avoid as much as possible living near a graveyard.
2. Keep the feet from wet, and the head well defended when in bed.
3. Avoid too plentiful meals.
4. Go not abroad without your breakfast.
5. Shun the night air as you would the Plague.
6. Tender people should have those much about them, sound, sweet and healthy.

When one became ill, there were instructions such as:

To break up a fresh cold. Nothing is better than a glass of hot flip on going to bed. Put the poker in

the fire to heat. Mix some ginger and molasses in a beer mug. Pour on some sour cider. Plunge in the red hot poker and stir it up till it foams well. This is a very agreeable cure. Warm the bed hot with the warming-pan and put in some hot bricks. A fine sweat will carry off the cold.

A slice of salt pork spread with pepper and bound on with a strip of red flannel will cure a sore throat. Or, in a pinch, a stocking taken warm from the foot and bound about the throat is efficacious.

If the cold persisted and the lower respiratory tract was involved, there was this type of remedy awaiting trial:

For a sudden attack of Quinsy or Croup, or a cold that is tight on the lungs, bathe the neck with bear's grease and pour it down the throat. Goose grease or any kind of oily grease is as good as bear's grease. Onions stewed in molasses are loosening. Put draughts of wilted horseradish leaves on the feet. A drop or two of skunk's oil or hen's oil on a lump of sugar will loosen up a cold.

This seems to be the period when lubrication of the "bronchial tubes" and the entire respiratory tract was advocated—when the heart of a baked onion placed in the ear drew out the "trouble" or "humour."

The major care of the sick was at home with home remedies. If they were unsuccessful, the local doctor was called. Many herb medicines made at home were basic prepara-

---

[2] *The Documtur Housewife*—The Fruit of Experience freshly gathered from Elderly Lips, and preserved in print. A Guide to Domestic Cookery as it is practiced in the Connecticut Valley, 1805, pp. 1–3.

tions, and many treatments such as poultices similar to the one previously mentioned, which was composed of "onions stewed in molasses," were resorted to frequently. Mustard footbaths seemed to be considered good for everything.

The medicines that were not concocted at home were procurable from the patent medicine man as he traveled from town to town, or obtainable as proprietary preparations in the apothecary shops. Burdick's Blood Bitters, Ayer's Cherry Pectoral and Lydia Pinkham's Vegetable Compound were popular examples of the latter. Traveling patent medicine peddlers sold such things as Snake Oil and Kickapoo Extract to gullible buyers, then they promptly left town.

Most families kept sick members at home. The well-known picture, "The Doctor," presents a sickroom vigil with the members of the family waiting for the crisis to be reached and passed (Fig. 8–5). Pneumonia was one of the most feared diseases.

Providing an adequate or well-balanced diet was difficult. Francois Appert's work in canning helped to add variety to the diet because now food could be preserved.[3] Appert felt

---

[3] Appert, F.: *Art of Preserving All Kinds of Animal and Vegetable Substances.* London, Black, Perry & Kingsbury, 1811.

that heat applied to food, sealed in a container in the absence of air, prevented food from spoiling. He was aware of the necessity of obtaining a proper seal. In America in 1819, the first canning establishment using Appert's technique was set up in Boston. Outbreaks of disease due to food spoilage occurred occasionally.

In 1853, Gail Borden perfected the process for manufacturing condensed milk that was immediately used in feeding babies and was responsible for saving many of their lives. (See Figure 8–6.)

The steam pressure autoclave was utilized from 1874, and the new science of bacteriology was applied to the food preservation industry. Refrigerators were unheard of, but ice chests or iceboxes were in vogue. Large chunks of ice were placed in these boxes. The ice melted and, consequently, food spoiled because of this inefficient method.

Proud mothers brought newborn babies to the local grocery shop to be weighed on the same scales that were used for weighing meat and produce (Fig. 8–7).

Keeping a sickroom warm and free from smoke from wood-burning stoves or fireplaces was a difficult problem. Furnaces with coal replacing wood as a source of fuel were available from around 1850.

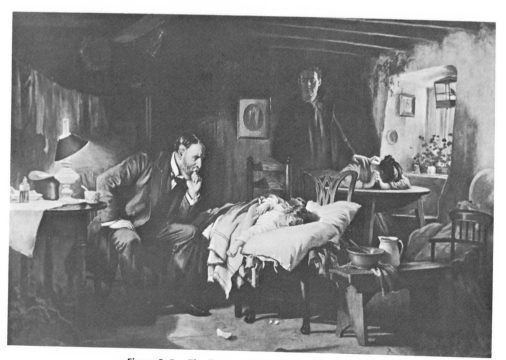

Figure 8–5. The Doctor. (Courtesy of Wyeth Laboratories.)

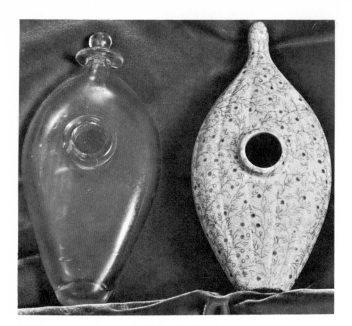

Figure 8–6. Nursing bottles used during the late eighteenth and early nineteenth centuries. One is of blown glass with glass nipple; the other is of porcelain that probably matched the family's china. (Author's collection.)

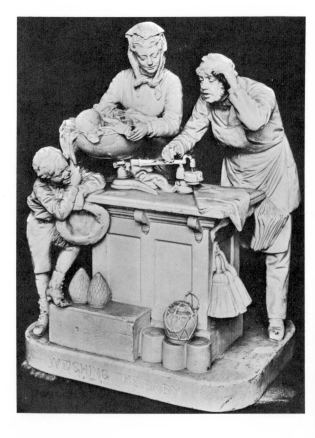

Figure 8–7. Weighing the baby. (Statuette by John Rogers, 1877. Author's collection.)

The *sanitary aspects* of living needed scrutiny. Outdoor toilet facilities (privies) were used commonly. Gradually, these were replaced by an indoor flush toilet by those people who could afford this improvement. Indoor plumbing was slow in reentering the historical picture. Water was brought into homes through a water system composed chiefly of wooden logs, the center of which had been removed. Eventually, cast iron replaced the wooden pipes. Many families set barrels out in the yard to catch rain water. They realized the value of conservation of natural resources. In outlying areas, wells provided the water for the household. All water supplies served as a rich potential source for the transmission of infection. The quality of the water needed improving because pollutants came in contact with the water supply and thereby caused contamination.

The removal of waste material, sewage, was another serious problem. Community water supplies to assist in the removal and disposal of sewage were slow to evolve. It was partially solved by draining this water through a system of sewerage pipes. In 1829, a slow sand filtration system to remove the major source of pollution was constructed in London. In time, filtration systems appeared.

Epidemics of cholera, yellow fever, smallpox, diphtheria, scarlet fever, dysentery, typhus and typhoid were devastating to the people of this century. Contaminated water played its role in the transmission of disease as did food, utensils and persons who were disease carriers.

An early public health reformer in this period was *Lemuel Shattuck* (1793–1859), a former teacher, who was engaged in the book selling business. In 1842, he was instrumental in achieving the passage of a law in Massachusetts that resulted in statewide registration of vital statistics.

In 1845, he compiled and published a *Census of Boston* that encouraged and stimulated accurate reporting of statistics in the United States. Shattuck's Census presented the shocking facts of a high mortality rate with an unbelievably high infant and maternal mortality rate.

His crowning achievement came in 1850 when the results of his efforts were published by the Massachusetts Sanitary Commission. The Shattuck Report, one of the first public health documents in the United States, was an important milestone in the evolution of the field of public health. Shattuck recommended state and local health departments or boards of health and emphasized the need for sanitary surveys.

Private Nursing. The care given to patients in their homes was very different from that in hospitals. Only the very poor or homeless went to hospitals. Respectable people felt it a disgrace to send one of their relatives to a hospital. With hospital conditions as they were, this feeling is understandable.

The most expert person in the family, usually the mother, cared for a sick person. Neighbors volunteered for "night watching," which, though unskilled, assured that medicines were given or new symptoms reported. In early days there were almost no doctors so that mothers prescribed for their families.

There were a good many "monthly" (obstetric) nurses in those days whose duties involved midwifery.

HOSPITALS

Hospitals were unattractive places in structural design and psychological milieu. Pest houses were part of the hospital complex. Most hospitals were subject to crowded conditions and were filled with the critically sick and dying. In many, adequate beds and pillows were the exception rather than the rule.

Bellevue in 1736 had only a small ward for the sick. It was situated where New York's City Hall now stands. For some time it was used only as a "pest house."

In 1811, the city purchased a tract of land which had been named Belle View. The cornerstone of this institution was laid in 1811 and the hospital was opened for occupancy in 1816. By a ruling of the Common Council in 1825 the name of *Bellevue Hospital* was adopted. The original plan provided for cells for unruly patients and prisoners, apartments for maternity patients and sixty rooms, forty-one of which were set aside for paupers. Women inmates of the Almshouse did the cooking, laundry and what nursing care was given.

In 1837 an investigation was made; conditions were found to be unspeakable, and the pest house, prison and later the psychiatric wards were removed to Blackwell's Island. The poorhouse continued under the same roof with the hospital until 1848. No better attention was given the sick; the dirt and neglect were shocking and the death rate was 25 per cent. Upon the creation of a medical board in 1847 matters improved slightly, but treatment of the sick remained most deplorable.

Blockley, of Philadelphia, was also a combination of poorhouse, quarters for mentally ill and hospital. (During the Revolution the inmates were freed by the British troops.) All the work of the place, including nursing, was supposed to be done by the inmates.

An investigation in 1793 brought to light shocking conditions, but they were not improved. In 1832, the problem was reviewed again, and Bishop Kendrick of Emmitsburg was persuaded to send a group of Sisters of Charity to undertake the task of reform. Their work so effectually transformed the hospital that they were asked to remain, but the bishop was not of like mind. After they left, conditions again grew unsatisfactory and remained so until *Alice Fisher,* a Nightingale nurse, arrived in 1884.

Hospital patients were penniless folk, usually homeless and friendless. In most of the city hospitals the nursing was done by inmates usually over 50 years old, many being 70 and 80. The doctors sent feeble old people to serve as nurses in the wards because they could get better food there.

There was practically no night nursing, except for a woman in childbirth or a dying person, when a "night watcher" would be provided.

An article in *Harper's Weekly* in 1859 presents an interesting picture of the *New Orleans Charity Hospital* (Fig. 8–8). Admissions that year were 11,337 with 8923 discharged while 2290 died. During the yellow fever epidemic of the preceding year, 2727 patients were admitted with this disease, 1313 were discharged and 1382 died. A miasmometer was used for detection of organic impurities.

Dr. Meigs, in *The Old Nursing and the New,* offers an explanation of these conditions:

Formerly little was known by the world in general of what took place in a hospital. The patients were largely cut off from communication with the outside [either because of restricted visiting days or because they were friendless], officers and employees of hospitals were jealous of intrusion.

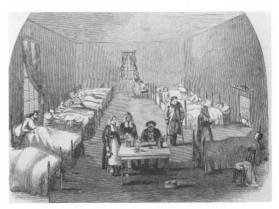

Figure 8–8. New Orleans Charity Hospital in 1859.

Visiting was not encouraged . . . Managers made tours of inspection, but saw little of the real internal workings. Visiting physicians and surgeons knew little of what the resident staff did. There was no real inspection of the work of the nurses, and if a physician had cause for complaint, the superintendent was too busy with other matters, was not used to disciplining nurses and so did nothing.

Dr. James J. Walsh, in *The History of Nursing,* adds:

Hospitals were as a rule in a disgraceful state of degradation. They were dirty and ill ventilated, they reeked with infection, so that patients who came in suffering from one disease, or from a wound, caught another disease or some virulent infection. The death rate was fearfully high, sometimes actually more than 50 per cent. In the days before Lister, hospital surgery was extremely discouraging. The only nurses that could be obtained for hospitals were women who did the menial work besides caring for the patients.

Prejudice against hospitals arose here, as it had done in Europe, because of the neglect and ill treatment of patients and because the death rate from infections was high. A writer as late as 1877, in speaking of maternity hospitals, remarked; "Experience has taught us that any kind of a home is a safer place for a woman to be delivered in than any hospital; but there are cases with no homes who must be provided for." The change in the attitude of the public toward hospitals indicates how radical has been the change in hospital conditions.

Religious Nursing Orders. Almost the only good hospital nursing was done by religious orders. "The beautiful order enforced by their gentle discipline, their self-denial, patience, skill and tact, were the effect of Christian charity on the sympathetic hearts of intelligent women."[4] Their gentle manner, dignity and poise were models for all nurses; the term "sister" seems to fit. Unquestionably their nursing surpassed any other in quality.

There was need for a highly respectable, well prepared group of women to nurse the sick. Because of the request of Archbishop Du Bourg of the Order of St. Sulpice, the first American religious order in the United States was founded by Mother Elizabeth Seton in 1809.

Elizabeth Bayley Seton (Blessed Elizabeth Ann Seton, Fig. 8–9) (1774–1821) was born in New York at a momentous time in history. Her father, Dr. Richard Bayley, was one of the leading physicians of his day and was the first professor of anatomy at King's College, now Columbia University. He was also the health officer of the Port of New York, was responsible for the development of the quarantine laws of the State of New York and was given authority to administer them.

Elizabeth, a beautiful and popular young lady, married William Seton, a banker, in 1794. The marriage was a most happy one

---

[4]Wise, T. W.: *Review of the History of Medicine.*

even when they were weathering family sorrows and financial reverses.

Elizabeth Seton had demonstrated an interest in helping people in times of need. In 1797 she and other society matrons formed the Widow's Society in New York. This organization, which was dedicated to public charity, was the Protestant equivalent of St. Vincent de Paul's Ladies of Charity. These women raised money for poor widows and visited them in their homes to nurse and comfort them.

The Setons traveled to Italy, leaving New York when an epidemic of yellow fever was raging. On arrival in Italy, all passengers were quarantined in a grim and loathsome lazaretto or pest house. Mr. Seton, already in a weakened condition, succumbed to a fatal infection.

When Mrs. Seton returned to America, she had to face financial ruin and its tragedies. Meanwhile she had joined the Catholic Church.

An interest in teaching prompted her to open a school for girls in Baltimore which marked the beginning of the parochial school system of education in the United States. A choice spot of land at Emmitsburg was selected for a school. Immediately, applications were received from young women who wished to join her and become sisters in this new teaching order.

In 1809, Mother Elizabeth Seton with her newly formed religious family, attired in a habit that resembled Mrs. Seton's own widow's dress, arrived in Emmitsburg. This group was interested in affiliating with the community of the Sisters of Charity founded by St. Vincent de Paul. Requests from Mother Seton's sisters for nuns to come from Paris to America to explain the Rule of St. Vincent and help them to become established properly was denied because of Napoleon. The Rule had to be adapted to the needs of the American group.

The beginnings of the *Sisters of Charity at Emmitsburg in 1809* divided into *seven different branches of the community.* This provided leadership opportunities in nursing education, delivery of nursing service and parochial education.

By 1850, the sisters at Emmitsburg officially united with the world-wide community of Sisters of Charity of St. Vincent de Paul, at which time the habit of blue with the large linen headdress or "cornette" was adoped.

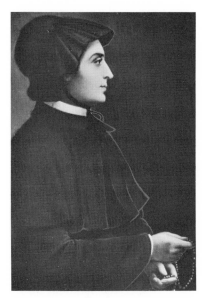

Figure 8–9. Blessed Elizabeth Bayley Seton. (Courtesy of St. Joseph's College, Emmitsburg, Md.)

The Sisters of Charity of New York, referred to as the Black Cap Sisters of Charity, wear the headdress and habit originally worn by the founding group. The Sisters of Charity of Greensburg, Pennsylvania, although a separate entity, have the black cap and habit as did the New York unit. The Sisters of Charity of New Jersey, Halifax and Cincinnati substituted a veil but wore the original dress or habit worn before the affiliation with the Paris Sisters of Charity of St. Vincent de Paul.

In 1812, the Sisters of Charity of Nazareth, Kentucky, were founded by *Mother Catherine Spalding*. The sisters incorporated the care of the sick in their homes into their daily work. They went on horseback to the homes of their patients. This order included both teachers and nurses.

In 1823, the Baltimore Infirmary, later the University of Maryland Hospital, was established by six professors as a private proprietary school in a clinical setting. There were four wards and two resident students. These medical resident students were required to pay $300 a year, in advance, for board, room and laundry. The visits of the medical and surgical staff men were paid for every day at noon. Only patients who were acutely ill were admitted, and they were required to pay a fee of $3.00 a week, which included room, meals and care. This hospital did not furnish any material assistance to the visiting doctors or professors. They had to use their own medicines, bandages, instruments and even their own leeches.

In short order, these professors sent a request to Emmitsburg for Sisters of Charity to staff the hospital. Their request was granted. The sisters were in charge of the hospital housekeeping, kitchen and laundry, supervised the wards and administered simple care and medications.

Treatments were carried out by the house doctor or resident—this was a learning experience for him.

In 1829, *the Sisters of Our Lady of Mercy*, of Charleston, South Carolina, undertook an unusual assignment—the Hospital of the Society of Working Men. The Brotherhood of Saint Marino was an association of mechanics and laborers who were the motivating force behind the inception of this hospital and assumed its financial support. The Society evolved because of the need for a place to house and take care of homeless men.

Demands for nursing care from the various religious orders became very great. Epidemics, though an added burden, were handled with courage and skill, and visiting nursing was an important function of their efforts. The Sisters of Mercy offered their services to the Board of Health during an outbreak of cholera and yellow fever.

When epidemics subsided, many children were left orphaned. Institutions were needed to care for these (Fig. 8–10). St. Vincent's Infirmary, in Louisville, Kentucky, opened mainly to house the orphans after a cholera epidemic.

Sisters staffed psychiatric hospitals, such as the state hospital, Maryland Hospital in Baltimore, which was under the supervision of the Sisters of Charity until 1840. Then, the Sisters opened an institution for psychiatric patients which was later called the Mt. Hope Retreat.

Many religious orders contributed their efforts to alleviate the sickness and tribulations of this period, which is evidenced in the many hospitals constructed and serviced by them.

Sister Mary Aikenhead, who was trained in England, founded the *Irish Sisters of Charity* about 1815. They did social work among the poor and public health and hospital nursing during epidemics of plague, cholera and typhus. At Cork in 1831, during a cholera epidemic, the people were afraid to enter hospitals until they learned that the Sisters of Charity were working there.

Mother Aikenhead wished for a sister's hospital in Dublin, and sent three nuns to be trained at the Hôpital de La Pitié in Paris. They remained there a year. Upon their return a hospital of twelve beds was established, which grew rapidly into an excellent institution. They organized other hospitals and an asylum for the blind. In 1857 they went to Australia and continued their work.

In 1831 Mother Catherine McAuley founded the *Sisters of Mercy* with a house near Dublin.

Many Roman Catholic nursing orders sent their members to America for missionary work. Nuns came from Ireland, France, Germany, Italy, Spain and Portugal. The *Sisters of Mercy*, the *Sisters of the Holy Cross* and others started communities and established hospitals. Some of them also did private nursing.

The *Sisters of St. Joseph*, the *Sisters of Charity*

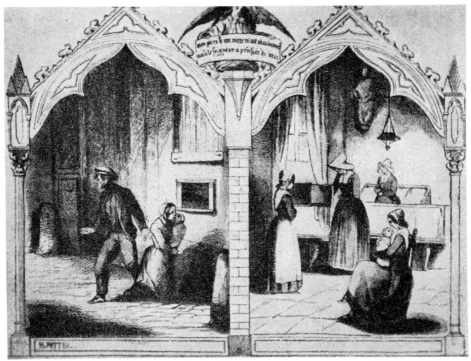

Figure 8–10. *Left,* A woman is secretly placing her child in the receiving box of a foundling asylum. *Right:* Glimpse into the interior of the foundling asylum with the box opened. (From the magazine *L'Illustration,* 1852. Ciba Symposia, 1940.)

of Nazareth and the *Ursuline* nuns had many houses and hospitals. The *Sisters of St. Mary,* who worked in St. Louis in the 1880's, were called the "smallpox sisters" because of their work with this dreaded disease.

At the time of the Civil War the larger and better hospitals were those staffed by Roman Catholic nuns. The Alexian Brothers were in hospital work by 1870.

A *social reformer* of note was *Mrs. Elizabeth Gurney Fry* (1780–1845) whose phenomenal work in prison reform has been recognized throughout the world. Elizabeth Gurney was a deeply religious Quaker who married Joseph Fry and settled in London. As an active member of the Society of Friends, she decided to seek admittance to *Newgate Prison* to attempt to reform the criminals; this was an early rehabilitation project.

In 1813, she visited Newgate and was horror-striken at the conditions and the treatment of the poor victims incarcerated there (Fig. 8–11). The prison was cold, dark, damp and poorly ventilated. The prisoners were meagerly fed, not properly clothed and not segregated. Thieves, murderers, sex

offenders, mentally ill, mentally retarded— all were housed together. Many children were inmates of this institution.

Mrs. Fry asked to talk to the women prisoners. Armed men were offered to protect her from this snarling mob. She refused their protection, and her quiet manner, somber dress and genuine interest in them calmed the unruly group. Later, she brought food and clothing, soap and towels for the children as well as adults; she commenced a program of instruction for the children that was later attended by the women; she provided the women with sewing materials so that they might earn a livelihood when released. She inspired some of her friends to come and read to them as they worked.

Elizabeth Fry was an eloquent and forceful speaker and after visiting prisons in the British Isles and in Europe, she endeavored to share her findings with the public. She made them aware of the need for reform in nursing and in hospitals as well as in prisons.

Mrs. Fry set an example of human kindness to people who had received relatively little of it from life. She urged careful trials

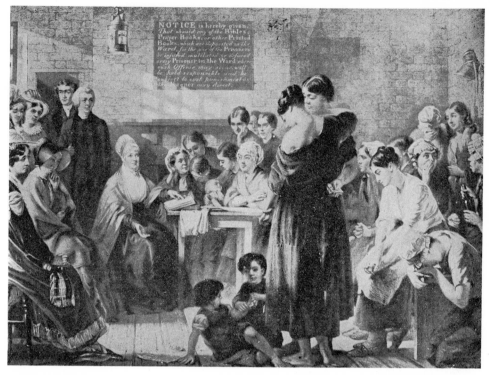

Figure 8–11. Elizabeth Fry reading to the prisoners at Newgate Prison, 1823. (Whitney: *Elizabeth Fry, Quaker Heroine.* Little, Brown & Co.)

for offenders, planted the ideas for reform schools, stressed the need for psychiatric cases to be separated from criminals and insisted that law offenders needed moral assistance in hospitals, rather than punishment in jails. Her concepts of rehabilitation were very sound.

In England in 1840, this group of ardent helpers who assisted her so capably in her crusade were organized and called the "Society of Protestant Sisters of Charity." Their primary objective was to supply nurses for the sick of all classes in their homes. This group was motivated by deep religious convictions but were secular in organization. They became the *Institution of Nursing Sisters.*

The work of Mrs. Fry had a profound influence on many people, including a young Lutheran minister, *Theodor Fliedner* (Fig. 8–12) (1800–1864). He was appointed pastor of a church in Kaiserswerth, Germany, in 1822. Shortly after his arrival, the main industry of this little community failed, and the people had financial difficulties. Pastor Fliedner set out on a tour to raise funds and returned with money and ideas for a pro-

gram of social work prompted by the efforts and results of the work of Mrs. Fry.

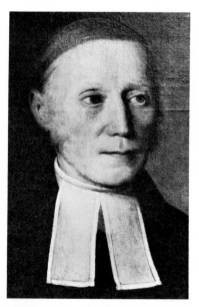

Figure 8–12. Pastor Theodor Fliedner. (Courtesy of Kaiserswerth Institute.)

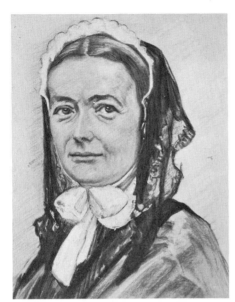

Figure 8–13. Frederika Münster Fliedner. (Courtesy of Kaiserswerth Institute.)

He married Frederika Münster (Fig. 8–13) in 1828, and they raised a family of ten children. Because of the inspiration of her husband, she organized a Woman's Society for visiting and nursing the sick poor in their homes. It was inadequate to meet the heavy demands. Women prisoners and children were being released from the jails and needed hospital as well as nursing care, and also schools. The Fliedners opened their home in 1833 for these returning prisoners.

Recognition of the need for female resources in the Protestant church sparked the restoration of the ancient order of Deaconesses. Pastor Fliedner and his wife Frederika became the crusading spirits and, in 1836, founded the *Kaiserswerth Institute for the Training of Deaconesses.*

They purchased the largest, finest house available in Kaiserswerth. By the end of the first year, seven hard-working young women were in training. Pastor Fliedner, like St. Vincent de Paul, wanted youthful, enthusiastic girls of refinement with healthy bodies, good moral standards, good character, twenty-five years of age or over, who were desirous of caring for the sick. The daughter of a physician, *Gertrude Reichard* was the first to become a deaconess. Each one was consecrated for her work by the laying on of hands and a blessing.

The Fliedners were well qualified to direct the educational endeavors of this order. They organized training centers for the teachers of nursery schools (called infant schools), elementary schools, vocational schools and high schools. They opened an orphanage and kindergarten, which provided learning experience for the student teachers. In addition, they directed the school for nurses and the hospital, which also served as a training and practice center for the students (Fig. 8–14).

The dress of the deaconess was a plain blue cotton gown with a white apron, large turned-down collar, white muslin cap with a frill around the face, tied beneath the chin with a large white bow. When they went outside, they wore a long black cloak and a black bonnet over their cap. (See Figure 8–15.)

The initial course of instruction consisted of housework, bookkeeping, letter writing and oral reading. The student made a choice between becoming a teacher or a nurse. In addition to her hospital experience, the student was given some instruction in visiting nursing in the village under Mrs. Fliedner's supervision. She very forcefully assisted her nurses in establishing independence with regard to doctors, the clergy and hospital governing bodies and authorities.

According to the original plan, these deaconesses took no vows, but made a simple promise "to work for Christ"; they received no salary, and were taken care of for life. This is the so-called *motherhouse* system, which, like the monastic system, provides its members with a permanent home so that when deaconesses are sent out to private duty, to other hospitals, to do visiting nursing or to distant mission fields, they are always under the protection of their home organization.

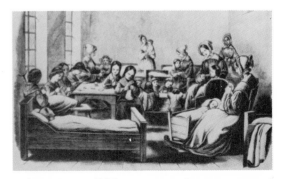

Figure 8–14. Child care was an important aspect of nursing for the Deaconesses of Kaiserswerth. (Author's collection)

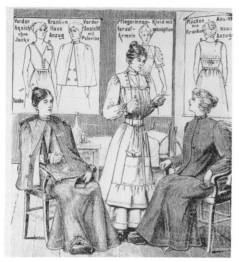

Figure 8–15. The teaching function of the nurse was emphasized by the deaconesses, and clothing design to fit the person's need seems to have played a significant role. (Author's collection)

Their work is centered chiefly among the poor. Deaconesses may work in almshouses, have charge of orphanages, teach children, work among prisoners or unfortunate women or do private nursing. They have helped in many epidemics and in many wars.

Many schools for nurses inherited much from the deaconess organizations and absorbed from Frau Fliedner items such as preliminary grouping (long called "proba-

tion"), the doctor's certificate of health, usually a clergymen's certificate, money allowance, regular classes and lectures, special etiquette and a woman superintendent in full charge. They did not admit "lady probationers," as did the English hospitals, but insisted that all nurses be on the same social level. They required that nurses sent out to private duty be treated as members of the family, not as servants, and they saw to it that they were allowed proper time for rest.

After Frederika Fliedner died in 1842, Pastor Fliedner married *Caroline Bertheau* who continued this very worthy project. It soon seemed essential to give some brief instruction in the care of the sick to the women of the community. This endeavor had two objectives: helping the women of the community to do a better job of caring for their families and providing a reservoir of lay nurse helpers.

Kaiserswerth remained the motherhouse of many deaconess institutes throughout the world, and the graduates of the deaconess program went to these areas bringing an atmosphere of peace and love to the sick and needy (Figs. 8–16 and 8–17).

Communities and doctors were becoming aware of the value of better prepared religious as well as lay women in caring for the sick. In 1841, a doctor asked for a nurse to work in his dispensary; her work was to be preventive in character. She was to instruct

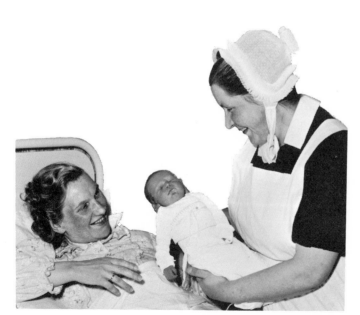

Figure 8–16. A deaconess rejoicing with a mother. (Courtesy of Kaiserswerth Institute.)

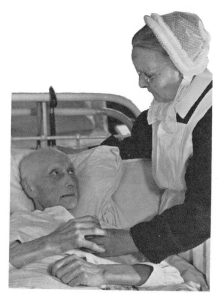

Figure 8–17. A deaconess empathizing with her patient. (Courtesy of Kaiserswerth Institute.)

mothers in the care of the sick in homes, to ask if all members of the family had been vaccinated, to report illnesses and to teach ways of cooking inexpensive foods.

Pastor Fliedner's influence extended to America when in 1849, with four deaconesses, he arrived in Pittsburgh. They were to assume responsibility for the *Pittsburgh Infirmary* (now *Passavant Hospital*). This was the first Protestant church hospital in the United States. The clergyman who requested the assistance of Pastor Fliedner in permitting the deaconesses to come to this country was *William Passavant*. A deaconess motherhouse was to be established here to educate sisters for this country. This became a reality in 1850. The first American deaconess was *Louisa Marthens* who was consecrated on May 28, 1850.

Jacobs[5] has indicated that Pastor Passavant's plan was too progressive for his parish to undertake so that it was never a large project, but the quality of the work of the deaconesses was noted in their efficient care of the sick during cholera epidemics, the Civil War and in the establishment of other institutions.

Amalie Sieveking of Hamburg, Germany,

whose humane concerns were reflected in many nursing projects, did volunteer nursing service during an epidemic of cholera. She and the society she formed, called the Friends of the Poor, were instrumental in assisting in the development of Kaiserswerth.

Sister Elizabeth Fedde was the first nurse to practice among the Norwegian sick poor of the United States. She came from Norway and was a trained nurse as well as a trained pharmacist. She established the Norwegian Lutheran Deaconess Home and Hospital in Brooklyn, as well as the Lutheran Deaconess Home and Hospital in Minneapolis, and she was active in caring for the sick in their homes.

The first nursing order that was established by the *Anglican Catholic Church* was the *Sisters of St. John's House* in England. They were founded in 1848 to give nursing care to the sick in hospitals and in the homes of the community. Preparation for this work was given at King's College Hospital.

The *Episcopal Church in the United States* established a group of sisters in the Diocese of Maryland. These deaconesses cared for the sick in a house called St. Andrew's Infirmary. This group had no previous training in nursing, but they were imbued with a zealous desire to be of service. Their efforts were rewarded.

The *Sisters of the Holy Communion*, founded in 1845, carried out both hospital and home nursing in addition to doing parish work and teaching parish school. *St. Luke's Hospital* in New York City was constructed because of the vision, inspiration and direction of its founder, first pastor and superintendent, *Dr. William Augustus Muhlenberg* (1796–1877). It first opened as The Infirmary of the Church of the Holy Communion in 1854 and then became St. Luke's Hospital in 1858. The Sisterhood of the Holy Communion under the leadership of *Sister Anne Ayres* accepted the responsibility of providing the superior nursing service in St. Luke's from its inception until 1888.

The architecture of St. Luke's Hospital was most interesting as is recorded.[6] It was built around the Church of the Holy Communion. "The patients lived in the House of the Lord. St. Luke's, as a church, has the chapel for its nave and the wards for its

[5]Jacobs, H. E.: *A History of the Evangelical Lutheran Church in America.* (The American Church History Series, IV), New York, The Christian Literature Co., 1893, p. 387.

[6]*History of the St. Luke's Hospital Training School for Nurses,* New York, 1938, p. 18.

transept." The prayerful atmosphere with its soothing organ music pervading the confines of the wards coupled with the willing service of the sisters must have been of great value in the healing process.

Dr. Muhlenberg emphasized that the patients were guests of the church and stressed the concept of the opportunity of the Christian family to entertain their guests, all of whom were sick. He mentioned that the nurses should consider the need for "a cheerful spirit, skillful devotion and appreciative interest in the patient individually."[7] This was a preview of the modern idea of considering the patient as a person! The motto of St. Luke's appears on the pin of the School of Nursing: *Corpus sanare, animam salvare* — to heal the body and to save the soul. Religious fervor accompanied scientific progress.

There are several anecdotes that give a picture of the times. In the instructions given to the sisters, Dr. Muhlenberg taught that they were to pour the patient's medication and bring it to the patient when it was due rather than follow the then currently accepted method, which was to require the patient to be responsible for taking his own medicine. He felt that this would eliminate many problems.

Patients cannot be trusted with their own medicine. They cannot be made to understand the fallacy of the argument, that if a teaspoonful of anything will cure a man slowly, the whole bottle will do it immediately. It is not an unheard of thing for an elegantly disguised and flavored medicine to be rubbed on an injured limb, and for the cooling lotion, ordered at the same time, to be faithfully taken in teaspoonful doses after meals. To avoid such gross mistakes as these, it is customary in hospitals for the nurse to administer the medicines according to distinctly marked directions on the bottle. This works well, and mistakes are rare. But to have the medicine given by one who is herself responsible for its proper administration and preparation, who is required by the rules of the Sisterhood to understand its nature, the ordinary dose, and its expected effect, and who is honest and faithful enough to report immediately any mistake which may occur, shuts up many sources of error and danger.[8]

Another interesting notation concerned the value of diet in the plan for care of the patient. He stated,[9] "Every physician knows that the only hope for a man in the third week of typhoid lies in the amount of nourishment he can be induced to take. In private practice, he administers food and stimulant with his own hand." He proceeded to discuss the impossibility of the physician's assuming this duty in a hospital and inveighed against any but the best prepared and most capable of nurses accepting this responsibility.

In this century and the early part of the twentieth, it was well known that only good nursing care brought a patient through a serious case of pneumonia, typhoid fever or other affliction of serious import.

In 1863, the Sisterhood of the Holy Communion reorganized; some of the sisters remained in the original order; others formed the Sisters of St. Mary; another segment established the Sisters of St. Luke and St. John.

The *Sisters of St. Mary* engaged in a special field of nursing that needed skilled nursing attention — venereal disease control. They managed a home for delinquent girls and women, and finally built and staffed St. Mary's Free Hospital for children in New York City.

In 1855, another very important Anglican order, *St. Margaret's Sisterhood*, was founded. The Sisters of St. Margaret were invited to come to the United States, and in 1871 they arrived from England. They participated in the nursing service administration of the Children's Hospital in Boston. This community of sisters remained in charge for 45 years. Their greatest contribution was effected at this hospital, but they opened and maintained several others through the years.

St. John's Sisterhood and the *Sisterhood of All Saints*, both Protestant, worked in Baltimore. It was from the latter that Sister Helen, the first superintendent of nurses at Bellevue, came.

Deaconesses were also found in the *Methodist Church* and nursing profited by their efforts. Many of the deaconesses' hospitals were maintained under the supervision of these deaconesses.

Still another group of *deaconesses* was organized by the *Mennonite Church*.

---

[7] *Ibid*, p. 20.

[8] *Ibid*, p. 23.

[9] *Ibid*, p. 24.

LAY LEADERSHIP IN NURSING

A compassionate young lady, Annie M. Andrews (Fig. 8–18), left her home in Syracuse, New York to assist the victims of yellow fever and their families in Norfolk, Virginia. She worked tirelessly to keep patients alive or to comfort, console and assist them toward a peaceful death. Her skill and valor have been documented[10] and her efforts and deeds have been compared to those of Florence Nightingale.

The Howard Association of Norfolk, grateful for the eminent services of Miss Andrews as well as the noble example she set, presented her with the gold medal usually awarded only to physicians. The Howard Association was formed in 1856 for the protection of the sick and suffering because of inhumanity to man.

---

[10] *Harper's Weekly*, Vol. I, June 6, 1857, pp. 353–354.

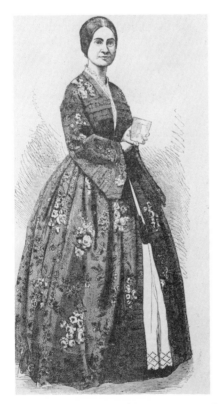

Figure 8–18. Annie M. Andrews, a recognized nurse heroine of the yellow fever epidemic in Norfolk in 1855.

PROGRESS IN PSYCHIATRIC CARE

Mental illness was generally thought to be incurable. Few persons realized that these patients needed humane treatment; the law classed them next to criminals. Up to 1820, the mentally ill were exhibited for payment for the diversion of the public. Iron manacles were used in asylums up to 1886, and the McLean Asylum of Massachusetts, established in 1817, was the first institution of the sort to treat its patients kindly. The Friends' Asylum at Philadelphia, of the same period, was one of the few hospitals that appreciated the patient's needs.

In America, the pioneer crusader for the reform for the mentally ill was *Dorothea Lynde Dix* (1802–1887). Her first contact with the mentally ill came in 1841 when a theological student who had been given a class assignment to teach Sunday school at the jail in East Cambridge, Massachusetts asked if she, a retired school teacher, would be willing to assume his assigned task. She was shocked by the environmental conditions in which the prisoners lived. Many of the prisoners were mentally ill. The treatment they received ranged from indifference through negligence to brutality. The assumption seemed to be that they were incapable of sensation; therefore no heat was provided for these tragic prisoners. Because of her persistence, logic and forcefulness in the court of East Cambridge, heat was provided in jail. This was the first milestone.

After surveying the needs of the mentally ill in Massachusetts, gathering data, securing the support of influential citizens, presenting the facts and then obtaining the results she desired, she moved on to the state of Rhode Island. Her phenomenal success continued as she gained the financial backing of a wealthy gentleman, Cyrus Butler, who provided for the establishment of *Butler Hospital*, an outstanding psychiatric institution.

The success of Dorothea Dix was due to the painstaking cataloging of facts that were repulsive to honest, forthright citizens. Such was her presentation of a patient in Rhode Island who had been literally entombed in a six by eight foot stone cell into which no sun, heat or companion could enter because the door was bolted. The poor helpless sufferer had frost and ice coating the walls, the bed and himself. The realization of the existence of this incredible cruelty won support for the patients for whom she fought so desperately. She had found patients "confined in cages, closets, cellars, stalls, pens, chained, naked, beaten with rods and lashed into obedience." Through her efforts, the first state psychiatric hospital was constructed in Trenton, New Jersey; Canada, as well as the United States and Scotland elevated their standards of care for the mentally ill. Her fiery crusade continued until at the time of her death more than thirty psychiatric hospitals had been established in the United States and other countries.

In the December 2, 1865 issue of *Harper's Weekly*, an article entitled "Dancing by Lunatics" described a dance at the Lunatic Asylum on Blackwell's Island, New York, at which the patients were the dancers (Fig. 8–19). The change in attitude toward the mentally ill at that time was reflected in the editorial: "Occasions of this sort no doubt tend in a great degree to relieve the sluggish melancholy which too close confinement or too monotonous surroundings are apt to produce in our institutions for insane people. It is often the case that isolation renders incurable diseases of the mind which a more considerate treatment might ameliorate, or perhaps entirely relieve."[11]

---

[11]*Harper's Weekly*, Vol. IX, December 2, 1865, p. 765.

Samuel Gridley Howe (1801–1876), the well-known social reformer, made a major contribution to patient care in the course of his work with the blind. Through his efforts, the New England Asylum for the Blind, later called *Perkins Institute*, was chartered in 1829 and opened in 1832. He directed this famous school for forty-four years. Two famous pupils were Laura Bridgman, who was deaf as well as blind, and Anne Sullivan Macy, who tutored Helen Keller. The education of individuals with the special problems of blindness and deafness was now a reality.

Dr. Howe was an ardent supporter of Dorothea Dix in her efforts on behalf of the mentally ill. His wife, *Julia Ward Howe*, joined him in the opposition of slavery.

Louis Braille (1809–1852), another pioneer in the crusade for assistance for the blind, became blind himself at the age of three as the result of an accident. He was admitted to a school in Paris when he was ten years of age, and later he became a teacher there. In order to augment the learning situation for his students, he improved the system of writing with dots that Charles Barbier had devised. The *Braille system of communication* by the use of this raised-dot method has been utilized by the blind for printing, writing and in musical notation. Louis Braille had an interest and developed skill in playing the organ, and he became an organist in a church in Paris.

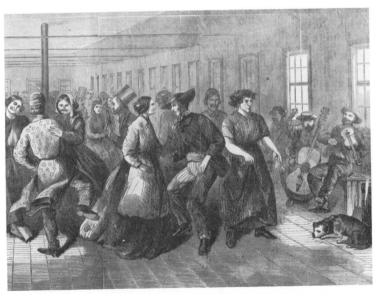

Figure 8–19. Ball given for the patients of the "Insane Asylum" on Blackwell's Island, November 6, 1865.

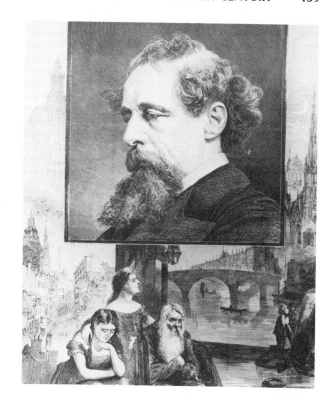

Figure 8–20. Charles Dickens, a catalyst for social reform.

The facile pen and ingenious skill of *Charles Dickens* (1812–1870) were forceful weapons for social reform in the nineteenth century (Fig. 8–20). He had the rare ability to portray in a startlingly revealing way the social evils of his day, to break the literary barrier by his selection of characters from the stratum of society that needed assistance and to provide a detailed and accurate description of many diseases. This was an unusual combination of faculties.

Disease was a constant and often catastrophic problem. It was strikingly in evidence because of the lack of institutions to house people with specific conditions. His powers of observation socially and medically were most acute and vie with those of the most gifted medical clinician of the period. Brain[12] develops, in an interesting way, the medical observations and recordings of Dickens.

Dickens waged a powerful crusade to make citizens aware of needs for social change. He portrayed the plight of the orphan and the need for more stringent child-labor laws; he exposed the unfair court trials, with imprisonment for minor offenses, and the unjust length of imprisonment, with members of the family incarcerated with parents;[13] he wrote of the birth of children in prisons and their lives there, of life in workhouses and the evils of the apprenticeship system,[14] of poor preparation of teachers and educators, of cruel treatment of the mentally retarded,[15] of brain washing of victims in prison,[16] of the unscrupulous tactics of lawyers, of inadequate preparation of doctors, of grave robbing to sell cadavers to medical students,[17] and of the ghastly level to which "nursing" had sunk.

Dickens' *Martin Chuzzlewit* (1844) focused attention on the nursing care given by pardoned criminals, women who were too old for harlotry and women of low moral standards with a lack of interest in or love for their fellow men. His immortal portrait of *Sairey Gamp* (Fig. 8–21) reflects the nature

---

[12] Brain, Russell: *Some Reflections on Genius.* Philadelphia, J. B. Lippincott Co., 1960, pp. 123–136.

[13] Dickens, Charles: *Little Dorrit* (1857).
[14] _____: *Oliver Twist* (1838).
[15] _____: *Nicholas Nickleby* (1838).
[16] _____: *A Tale of Two Cities* (1859).
[17] *Ibid.*

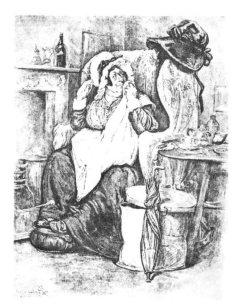

Figure 8–21. Sairey Gamp. (From Dickens' *Martin Chuzzlewit.*)

of these unfeeling, unsympathetic, alcohol-imbibing characters who contributed their share to the sufferings of mankind.

DEVELOPMENTS IN BIOLOGICAL AND PHYSICAL SCIENCES AND MEDICINE

Physiology

It is to *René T. H. Laënnec* (1781–1826) that we owe the contribution of the *stethoscope.*

Tuberculosis, also called the White Plague, was an ever-present affliction in this century, and the incidence of this disease was very high. It has been stated that one third of all the patients in Paris hospitals had tuberculosis. It seemed to consume a person and, in fact, was called "consumption."

In treating patients with this condition, Laënnec had resorted to palpation and percussion but was dissatisfied with the ineffectual method of listening to chest and heart sounds. It was the custom in this period for the physician to place his ear over the patient's chest in order to hear these sounds. Many physicians were reluctant to use this method because of the uncleanliness of the patient; the coughing of the patient; the modesty of the patient; or the obesity of the patient which muffled the sounds.

In 1816 while walking near the Louvre, he observed children on one end of some wooden beams tapping out messages to children who were listening intently at the other end. Immediately, Laënnec had an inspiration; he returned to the hospital, rolled some paper into a tube, placed one end over the chest of an obese patient and rested his ear against the other end. He heard heart sounds more clearly than ever before.

This chest examiner he called a stethoscope. At first, it consisted of the rolled paper tied with string and then he devised a cylinder made of light wood—about twelve inches long—that could unscrew into two parts. (It was Dr. Cammann of New York who developed the binaural stethoscope.)

Laënnec believed that tuberculosis was contagious, that it was curable, that the disease might be quiescent without manifest symptoms and then later blossom into an acute phase. Laënnec felt strongly that scrofula, called "King's Evil," was tuberculosis of the lymph nodes of the neck. This form of the disease as well as several other varieties occurred at a time in history when milk was not pasteurized.

The cause and cure of this disease still needed to be discovered, but Laënnec contributed to the advancement of medicine and thereby benefited society with his stethoscope.

William Beaumont (1785–1853) was the son of a prosperous farmer in Lebanon, Connecticut. He enlisted in the United States Army as a surgeon's mate and later was assigned to a lonely outpost on Mackinac Island. Here he met the man who was to become Beaumont's physiological laboratory.

Alexis St. Martin was a young trapper who had been wounded accidentally by a gunshot blast. This injury left an opening through which Dr. Beaumont studied the reactions of the stomach to various types of food, liquid and emotions. The wound never healed.

In his study of this most unusual affliction, Army Surgeon Beaumont shed much light on one of nature's most baffling mysteries, the process of digestion. In 1833, he wrote *Experiments and Observations on the Gastric Juice and the Physiology of Digestion.*

Claude Bernard (1813–1878) was said to be

responsible for introducing the use of the scientific method into the field of medicine. It is recorded that before Bernard, medicine was purely empirical. His skill in the use of the experimental method of scientific investigation led to an expansion of the knowledge of body organs.

The fruits of his labors included: studies of digestion, concentrating on a study of the breakdown of sugar in the body as well as the part played by pancreatic juice; explanation of the role of glycogen in the liver; demonstration of the vasomotor mechanism in governing bodily activities, with the conclusion that irritation of the vagus nerve could cause an increase in sugar production, resulting in sugar excreted in the urine (glycosuria); the discovery, through studies of carbon monoxide poisoning and experimentation, that carbon monoxide could displace oxygen in the red blood cells; the proof through experimentation that curare destroyed the contact between nerves and muscles. He found that the muscles reacted to artificial stimuli. He proved that disease could be produced artificially by biochemical experiments.

Bernard's efforts were published in 1865 in his classic work, *An Introduction to the Study of Experimental Medicine*. As a result of his labors, the fields of physiology and physiological chemistry have been enriched.

In 1865 an Augustinian monk, *Abbot Gregor Johann Mendel*, of Brunn, Moravia, announced the results of his research in a publication that went unnoticed for almost half a century. *Mendel's law* of dominant and recessive characteristics has had applications in biology, eugenics and in the understanding of heredity, even the hereditary aspects of some diseases.

Hermann von Helmholtz (1821–1894) utilized his background in physics and mathematics and made practical applications in the field of medicine, especially in the fields of physical optics and acoustics.

Among his achievements were the invention of the *ophthalmoscope* and the *ophthalmometer* and an understanding of the transmission of sound through the middle ear, which he described, to the brain. He presented a delineation of the law of conservation of energy as well as fundamental principles relating to the over-all field of dynamics—hydro-, thermo- and electrodynamics.

Anesthesia

Pain has been one of the greatest afflictions in the history of mankind. There were many attempts to find soporific potions to deaden pain. Earlier groups resorted to the use of wine, opium, mandrake and many other substances that were more merciful than the cruel methods of either rendering the patient unconscious or obtaining strong individuals to restrain the patient by force. The world desired something to dull the senses and permit the blissful state of unconsciousness needed so desperately by both surgeon and patient.

The answer came in the discovery of *anesthesia,* one of America's greatest gifts to the world.

In 1766, Joseph Priestley isolated nitrous oxide. A physician from Georgia, *Crawford W. Long* (1815–1878), used ether for surgical operations and in obstetrics. During the 1840's, the famous circus owner, P. T. Barnum, sent traveling bands of entertainers around the country to give the "ether frolics." In 1842, some of Long's young medical friends inhaled ether for a bit of fun and amusement. Long also joined as a participant in this "ether frolic." He realized that ether gave a person more than a feeling of euphoria and that its use might be tried for surgical purposes. This he did successfully, but did not report his success until 1849.

A dentist of Hartford, Connecticut, *Horace Wells* (1815–1848), administered nitrous oxide while extracting teeth, and it was a successful venture. He, too, had witnessed a public demonstration of "laughing gas"; the demonstration was attended largely by young men in the field of medicine as a form of amusement.

Dr. Wells obtained permission to give a clinical demonstration before a class at Harvard Medical School. Unfortunately, the patient was not anesthetized completely and screamed during the operation. The medical students jeered and shouted humbug; the demonstration was considered totally unsuccessful, and Wells was humiliated.

A dentist in Massachusetts, *William T. G. Morton* (1819–1868), was present at the unfortunate demonstration of his friend, Dr. Wells, and felt that something else was needed that would be more reliable.

Sulfuric ether had been known and used.

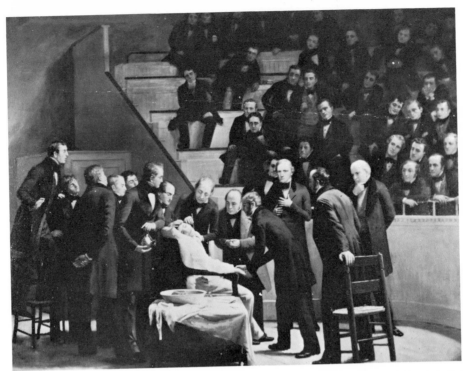

Figure 8–22. The first public demonstration of the use of ether at the Massachusetts General Hospital. (Painting by Robert Huckley, Boston Medical Library. Courtesy of Massachusetts General Hospital.)

In 1846, after experimenting with ether upon himself, Dr. Morton administered ether to a patient of the famous surgeon, John Collins Warren, professor of anatomy and operative surgery at Harvard Medical School and chief of surgical service at Massachusetts General Hospital. When the patient became unconscious, Dr. Warren, turning to the surgical staff, said, "Gentlemen, this is no humbug." It was administered in the operating room amphitheater, called the Ether Dome, of the Massachusetts General Hospital (Fig. 8–22). The patient was placed in the operating chair, which was upholstered in red plush with an adjustable back. This operating chair is still part of the background of the famous Ether Dome of "M.G.H."

Surgical operations could now be performed that would have been impossible without anesthesia. The terms anesthesia, anesthetic and anesthetist are supposed to have been proposed by Oliver Wendell Holmes.

Obstetrics and Gynecology

The world owes a tremendous debt of gratitude to *Ignaz Semmelweis* (1818–1865), a brilliant Hungarian physician who was an independent thinker, an earnest, careful investigator and an ardent reformer interested in improving medical practice and thereby saving lives. He possessed earned degrees of doctor of medicine, master of midwifery and doctor of surgery.

He received an appointment as assistant director of the Obstetric Clinic at the Lying-in Hospital in Vienna. He was appalled at the high maternal mortality rate due to *puerperal sepsis* or *childbed fever*. People dreaded going to hospitals in this century because the chances of survival were poor.

He began to use his powers of observation and to analyze patient care. He noted a marked difference in the maternal mortality rate between two of the clinics. In the one in which the midwives practiced, the incidence of childbed fever as well as the mortality rate were decidedly lower than in the clinic in which the medical students practiced. The transfer of infection, Semmelweis determined, was due to the filthy habits of medical students who dissected bodies on the autopsy table and then went directly to deliver a baby or to examine a prenatal or postpartum patient. He confronted medical students with his observations and indicted them for transferring infection by not washing their hands. He was derided by his colleagues who protested explosively against his requirements.

He demanded that medical students wash their hands with soap and water, then chlorinated lime and finally scrub their hands with fine sand. The drop in the death rate of maternity patients was astounding. One further fact was suspected by Semmelweis: that doctors carried infections from one patient to another. Thus, it was essential to wash hands after treating every patient. In 1861, he published an account of his valuable research efforts in *The Cause, Concept, and Prophylaxis of Childbed Fever*.

His theory was revolutionary and was not accepted by his contemporaries. Their treatment of him and his work was responsible for his eventual mental illness. He died in 1865 of a wound infection that caused blood poisoning, the disease he fought to eliminate.

Another leader in the fight to eliminate childbed fever was *Oliver Wendell Holmes* (1809–1894). After graduation from Harvard in 1829, Holmes abandoned the study of law for that of medicine.

In 1842, he wrote an essay on homeopathy that was a forceful exposition of the fallacies of that form of healing.[18] In 1843, he composed a brilliant essay, *The Contagiousness of Puerperal Fever*, which was a medical classic. It

was published five years before the work of Semmelweis appeared. His views were bitterly attacked by his medical colleagues, but, like Semmelweis, his opinions and theoretical concepts were correct. In 1855, he republished this paper, adding an introduction in criticism of these unjust remarks. Many years later he wrote a letter to a friend with this comment: "I do know that others had cried out with all their might against the terrible evil before I did, and I give them full credit for it. But, I think I shrieked my warning louder and longer than any of them and I am pleased to remember that I took my ground on the existing evidence before the little army of microbes was marched up to support my position."

As may be noted, Pasteur's work (1879) showing the connection between streptococci and the disease of puerperal fever had received wide publicity after Holmes's foregoing letter had been written.

MEDICAL EDUCATION

In early nineteenth century New England medical practice, more than half of the practicing doctors were not graduates of a medical school—however brief the medical school courses were. Preceptors taught students of medicine by observation and practice, either in the doctor's office or on his home visits, and by reading. There were no formal medical schools in New England until 1782 and as late as 1840 probably no more than one third of the physicians in practice had graduated from medical schools. The preceptor-apprentice system of medical education was firmly entrenched; it was common practice for a young man to have spent as many as 144 weeks or almost three years as an assistant to the preceptor-doctor. This vested interest group, preceptor-doctors, became a powerful force for prevention of progress in medical education and medical care. The medical apprentice helped with farm and home chores and, in addition, paid a tuition averaging $100.

There were no uniform New England laws governing medical qualifications, practice and licensure. Many doctors expressed the need for a liberal arts foundation, for anatomical dissecting materials, for clinical facilities in which to practice and for a much upgraded plan for medical education.

---

[18]The nineteenth century, which witnessed such phenomenal progress in medicine, also observed several unusual developments. One of these was the founding of *homeopathy* by *Samuel Hahnemann* (1755–1843) in the early years of this period. His theories were that a medication that produces symptoms similar to the ones causing the disease could cure the patient—"like cures like"; that the more medicines are diluted the more potent they become; that all nervous diseases cause or are caused by an itch. He inveighed against emetics, purging, cupping, bloodletting, and blistering. He had many opponents, but also many supporters even in the United States. Homeopathic medical schools and homeopathic hospitals were opened. Homeopathy has practically disappeared.

In scrutinizing this period, reflected against a background of social distress, the need for well-prepared nurse practitioners for every age group, in a variety of settings and with a myriad of health problems, has been presented. The contributions of many religious orders as well as strong individual leadership have been recognized.

REFERENCE READINGS

Armstrong, George. *The Summer of Pestilence—A History of Yellow Fever.* Philadelphia, J. B. Lippincott & Co., 1856.

Bailly de Barberey, Helene: *Elizabeth Seton.* Trans. from sixth French ed. by J. B. Code. New York, The Macmillan Co., 1927.

Dickens, Charles: *Martin Chuzzlewit.* Boston, Estes & Lauriat, 1896.

Eaton, Evelyn, and Moore, Edward R.: *Heart in Pilgrimage.* New York, Doubleday & Co., 1948.

Marshall, Helen E.: *Dorothea Dix, Forgotten Samaritan.* Chapel Hill, University of North Carolina Press, 1937.

Packard, Francis R.: *Some Accounts of the Pennsylvania Hospital from 1751 to 1938.* Philadelphia, Engle Press, 1938.

Robinson, Victor: *Victory over Pain.* New York, Henry Schuman, 1946.

Rosenberg, Charles: *The Cholera Years.* Chicago, The University of Chicago Press, 1962.

Slaughter, Frank G.: *Immortal Magyar.* New York, Henry Schuman, 1950.

Thompson, Morton: *The Cry and the Covenant.* New York, Doubleday & Co., 1954.

Thorwald, Jurgen: *The Century of a Surgeon.* New York, Pantheon Books, 1956.

Tilton, Eleanor: *Amiable Autocrat: A Biography of Dr. Oliver Wendell Holmes.* New York, Henry Schuman, 1947.

CHAPTER 9

Nursing Leadership in Educational Preparation and Practice of the Mid-Nineteenth Century

Nursing is an art; and if it is to be made an art, requires as exclusive a devotion, as hard a preparation as any painter's or sculptor's work; for what is the having to do with dead canvas or cold marble, compared with having to do with the living body—the temple of god's spirit... it is one of the fine arts; I have almost said, the finest of fine arts.

Florence Nightingale

THE STATUS OF WOMEN

The midpoint of the nineteenth century was marked by the blossoming of Victorian society and a demand for emancipation of women, who were forced to live a life devoid of educational and career opportunities.

The wealthy young lady frittered away her time in sewing, painting or musical activities; however, there were those who inveighed against such a stultifying existence.

The leadership of many women, such as Susan B. Anthony, Lucretia Mott, Elizabeth Blackwell and Florence Nightingale, should be remembered with gratitude by women of succeeding generations.

In London in 1840, women were refused admission to the first world convention to abolish slavery. The issue of segregation of women was not recognized. In 1848 in Seneca Falls, New York, there was a convention for *Woman's Rights*. This crusade was of monumental proportions and great historical significance. Susan B. Anthony and many others fought for the rights of women as human beings: suffrage, an opportunity for higher education and an opportunity to practice the professions, which included law and medicine.

Throughout the course of history women had been midwives; now men were midwives. There was no question in Victorian society of the indelicacy of men delivering women in labor, but it was unthinkable for a woman to practice medicine or to study anatomy or physiology.

Still another milestone was reached when *women were readmitted* into the medical field. The well known pioneer was *Elizabeth Blackwell* (1821–1910). Miss Blackwell's struggles to gain admission to medical schools are well known. She was informed that she might as well lead a revolution as try to be a physician. Geneva Medical College in Geneva, New York, consented to admit her in 1847. After some tribulation, she received her degree of doctor of medicine. Her troubles were just beginning because she was unable to secure a hospital staff appointment, and patients seemed disinterested in a woman doctor even though women midwives had been an accepted custom for years.

In 1853, Dr. Blackwell set up a dispensary, and in 1857 she was able to establish the New York Infirmary for Women and Children. This was to be the clinical setting for practical experience for women students of medicine. In 1865, she was responsible for founding the *Women's Medical College of the New York Infirmary for Women and Children.* The hospital was staffed by women doctors, and their service extended into the community. They employed a doctor to visit homes in order to care for the sick poor as well as a physician to give instruction to women on the subjects of health, hygiene and sanitation.

Dr. Blackwell was a close personal friend of Florence Nightingale, and they shared many interests and desires for the welfare of mankind.

The die had been cast, the readmission of women into the field of medicine, even in small numbers, was now assured. The Woman's Medical College of Pennsylvania was opened in 1850. There were eight candidates for the degree of doctor of medicine in the first class. The course consisted of two college semesters of three months each or one academic year.

Lucretia Mott announced in her *Discourse on Women* that "a new generation of women is upon the stage." Indeed, the world was aware of a gifted and forceful woman leader in the field of nursing and health who set in motion the great reform that was to revolutionize nursing.

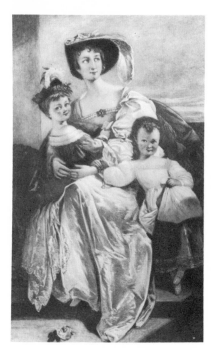

Figure 9–1. Mrs. Nightingale and her daughters Parthenope and Florence.

FLORENCE NIGHTINGALE

The social reformers of the early nineteenth century had focused attention on the plight of the poor and on the needs for reform in prisons, hospitals and nursing. Leadership in the social aspects of living and in nursing was needed. The person who responded to this exigency was *Florence Nightingale*, who cannot be considered as the product of her time but rather must be regarded as one of those rare and gifted people who transcend the period of their own existence and whose plans and accomplishments represent the thinking of a much later period of history.

She was the contemporary of such gifted individuals as Pasteur, Lister, Koch, Roentgen, the Curies, Darwin, Mendel, Wordsworth, Byron, Shelley, Keats, Swinburne, Dickens, Longfellow, Emerson, Beethoven, Schubert, Mendelssohn and Brahms.

Florence Nightingale was born on May 12, 1820. Her parents, Mr. and Mrs. William Shore Nightingale of Lea Hurst, Derbyshire and Embley Park, Hampshire, were traveling in Italy when Florence was born and named

her for the city of her birth. (See Figures 9–1 and 9–2.)

Her youthful surroundings included living in many places on the continent as well as in the warmth and gaiety of an English manor in nineteenth-century England. In a period when young women were subjected to the constricting influences of Victorian society, Miss Nightingale welcomed her father's guidance and under his influence gained a liberal education, not only in Latin, mathematics, philosophy, religion, and modern languages but also, as one who knew her records,

by the surroundings of life itself — by travel and the study of people, cities, public movements and institutions, and, . . . by intellectual and cultured companionship under the home roof. Those who can remember still look back on the peculiar charm of the family life at Embley and at Lea Hurst; on Embley summer mornings filled with what Walter Scott somewhere calls 'mututinal inspiration;' when the talk over the breakfast-table was so vivid with interests and sympathies that sometimes, before the meal was over, the very bookshelves would be called into requisition to provide statistics and quotations . . . and Blue-books would find their way among the silver and

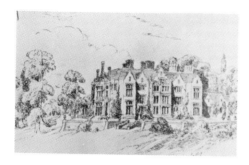

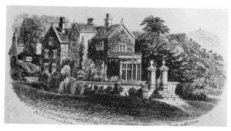

Figure 9–2. *Above:* Embley Park in Hampshire, Florence Nightingale's summer estate from a sketch by her sister Parthenope. *Below:* Lea Hurst, the winter home of Miss Nightingale in Derbyshire near Mattock.

china on the breakfast-table and huge tomes of reference be heaped on the carpet at Mr. Nightingale's feet.[1]

Florence's sister, Parthenope, who later became Lady Verney of Claydon, presents charming descriptions of one of their memorable visits in Paris in 1839–40, where in the mansion of Mrs. Clarke, the mother of Madame Mohl, the Nightingale family met the best political, literary and scientific society of that period. It is hardly surprising that Florence Nightingale evolved into an attractive, charming, brilliant, dynamic, gifted and forceful leader whose thoughts and desires were channeled into action (Fig. 9–3). Her intelligence and education were recognized by many of the scholars of the last century.

An important contact between Florence Nightingale and a gentleman in the United States had a profound influence on her decision to pursue the life of a nurse. In 1844, Dr. Samuel Gridley Howe and his wife, Julia Ward Howe, were visiting the Nightingale family at their summer estate at Embley in

Hampshire. Florence, at the age of 24, was undergoing a particularly frustrating experience: she wanted to be useful to humanity instead of being waited on herself. She turned to Dr. Howe for counsel:

Dr. Howe, you have had much experience in the world of philanthropy; you are a medical man and a gentleman; now may I ask you to tell me, upon your word, whether it would be anything unsuitable or unbecoming to a young English woman, if she should devote herself to work of charity in hospitals and elsewhere as the Catholic Sisters do?

My dear Miss Florence, Dr. Howe replied, it would be unusual, and in England whatever is unusual is apt to be thought unsuitable; but I say to you, go forward, if you have a vocation for that way of life; act up to your aspiration, and you will find that there is never anything unbecoming or unladylike in doing your duty for the good of others. Choose your path, go on with it, wherever it may lead you, and God be with you![2]

This auspicious occasion has been described by Mrs. Howe in her *Reminiscences* and by their daughter, Laura E. Howe Richards, in two of her books. This discussion seemed to have had a catalytic effect on the inner de-

[2] Bishop, William J.: "Florence Nightingale's Message for Today." *Nursing Outlook,* 8:246–247, 1960.

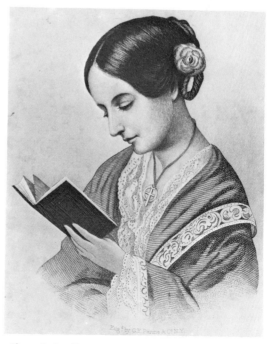

Figure 9–3. Florence Nightingale. (Author's collection.)

[1] "Florence Nightingale — By One Who Knew Her," *The Nursing Mirror and Midwives' Journal,* August 20, 1910, pp. 311–312.

sires of Florence Nightingale and prompted the action she later took.

She was drawn to philanthropic endeavors, always analyzing and planning a program of care for the welfare of others. She applied theoretical concepts to practical ends. When she delineated a systematic study of the "ameliorative treatment of physical and moral distress," she gathered her data by visiting many institutions and enrolled in the program for nursing under the direction of Pastor Fliedner at Kaiserswerth. Although she did not become a Lutheran Deaconess, she finished the three months' program and later reflected with gratitude about her experience at Kaiserswerth. She then went to Paris to study and learn in the historic institutions and under the guidance of the Sisters of Charity of St. Vincent de Paul. She was determined to replace the ill-prepared, sadistic nurses of the period so well depicted in Charles Dickens' *Martin Chuzzlewit*, with intelligent, kind, well-prepared nurses.

Miss Nightingale's first position was superintendent of the *Establishment for Gentlewomen During Illness*. She planned for the patients and the doctors with great skill, and was successful and happy. Within a short time she was asked to become superintendent of nurses at King's College Hospital, and had begun to plan her work there when the call came to go to the *Crimea*.

Russia's desire for Constantinople, dating from the time of Peter the Great, culminated in the outbreak of the Crimean War in 1854. England and France came to the defense of endangered Turkey in March of that year. For the first time in modern warfare, a civilian correspondent presented the news coverage. Before this war, the general simply gave out the report of success or failure. Now a vivid picture of the conditions for the poor soldier was presented to the public.

In addition to astronomically high battle wounds and deaths from uncontrolled spread of infection, cholera broke out among the troops and spread with frightening rapidity. On September 20 at the battle of Alma, England's losses were 2,860 wounded and 619 dead. The news did not reach London until September 30. The next news was of the famous battle of Balaclava, immortalized by the charge of the Light Brigade. The battle of Inkerman later resulted in British casualties of 2,612 killed and wounded.

It is related that "between the battle of the Alma and the battle of Inkerman something had happened to the conscience of the British nation . . . we find recorded 'the arrival of Miss Florence Nightingale with her nurses at Scutari, on their mission of mercy to the wounded soldiers.' "[3]

The memorable letter of Sir Sidney Herbert, the Secretary of State for War, contained a plea and a recognition of Florence Nightingale's unique qualifications for such an assignment:

There is but one person in England that I know of who would be capable of organizing and superintending such a scheme. . . . My question simply is, would you listen to the request to go out and supervise the whole thing? You would, of course, have plenary authority over all the nurses, and I think I could secure you the fullest assistance and cooperation from the medical staff, and you would also have an unlimited power of drawing on the Government for whatever you think requisite for the success of your mission. . . . I must not conceal from you that upon your decision will depend the ultimate success or failure of the plan. Your own personal qualities, your knowledge and your power of administration, and among greater things, your rank and position in society, give you advantages in such a work which no other person possesses.[4]

At a time in history when schools of nursing were unknown, she assembled a staff of workers in less than a week. In the quiet of an October evening it is reported that the dedicated group embarked upon its historic mission. She had in her group Roman Catholic and Anglican sisters, lay nurses from St. John's House and others, 38 in all.

Many of the medical officers of the Army were opposed to the idea of women nurses. They felt that the nursing care given by untrained orderlies was as good as could be expected in war and that women would be burdensome.

Miss Nightingale and her band were assigned to the base hospital at *Scutari*, across the strait from Constantinople (now Istanbul). Here in a beautiful setting was the great Barrack Hospital, supposed to accommodate 1700 patients (Fig. 9–4.) At that time there were between 3000 and 4000 sick and wounded, and *four miles of beds*. Miss Nightingale and her 38 nurses were given charge of 1500 patients.

---

[3]*Ibid.*, p. 312.
[4]*Ibid.*, p. 313.

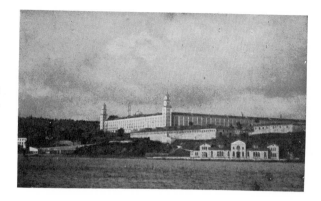

Figure 9–4. Barrack Hospital at Scutari, as seen from the American Hospital, Constantinople, 1927. (Courtesy of International Council of Nurses.)

Upon their arrival the chaos they surveyed was inexpressible. The miraculous change which was wrought by Miss Nightingale and her team of nurses is incredible. This endowed leader drew upon her warm human sympathies, her brilliant mind, her rare administrative skills, her abilities in writing, publicity, political and social statesmanship to achieve her successes (Fig. 9–5).

The *hospital conditions* were indescribably poor. The crowded wards had unspeakable toilet and sanitary accommodations. There were not enough beds, and those that did exist were of straw. Many patients lay on the floor. There were few sheets and practically no hospital clothing; most of the patients were still in their uniforms, stiff with blood and covered with filth.

There were no basins, few utensils of any sort, no soap and no towels. There were no knives or forks so that the men ate with their fingers. It took four hours to serve a meal, and most of it was not edible. There was practically nothing that a very sick man could eat. There was no night nursing; the men, left alone in the dark, spoke of the terror of it. With these conditions, the death rate was *42 per cent.*

Miss Nightingale began by opening five diet kitchens and setting up a laundry. At the Barrack Hospital in Scutari, a missionary from New England, *Rev. Cyrus Hamlin,* contributed his services by baking bread and washing clothes for Miss Nightingale.[5] She had been told that there were plenty of supplies, but they could not be found; some had been sent to wrong ports, and some were buried under munitions. Using her own funds for emergencies, she asked friends at home to provide more.

---

[5] Widmer, Carolyn L.: "Grandfather and Florence Nightingale." *American Journal of Nursing,* 55:569–571, 1955.

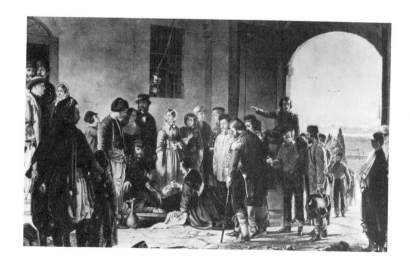

Figure 9–5. Florence Nightingale at Scutari, assessing patient needs and giving directions for care. (Courtesy of *Nursing Mirror.*)

Her evaluation of this unbelievable and unnecessary situation was that of "calamity unparalleled." For years, many have marveled at her ability to analyze need and propose ways of solving problems. The opposition she faced and eventually conquered is a matter of record.

Not only was she a brilliant woman who was intellectually honest, but she was also courageous and exacting in achieving that which would make the world a better place in which to live.

Florence Nightingale's contributions to the field of dietetics have been recognized. She agreed that the physician should prescribe the diet for the patient, but she considered that the science and art of feeding the sick was an essential *part of nursing*.[6] In her plan for reorganization of nursing she emphasized the importance of food selection, preparation and service.

As a child she had visited the families of the poor with her mother, as was the custom in this period, and had learned the food habits and customs of many people. She constantly catalogued information in her mind; thus, she could produce data at a propitious moment and use it for the benefit of society.

The physical care and comfort of the patients reflected her interest and sympathy. Her duties included correspondence with their friends and families containing special messages for their wives and children. She recognized the need for organized occupation and wholesome recreation for soldiers in hospitals and encouraged the establishment of coffee-houses which provided music and recreation. Teachers were assigned to give courses to those interested in increasing their schooling.

In addition to recognizing the needs of persons and the role of the nurse in ministering to these needs, she recognized that the organizational framework in which one functioned affected patient care. Miss Nightingale was unsurpassed as a hospital administrator and hospital reformer. Dr. Schrimpton[7] comments on her book *Notes on Hospitals:* "This is the most practical, scientific work on the construction, management and administration of

Hospitals." A choice comment that depicts Miss Nightingale's gift for identifying incomplete instruction is the following: "We have gone over your draft very carefully and find that although it includes almost everything necessary, it does not define with sufficient precision the manner in which the meat is to get from the commissariat into the soldier's kettle."

In two months she had transformed the hospital into an efficiently managed institution. In six months she had reduced the death rate to *2 per cent*, and had won the respect of most of the surgeons; Lord Raglan, the Commander-in-Chief, gave her his cordial support. Because of her sanitary improvements and the provision of good nursing care for patients, Miss Nightingale reduced the mortality rate from 427 per 1000 in February, 1855, to 22 per 1000 in June, 1855. She utilized the scientific method of gathering data and was skilled as a statistician, presenting the factual evidence in a most graphic way. Dr. C. E. A. Winslow[8] referred to her as the "Lady with the Slide Rule," as well as a lady provided with the lamp of compassion and the broom of efficiency. (See Figure 9–6.)

[8] Winslow, Charles-Edward A.: "Florence Nightingale and public health nursing," *Public Health Nursing, 46:* 331, 1946.

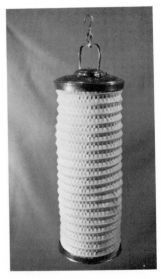

Figure 9–6. A lamp of the type carried by Florence Nightingale in the Crimean War. The outer case collapsed into the brass top and bottom, which held a removable candleholder and a candle. (Author's collection. Photo by DeLores Paul.)

[6] Cooper, Lenna F.: "Florence Nightingale's contribution to dietetics," *Journal of the American Dietetic Association, 30:* 121–127, 1954.
[7] Schrimpton, C.: *The British Army and Miss Nightingale.* Paris, A. and W. Galignani, 1864, pp. 30–34.

Miss Nightingale's interest in statistics and ability in using statistical scientific techniques won her election to the Royal Statistical Society in 1858. This was later followed by an honorary membership in the American Statistical Association in 1874.

The remarkable accomplishments of this great exponent of good nursing care earned her the deepest respect of all who knew of her work. During those first days of her charge, Miss Nightingale stood sometimes twenty consecutive hours superintending personally the distribution of stores and the gradual development of order. She herself, so far as was humanly possible, was with the worst and most terrible cases of wounded and with the dying.

"Before she came," said a soldier, "there was such a cussin' and swearin'; and after that it was as holy as a church." She made rounds with her famous lantern, whose wind shield prevented the candle in the candlestick within the lantern from being extinguished. She brought light and peace to her patients. "She could speak to one and to another, and nod and smile to as many more,... but she couldn't do it all, you know; we lay there by hundreds; but we could kiss her shadow as it fell, and lay our heads on the pillow again content."

Longfellow was moved to a poetic reflection on her wonderful human compassion in his "Santa Filomena:"

> Lo! in that house of misery
> A lady with a lamp I see
>   Pass through the glimmering gloom
>   And flit from room to room.
> And slow as if in a dream of bliss
> The speechless sufferer turns to kiss
>   Her shadow as it falls
>   Upon the darkening walls.
> As if a door in heaven should be
> Opened and then closed suddenly
>   The vision came and went
>   The light shone and was spent.
> A lady with a lamp shall stand
> In the great history of the land
>   A noble type of good
>   Heroic womanhood.

To reflect upon the way in which Miss Nightingale was viewed by her colleagues in the Crimean War, a story has been recorded of a special banquet celebrating the conclusion of the war.

It was given to a number of the more prominent officers who had served in the Crimea, and the talk turned on the different exploits of the war. Lord Stratford de Redcliffe suggested that it would be interesting to discover whose name, in the opinion of all these assembled, would be longest remembered in British history in connection with the war. As it was not possible to discuss the merits of officers present, Lord Stratford de Redcliffe proposed that each officer should write on a slip of paper the name of which he thought, and that he himself should receive and read the slips and announce the name which had gained the majority of votes. . . . when the slips of paper were unfolded, it was found that each officer present had written the same name—Florence Nightingale.

The Irish Sisters of Mercy, fifteen of whom had come about the same time as Miss Nightingale, were working in nearby Kulelie hospital. Conditions were similar, and the sisters had great difficulty in getting supplies or food for their patients. One of them wrote, "The hospital consists of long corridors as far as the eye can reach, with beds at each side; also poor soldiers, both wounded and frost-bitten, lie on the floor. . . . The men had only thin linen suits for a Crimean winter. . . . We are in the wards early and late. When we go to take two hours rest, we groan at the thought of what we leave undone."

A War Office report said of them, "The superiority of an ordered system is beautifully illustrated in the Sisters of Mercy. Their intelligence, delicacy and conscientiousness invest them with a halo of extreme confidence. One can safely consign his most critical cases to their hands."

The next summer, when the work was lighter, Miss Nightingale went with some of the Catholic sisters to the Crimea itself. There she contracted Crimean fever, probably typhus, and was desperately ill. The soldiers wept when they heard that she was ill. England anxiously awaited the outcome. She did not give herself time for proper convalescence and went back to Scutari.

Early in 1856, peace was concluded; the hospitals were closed one by one and the nurses went back, Miss Nightingale last of all, returning in July, 1856. By now she had become the popular heroine. Her name became a synonym for gentleness, efficiency and courage. Despite her retiring disposition, and her efforts to escape publicity, many honors were bestowed on her.[9]

---

[9] Queen Victoria and the Sultan of Turkey had given her beautiful jewels that she wore occasionally in Scutari to please the soldiers, but never at home.

Florence Nightingale's war work encompassed far more than reorganizing nursing and saving lives. It had broken through the age-old prejudice against women in the army, and it led in the end to a new attitude toward nursing and the establishment of a new occupation for women.

Before departing from the Crimean theater of operations, Miss Nightingale visited the cemetery where so many of the soldiers had been buried. She would never forget or ever forgive the fact that so many lives had been lost needlessly by carelessness and ignorance. In her diary she noted, "I stand at the altar of those murdered men and while *I* live I fight their cause."

It has been said that Florence Nightingale was not only "The Lady with the Lamp" carrying light into dark places, but that she was a sort of galvanic battery, stirring and frequently shocking the apathetic public into action. Due to her prodding, Parliament, through the actions of Sir Sidney Herbert, reformed the whole army medical system. Her *Notes on Matters Affecting the Health Efficiency and Hospital Administration of the British Army* formed the basis for these reforms. It took five years of hard, bitter fighting to carry them through, but the pledge she made to the dead soldiers at the Crimea had been fulfilled. Army hospitals and barracks were entirely reconstructed on a sanitary basis. A new code of sanitary regulations was adopted. An army medical college was founded and recreation clubs were established.

Even the health of the soldiers in India received her attention, and vast sanitary and irrigation projects as well as economic reforms were carried out by the government on her recommendations. Two of her reports, *Observations on the Sanitary State of the Army in India* (1863) and *Life or Death in India?* (1873), were forceful levers in this campaign.

The revolution which she initiated in military hospitals was carried over into civilian hospitals. Her book, *Notes on Hospitals* (1859), presented the most exhaustive study that had ever been made on hospital planning and administration. It contained clear, practical wisdom on every phase of hospital work.

Dr. Cope, in his book *Florence Nightingale and the Doctors*, comments:

Few of Miss Nightingale's contemporaries knew so much about hospitals as she did. When she was asked by the members of the Sanitary Commission in 1857 what British and foreign hospitals she had visited, she made this astonishing answer:

I have visited all the hospitals in London, Dublin, Edinburgh, many county hospitals, some of the naval and military hospitals in England; all of the hospitals in Paris and studied with the Sisters of Charity; the Institute of protestant deaconesses at Kaiserswerth on the Rhine where I was twice in training as a nurse; the hospitals in Berlin and many others in Germany, at Lyons, Rome, Alexandria, Constantinople, Brussels; also the war hospitals of the French and Sardinia.[10]

Dr. Cope further emphasizes that to Miss Nightingale a visit to a hospital was not merely a formality but rather a time of concentrated observation. He comments on her skilled observational techniques and her "interest in the general layout of a hospital, as well as in the details of ward construction, sanitation and general administration" in addition to the importance of nursing care. He continues: "It is no wonder that she was consulted about the plans for new hospitals. Doctors everywhere recognized her as an authority, and she obtained an unrivalled acquaintance with the plans of hospitals" in England, Canada, Australia and the United States. The plans for the Johns Hopkins Hospital at Baltimore were taken over to England for her criticism before the first buildings were built.

In December, 1859, a modest black volume containing only 77 pages was published entitled *Notes on Nursing*. The fame of the author made it, in the vernacular of our day, a "best seller." Within a month of publication 15,000 copies had been sold while at the time of her death well over 100,000 had been purchased.

The complete title of this classic is *Notes on Nursing: What It Is and What It Is Not*. The following year Miss Nightingale rewrote it and enlarged its content. It was then published in New York and translated into Italian, German and French.

In 1946, concern for the scarcity of copies of this priceless book prompted a reprinting for modern day appreciation. Dean Emeritus Annie W. Goodrich of Yale University School of Nursing wrote the Foreword.

The timeliness of the revival of *Notes on Nursing*, the plan and purpose of which is so clearly stated in Miss Nightingale's preface, cannot be questioned.

Nearly a century has passed since this woman of

---

[10]Cope, Zachary, M.D.: *Florence Nightingale and The Doctors*, Philadelphia, J. B. Lippincott Company, 1958, pp. 18–19.

great vision and wide experience, as her last contribution to humanity, epitomized in terse, sometimes caustic, but always convincing language, a message to the womanhood of the world.

It is a book which should be owned not only by every member of the nursing profession, but which should find its place in every home, not to replace the ever-increasing body of knowledge relating to the development of that priceless possession of every nation, its child-life, but because it interprets in simple terms the age-old principle of healthy living.

It should be noted that Florence Nightingale makes very clear the distinction between persons professionally qualified for the practice of nursing and the knowledge essential for every woman to whom may come at any time a call to render nursing service in some form.

Though the message of this little book is for all, to none should its appeal be stronger than to the American nurses of the twentieth century who, as teachers, as citizens, and oft-times as mothers, have, through their acquired knowledge, the responsibilities that citizenship in a democracy implies. It is a tragic fact that, despite almost phenomenal advances in the art and science of living, ignorance, poverty and disease still obtain in great degree. Let us hope that this little book will, in this present edition, continue its career of usefulness.

Students today marvel at the current pertinence of these basic principles of good nursing care and how clearly Miss Nightingale delineated the role identification for nurses.

A good nursing staff will perform their duties, more or less satisfactorily, under every disadvantage. But while doing so, their head will always try to improve their surroundings in such a way as to liberate them from subsidiary work and to enable them to devote their time exclusively to the care of the sick. This is, after all, the real purpose of their being there at all, not to act as lifts, water carriers, beasts of burden or steam engines—articles whose labour can be had at vastly less cost than that of educated human beings.[11]

Florence Nightingale was not interested in simply keeping people alive; she stressed that "Nursing is helping people to live."

Long before Dr. Osler pronounced his famous statement, "it is better to know the person who has the disease rather than the disease the patient has," Miss Nightingale had emphasized that one must "Nurse the sick not the sickness."

William J. Bishop of London put Florence Nightingale in proper perspective with today's world when he commented:

Miss Nightingale had always seen to the heart of things that the sick person must be treated and not the disease, that prevention is infinitely better than cure, and that nursing must hold to its ideal but must change some of its methods. And now after a hundred years the ministers of health, the global epidemiologists and the psychosomatic experts are just beginning to catch up with her.

Her ideas and ideals for nursing have not been completely understood or realized.

Florence Nightingale's remarkable demonstration at Crimea first showed the world that thousands of lives which were being wasted could be saved by good, intelligent nursing care, and that skilled nurses were essential in military hospitals. Her insistence from the beginning was that the most intelligent and competent kind of women were required for such work and that they must be especially prepared for it. She would accept no inadequately prepared people on her team, no matter how willing or obedient they might be.

It is no wonder, then, that when the Duke of Cambridge presided over a meeting to organize a plan for presenting a testimonial to Miss Nightingale after the Crimean War the resolutions were:

That the noble exertions of Miss Nightingale and her associates in the hospitals of the East, and the invaluable services rendered by them to the sick and wounded of the British forces, demand the grateful recognition of the British people;

that it is desirable to perpetuate the memory of Miss Nightingale's signal devotion, and to record the gratitude of the nation, by a testimonial of a substantial character;

and that, as she expressed her unwillingness to accept any tribute designed for her own personal advantage, funds be raised to enable her to establish an institution for the training, sustenance, and protection of nurses.

The nation's testimonial of fifty thousand pounds was channeled into the Nightingale Fund Training School for Nurses.

THE NIGHTINGALE SCHOOL FOR NURSES

The Nightingale Training School for Nurses, which opened in 1860, was a completely independent educational institution. St. Thomas's Hospital was selected for the clinical learning experience but a hospital

---

[11] Report of the Committee on the Cubic Space of Metropolitan Workhouses with Papers Submitted to the Committee, 1867, p. 72.

alone was not to be the center for the education and practice of nursing. They were to go also into homes where there was an emphasis on teaching patients and families about the preservation of health. In 1865 Florence Nightingale contributed to two books on nursing in a community setting. She is purported to have written an eloquent appeal for its extension in London. Miss Nightingale helped to found the first Community Nursing Association in Liverpool and outlined the whole basis of our modern public health nursing movement.

There were two major components to nursing in her thinking—"sick nursing" and "health nursing." This involved the preservation of "wellness" as well as the care of illness. She said that "Nursing proper is therefore to help the patient suffering from disease to live, just as health nursing is to keep or put the constitution of a healthy human being in such a state as to have no disease." Community health home care services have continued under the aegis of nursing to the present. It is gratifying to note that she was appalled at the criminal wastefulness of preventable disease.

The school of nursing which she founded prospered. Because she was a highly educated woman, she exemplified vividly what higher education could do for a person preparing for public service. She was probably better educated than many men of her period, even most doctors. She was a champion of educational opportunities for other groups. In the army she founded schools for soldiers, courses for the orderlies and cooks, and even fostered the founding of a medical school for officers.

The *aims* of the *Nightingale School* were to train hospital nurses; to train nurses to train others; and to train district nurses for the sick poor. The length of the program was one year. The size of the classes was small, which permitted a high degree of selectivity—between 1000 to 2000 applications were received, but only 15 to 30 students were admitted.

Of the two classes of students admitted, one was made up of educated probationers. This class paid a tuition fee. The other group of students was not required to pay a fee; their expenses were taken care of by the Nightingale Fund.

In 1875, a home sister or clinical instructor was appointed. She was *Mary Crossland*, who appears to have done a creditable piece of work in planning a program of clinical instruction. (See Figure 9–7.) Her efforts have been preserved in the letters that she wrote to Miss Nightingale of her progress. Her enthusiasm inspired several doctors to join in taking the students on clinical rounds. Mrs. Seymer[12] gives an example from a letter written on November 8, 1879:

Mr. Croft gave us rather a new style of clinical lecture this morning—some had expressed a desire to understand about aneurisms—so instead of beginning to tell, Mr. Croft asked questions: asked Miss G. if she had ever come across a case in the wards. She had, in a Medical ward. He then asked her to state what she had observed about the case, such as symptoms of pain, difficulty of breathing—cough—position of patient—diet—treatment, to

_____

[12]Seymer, Lucy R.: "Mary Crossland of the Nightingale Training School" *American Journal of Nursing, 61*:86, 1961.

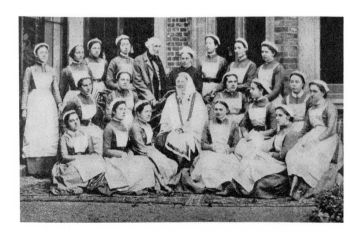

Figure 9–7. Miss Nightingale (center) and nurses of St. Thomas' Hospital, London, 1887. Lord Verney and Miss Crossland appear behind her.

all of which she gave good answers. Then Mr. Croft explained the cause of the different symptoms—the effect of diet and treatment and what share a nurse had in seeing the treatment was carefully carried out.

As early as 1867, Miss Nightingale's contractual agreements provided that in addition to her salary received from the hospital, the ward sister (head nurse) was paid by the Nightingale Endowment Fund for assisting in the training of students. The medical instructors were to be paid in a similar fashion. The arrangement with the hospital specified that there must always be a staff of experienced nurses for the care of the patients and in addition that there must be a well qualified graduate charge nurse to direct or teach those under her aegis. The head nurses were to keep weekly summary records of the work of each student; the matron recorded monthly summaries. Students were to keep diaries of their educational experiences. The students were to be taught to detect symptoms and the reasons for these symptoms and were to be given sufficient time to understand the reasons. She stressed the need for guidance for the student.

Miss Nightingale, in her *Suggestions for the Improvement of the Nursing Service of Hospitals*, inveighed against using nurses for cleaning and scrubbing. Her words were: "A nurse should do nothing but nurse. If you want a charwoman, hire one. Nursing is a specialty." It was her feeling that the hospital environment should encourage the nurse to nurse rather than to frustrate and thwart her efforts. Premature responsibility and overwork were recognized as dangers to sound growth and frequently encouraged the student to become disinterested in nursing. She encouraged step savers such as hot water piped up to the patient's floor, a lift or elevator to bring up the patient's food, a system of bells with valves that flew open and remained open until nurses could detect which patient needed her, a nursing environment that keeps pace with progress and an attitude of willingness on the part of the matron (director of nursing service) to see that nothing prevented the students from nursing. Her brilliant mind could not envision anything stereotyped or inflexible. For this reason, she did not approve of graduation for she stated: "Nursing is a progressive art in which to stand still is to have gone back." To have the idea that one had mastered a field of learning was abhor-

rent to one who had said: "Progress can never end but with a nurse's life."

Refresher courses were recommended by Miss Nightingale to keep nurses up to date in their field.

Miss Nightingale's plans met with opposition, chiefly from doctors. Of a hundred doctors whose opinion was asked, only four favored the idea. They themselves had given the nurses at St. Thomas' their training, and felt it was very good. One said, "Nurses are in much the same position as housemaids, and need little teaching beyond poultice-making and the enforcement of cleanliness and attention to the patient's wants." Another doctor said publicly, "A nurse is a confidential servant, but still only a servant. . . . She should be middle-aged when she begins nursing; and if somewhat tamed by marriage and the troubles of a family, so much the better."

A few doctors did understand what the movement might mean. One said, "A trained and educated nurse would soon become most popular and trusted. She would cooperate with the physician, her presence would inspire confidence in the patient, and she would restore peace and order to a distracted household."

Miss Nightingale envisioned a collaborative role for the nurse with the doctor. The English physician, Dr. Saleeby, has reflected that "if Lister was the father, then Florence Nightingale was the mother of modern surgery." Certainly without the reforms in nursing and hospital work which she introduced, the triumphs of modern medicine and surgery would have been impossible.

It was hoped that Miss Nightingale would take charge of the school, but her health was not equal to it. At this time she rarely went out, though she saw many persons on business relating to hospitals or nursing. It was very difficult to get an appointment with her, and could be done only if she were convinced that the one who sought it was in earnest. *Mrs. Wardroper*, who had been for some years at St. Thomas' and had used the untrained personnel, was chosen to take charge. For many years, however, Miss Nightingale selected the students and advised on details.

Miss Nightingale herself, keen at judging character, chose the students for their personal qualities as well as for their ability. They were required to read and write *well*. Those who saw the early Nightingale nurses were impressed with "the bright, kindly and pleasant spirit which seemed to pervade them." The ward "sisters," i.e., those in charge of departments or wards, were chosen for their teaching ability; they were expected to instruct the students on the wards. Miss Nightingale insisted that students be taught *why* things were so, and that they be given *time* to learn.

Despite its founder's prestige, the school faced many difficulties in its first ten years. One by one the doctors were convinced, and slowly the public came to see what an educated nurse meant.

Miss Nightingale was personally acquainted not only with the Queen and her Cabinet, but with every Prime Minister of her time, and many of the royalty of other nations. Eminent men came to her for advice.

She was an advocate of equal suffrage. She said, "I am convinced that political power is the greatest it is possible to wield for human happiness, and until women have their part in it in an open, direct manner, the evils of the world can never be satisfactorily dealt with." She opposed registration for nurses, and prevented the passage of a registration act in Great Britain for many years.

In 1859, Miss Nightingale published *Notes on Hospitals*, considered the most valuable work of its kind. Before her time, most hospitals had imposing and beautiful buildings, but lacked things pertaining to the comfort of the patients. Her practical mind and deep sympathy made her persevere until she convinced some that sanitation and convenience are more important than architecture. Her book, *Notes on Nursing*, has been an invaluable aid for all nurses. A few quotations from it are worth studying.

Health is not only to be well but to be able to use well every power we have.

Nursing proper is therefore to help the patient suffering from disease to live, just as health nursing is to keep or put the constitution of the healthy . . . being in such a state as to have no disease.

The suffering considered to be due to disease is often not disease at all, but due to want of fresh air, of warmth, of cleanliness, of quiet, of care in the administration of food.

Volumes are written upon the effect of the mind upon the body. I wish that more thought was given to the effect of the body upon the mind.

Merely looking at the sick is not always observing. It needs a high degree of training to look so that looking shall tell the nurse aright. A conscientious nurse is not necessarily an observing nurse, and life or death may lie with the good observer.

The matron [director of nurses] should be one whose desire is that her students shall learn — a rarer thing than is usually supposed. . . .

She defined nursing as that care which put a person in the best possible condition for nature to restore or to preserve health, to prevent or to cure disease or injury. Miss Nightingale stressed that the sick person must be treated and not the disease, she identified a "nurse the sick not the sickness" philosophy many years before Dr. Osler pronounced his famous statement: "It is better to know the patient who has the disease than the disease the patient has."

Florence Nightingale died in August, 1910, at the age of 90. Her family was asked to allow her to be buried in Westminster Abbey, but they knew her wishes and refused. Her grave is in the family plot at East Wellow, near Romney, in Hampshire, and its only mark is a small cross with her initials and dates. (There are monuments to her in London, Derby, Milbank, Florence and Calcutta, India, and beautiful memorials in St. Paul's Cathedral, London and at St. Thomas' Hospital.)

Florence Nightingale had raised the status of nursing to a dignified occupation, improved the quality of nursing care and was the founder of modern nursing education.

Few women in history have been endowed with her rare intellect and driving force and few women have exerted so far-reaching an influence on so many.

John Greenleaf Whittier dedicated a poem to "Florence Nightingale of England" in May of 1882.

Where pity, love and tenderness
Are found, (there) Christ must be;
So wheresoe'er thy footsteps press
His presence walks with thee.

In summary, Florence Nightingale was intellectually and academically, as well as financially, wealthy. She was probably better educated than most men of her period, especially most doctors. Miss Nightingale knew how to analyze situations, to present facts and to direct others and was gifted in interpersonal relationships and qualities of leadership. Her students of nursing were receiving a better preparation than most students of medicine. Miss Nightingale had an indomitable spirit behind an attractive and gracious exterior. She was not a submissive, sweet, smiling, quiet person but a gifted, brilliant, dynamic, forceful leader whose thoughts and desires were channeled into results. She had two aspects to her nature: a tremendous will power that wilted those who opposed her and a fantastic compassion for all who suffered. She was admired by scholars the world over.

Florence Nightingale foretold the transition of nursing as it moved from the prescientific to the scientifically oriented society in which it now functions.

How different might nursing education and nursing service have been if Florence Nightingale's philosophy had really been understood and practiced by all nurses; for her ideas and plans have not yet been fully realized. The world is richer because of her wisdom, brilliance and action.

Florence Nightingale's vision set into motion a most creative, social force which exemplified man's concern for his fellow man. She became a legend in her own time and a living memorial to the fact that nursing has a vital independent, as well as a collaborative, role.

THE WAR BETWEEN THE STATES (1861–1865)

On April 14, 1861, when *President Lincoln* summoned 75,000 volunteers for the Union Army, there was no army nurse corps, organized medical corps, or ambulance or field hospital service.

Members of many religious orders promptly volunteered and gave superior care to soldiers in their own hospitals, in army hospitals and on the battlefield (Fig. 9–8). One form of recognition of their outstanding contribution to both the Union and Confederate troops was the erection of the memorial monument, "Nuns of the Battlefield," in Washington, D.C. This remains a tribute to the nearly 600 sisters of 12 religious orders who served so heroically during this crucial period.

The nursing of some of the largest government hospitals was assigned to them. "There was an immense enthusiasm among the laity, but a total lack of experience and efficient organization. . . . The first hospitals were mostly empty barns or warehouses . . . but in the hands of the Sisters they became finally a model for European military sanitation."

All the Catholic nursing sisters received many compliments from the government because of their efficiency. Jefferson Davis paid them highest tribute and Abraham Lincoln gave them permission to purchase all supplies needed for their work. The sisters neither asked for nor received any compensation for their labors.

Yet these hundreds of devoted sisters were not enough to care for so many wounded and sick. Hundreds of lay nurses were needed to supplement them.

Outside of the religious orders, there were

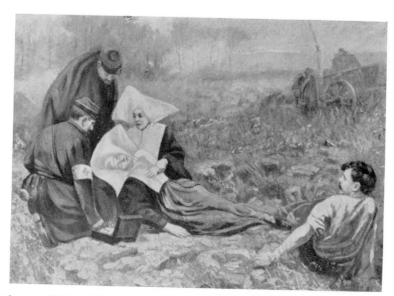

Figure 9–8. The Innocent Victim. A Sister of Charity killed on a Civil War battlefield while ministering to the wounded.

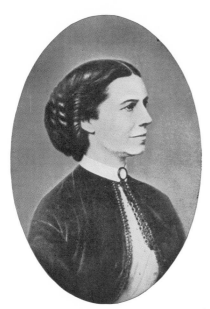

Figure 9–9. Clara Barton. (From a photograph taken during the Civil War.)

almost no other nurses with any real training. Women did request permission to be of assistance, and two such women were Clara Barton and Mother Bickerdyke.

Clara Barton (Fig. 9–9) (1821–1912), of North Oxford, Massachusetts, was born Clarissa Harlowe, but later changed her name to the simpler one by which she has been known and remembered.

When the Sixth Massachusetts Regiment arrived in Washington on April 19, 1861, she was there to dress the wounds of the men and feed them. Another project she undertook was supervising the shipment of field supplies in the wagon train that had been sent down for the soldiers. It is recorded that on one of her journeys with the wagon train, a herd of cattle to be used for food for the army was being driven ahead of the train. As this wagon train passed a Confederate hospital, the surgeon begged for assistance for his patients who were starving. The officer in charge of the cattle asked Miss Barton, "What can I do? I am a bonded officer and responsible for the property in my charge." "You can do nothing," she replied, "but ride on ahead. I am neither bonded nor responsible." Soon an ox was extricated from the herd and went to the grateful surgeon of the Confederate army.

Mary Ann Bickerdyke (1817–1901), affectionately called *Mother Bickerdyke*, responded to an urgent plea by her minister, Henry Ward Beecher (the brother of Harriet Beecher Stowe), for some women in his congregation to go to the government hospitals and battlefields and care for the sick and wounded (Fig. 9–10). She was a dynamic and

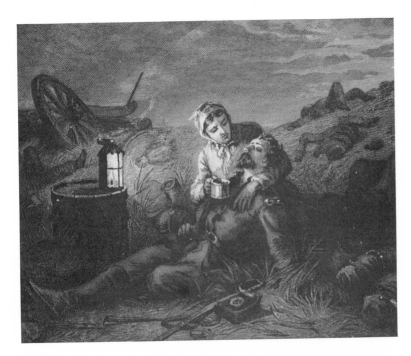

Figure 9–10. Mother Bickerdyke searching the battlefield at midnight to comfort the neglected or forgotten patient.

kind-hearted woman who gave the soldiers very good care. Mother Bickerdyke was of humble origin and moderate education, a widow, with two little sons. She had taken Dr. Hahnemann's short course in homeopathy and received a degree of Doctor of Botanic Medicine.[13] This background was useful in her nursing care of the wounded.

Dr. Brockett[14] describes the devoted attention she showered upon the enlisted men with but a private's pay, a private's fare and a private's dangers. She stressed that these boys were dear to somebody, and she would be a mother to them and fight for their rights and comfort. She is remembered as the "Soldier's Friend." The soldiers idolized her. Indeed, Dr. Brockett states: "woe to the surgeon, the commissary or quartermaster, whose neglect of his men and selfish disregard for their interests and needs came under her cognizance." (See Figure 9–11.)

Her efforts were remembered by the government when they launched the hospital ship, the S.S. *Mary A. Bickerdyke*, at Richmond, California, in 1943.

Although there were women such as these

two outstanding persons, there was still a need for more nurses. The public had been stimulated by the newspaper accounts of the medical treatment at some military camps, the lack of care for sick soldiers at these centers, the insufficiency of supplies and inadequacy of transportation so that surgical dressings or drugs were absent when most needed.

On June 10, 1861, *Dorothea Lynde Dix* (Fig. 9–12) was appointed *Superintendent of the Female Nurses of the Army*. From the Secretary of War, she was given the responsibility and authority to recruit and equip a corps of army nurses.

Document 213
To Volunteer Nurses
War Department, Military Hospital

Be it known to all whom it may concern that the free services of Miss D. L. Dix are accepted by the War Department, and that she will give at all times all necessary aid in organizing military hospitals for the care of all sick and wounded soldiers, aiding the chief surgeons by supplying nurses and substantial means for the comfort and relief of the suffering; also, that she is fully authorized to receive, control and disburse special supplies bestowed by individuals or associations for the comfort of their friends or the citizen soldiers from all parts of the United States.

Given under the seal of the War Department this twenty-third day of April, in the year of our

---

[13]Baker, Nina B.: *Cyclone in Calico.* Boston, Little, Brown & Co., 1952, pp. 18–20.

[14]Brockett, L. P.: *The Camp, the Battle Field, and the Hospital;* or *Lights and Shadows of the Great Rebellion.* Philadelphia, National Publishing Company, 1866.

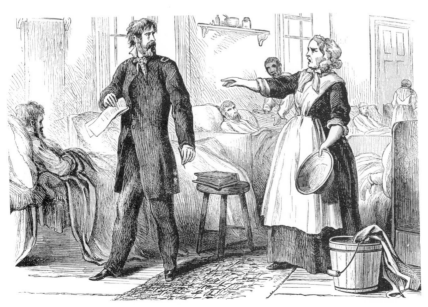

Figure 9–11. Because of her deep concern for the soldiers, Mother Bickerdyke often castigated a neglectful surgeon. (Author's collection.)

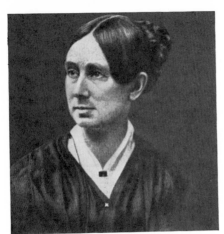

Figure 9–12. Dorothea Lynde Dix. (Courtesy of *The Trained Nurse and Hospital Review.*)

Lord one thousand eight hundred and sixty-one, and of the independence of the United States the eighty-fifth.

S/Simon Cameron
Secretary of War.

Military rank, so very important, was not given to her or the members of her corps. Miss Dix did not have a background of nurse's training as Miss Nightingale did, but she had established a record of organizational skill in her previous humanitarian achievements.

The qualifications of the army nurses stated that the women who were recruited must be over 30 and preferably 35, plain-looking women, dressed in brown or black with no ornamentation—no bows, no curls, no jewelry and no hoop skirts. Miss Dix soon had 2000 capable, enthusiastic women ready to serve the armed forces. Women from all parts of the country offered their services.

UNITED STATES SANITARY COMMISSION

In the late spring of 1861, handbills were distributed in New York City signed by over 90 respected ladies announcing a mass meeting at Cooper Union. More than 4000 determined women attended. They organized *The Women's Central Association for Relief.* This group and others of similar interest and organization banded together. The leaders of this newly formed group cajoled a Unitarian clergyman, Henry W. Bellows, D.D., of New England; a physician, Elisha Harris; and three other doctors into going to Washington to plead for the establishment of a Sanitary Commission.

The United States Sanitary Commission was established by order of President Lincoln on June 13, 1861. (See Figure 9–13.)

One of the reports of the Sanitary Commission revealed that 15 per cent of the physicians in the Northern regiments were either poorly qualified or totally incompetent for their task. Needless to say, the medical officers of the Army were resentful of the interference of the Commission in attempting to improve the medical care of the soldiers. Much is now known that might not have been disclosed but for their constant vigilance, and much was prevented that might have been disastrous for the welfare of mankind. The results of their endeavors included pavilion hospitals that could be dismantled and moved, standards for camp water supply systems, latrines and garbage disposal.

After the first battles of the war, the wounded had practically no care. "Common soldiers, untrained, lazy, and indifferent or brutal, were cooks and nurses for the war hospitals, the largest of which had forty

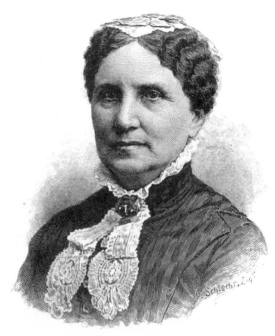

Figure 9–13. Mary A. Livermore (1820–1905), the devout advocate of suffrage and education for women, served with the United States Sanitary Commission during the Civil War.

beds. There were no medicines, no stores, nor ambulances. The camps were dirty and unsanitary." Those who knew of these conditions were filled with shame and resolved to do something about it. When they first offered supplies and service, the Government Medical Bureau looked upon the proposal with suspicion, but dire need soon forced it to accept. The Commission collected and distributed supplies of all sorts, planned camps and attended to their sanitation, tended the wounded on the field and in hospitals; in short, the Commission undertook a large share of the health work for the army. It provided such things as green vegetables, given by the farmers for the soldiers; thus, they prevented scurvy, the great army scourge. (Dehydrated vegetables were used, on the suggestion of a Harvard professor, in 1864.) In 1862, the Commission equipped a hospital train, an entirely new idea (Fig. 9–14). Called "the largest army charity the world has ever seen," the Commission collected and spent over $5,000,000 in cash and $15,000,000 in supplies, an unprecedented amount for those days.

The Women's Central Association eventually became a branch of the U.S. Sanitary Commission. An important activity which was assumed by the Women's Central Association for Relief was that of sending nurses to war areas where the need seemed most crucial (Fig. 9–15). Preparatory to their departure, an experience was planned for them at New York Hospital and Bellevue Hospital, as well as several Boston hospitals, for one month's observation and work.

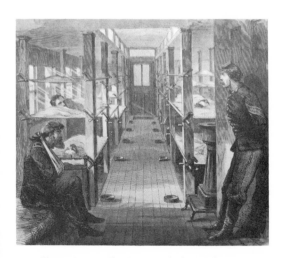

Figure 9–14. The interior of a hospital train.

RESPONSE OF NURSE VOLUNTEERS

Many members of the *Woolsey family* participated in nursing. Miss Austin[15] presents a fascinating account of a well-to-do family's involvement in the Civil War as well as in the development of a new approach to nursing education. Mrs. Woolsey together with her daughters Abby, Jane, Carry, Hatty, Georgy and Eliza contributed their talents in either nursing care or in making hospital supplies.

Georgeanna (Georgy) Woolsey was one of the first young ladies to be admitted to New York Hospital for a brief instruction and to "walk the wards." She then requested to join the ranks of Dorothea Dix. Georgy and her sister *Eliza Woolsey Howland* went to Washington to care for the army of the sick who were housed in every conceivable building. After a conference with Miss Dix, they commenced their volunteer nursing activities at Georgetown Hospital. While carrying out their nursing duties it became obvious that chaplains were needed. Thereupon Georgy wrote to President Lincoln requesting the appointment of chaplains to hospitals. She even delivered the letter to the back door of the White House. The President responded by the appointment of seven chaplains.

The opposition of physicians to women nurses and the lengths to which they resorted to encourage their return home are well documented by many of the volunteer nurses including Georgeanna Woolsey.[16] The almost insurmountable task faced by Miss Dix can thus be understood.

In 1864 Georgeanna Woolsey wrote:[17]

No one knows, who did not watch the thing from the beginning, how much opposition, how much ill-will, how much unfeeling want of thought these women nurses endured. . . . Government had decided that women should be employed, and the army surgeons . . . determined to make their lives so unbearable that they would be forced in self-defense to leave. . . .

Some of the bravest women I have ever known were among the first company of army nurses. They saw at once the position of affairs, the attitude assumed by the surgeons and the wall

[15]Austin, Anne L.: *The Woolsey Sisters of New York — 1860–1900.* Philadelphia, American Philosophical Society, 1971.
[16]*Ibid.,* p. 50 and p. 112.
[17]*Ibid.,* p. 112.

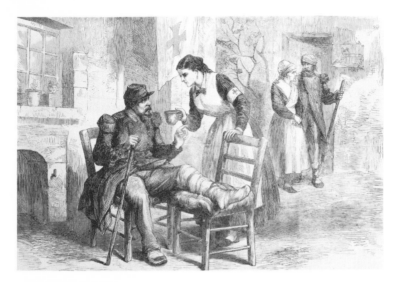

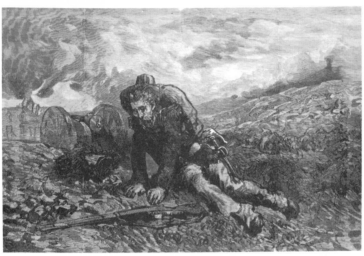

Figure 9–15. These pictures appeared in *Harper's Weekly* in 1871 and were marked "Cared For" and "Uncared For." They reflect the importance of the nurse in helping people to live. (Author's collection.)

against which they were expected to break and scatter; and they set themselves to undermine the whole thing.

None of them were "strong-minded." Some of them were women of the truest refinement and culture; and day after day they quietly and patiently worked, doing, by order of the surgeon, things which not one of those gentlemen would have dared to ask of a woman whose male relative stood able and ready to defend her and report him. I have seen small white hands scrubbing floors, washing windows and performing all menial offices. I have known women, delicately cared for at home, half fed in hospitals, hard worked day and night, and given, when sleep must be had, a wretched closet just large enough for a camp bed to stand in. I have known surgeons who purposely and ingeniously arranged these inconveniences with the avowed intention of driving away all women from their hospitals.

As the casualties increased, provision for their return to hospitals for care involved the use of transport steamers, in effect, *floating hospitals* (Fig. 9–16). Four nurses were assigned the duty of caring for patients on transports—Georgeanna Woolsey, her sister Eliza Howland, *Katherine Wormeley* and *Christine Griffin*.

Jane Stuart Woolsey, after receiving experience in nursing in hospitals in New York City, commenced her activities in the theater of war operations. Her refreshing reflections of this experience are presented in *Hospital Days*.[18] She praises the thoughtful inclusion of game-boxes or books for patients who might enjoy them; the green shades that were

[18]Woolsey, Jane Stuart: *Hospital Days.* New York, Van Nostrand, 1868, p. 47.

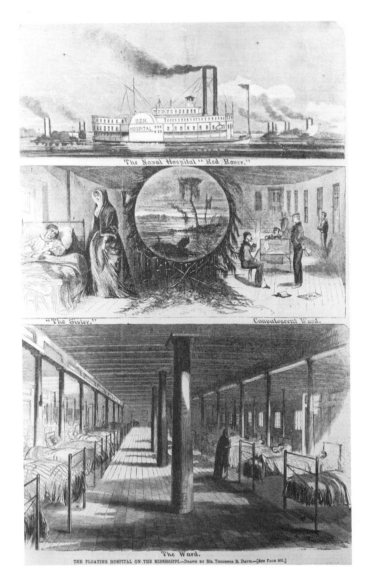

Figure 9–16. Hospital steamers, floating hospitals, transported many soldiers from the war theater. Nurses were in charge of the care given. (Author's collection.)

lowered to protect the eyes of feverish patients; the prints on the wall for diversion; and the rocking chairs with their swinging motion to relieve nervous tension. Soft, light slippers were provided for the men-nurses in the ward because it was understood that the heavy thud of a boot is "almost as intolerable to a patient as a 'sympathizer' sitting on the edge of his bed."

Indeed she opines:

No one can count up the value of these things, not only in the flannels for discharged, broken-down men, and woolen socks and mittens for convalescents going on guard in puddles of snow-water, but the distraction from pain in wounded men, the occupation and interest furnished to

wretches, bored, half sick, half well, wholly demoralized men who huddle in a hopeless way round the red-hot sheet-iron stoves.

Her concepts of nursing permeate her book. She describes her plan for learning about each patient's fancies and home habits; the changes in physical and mental condition; talking *with* them, listening to them, and writing for them; helping them invent occupations and amusements to while away the hours; and remembering that "many sad wives and poor children depend on my promptness" in analyzing each patient's need and carrying out the best possible regimen to hasten his return to health.

Miss Woolsey relates an incident in which her sister Georgy interacts with the doctor for a better approach to patient care.[19]

On one of these nights a nurse came hurriedly up with the word, "There's a man dying in Ward _____; we can't do anything for him."—"Has he taken anything since he came in?"—"No'm, can't eat nothin', doctor says musn't give him no stimulants, stomach's too weak." "I'll have a look at him," says G (Georgy)—and after the nurse goes out—"the surgeon doesn't know a bronchitis from a broken leg. There's not a man in that ward who ought to die.—If he is dying, he is dying of starvation." She hunts up the doctor and asks if wine-whey, the lightest of stimulants, may be tried. Doctor didn't know what it was, but had no objection; "man couldn't live anyhow." The man took the cup full eagerly, was "out of danger" in the morning, got well,—the doctor directing the nurse to be very particular to "give him his wine-whey 'reg'lar"—went back to the field and helped to take Richmond.

Miss Woolsey stressed that she followed "those who were assigned to carry trays" and she served those who were unable to serve themselves, and checked to see that every person had enough food or obtained more suitable food. She carried a memorandum book with her as she watched patients and made notations. For example: "Mr. M_____ has expressed a longing for some Boston brown bread. Memo: try and get him some. For a patient whose appetite was on the wane and who didn't feel the effort to eat was worthwhile. Memo: try champagne in a long-spouted cup."

This most remarkable family received much gratitude from nurses, patients and their families for devotion and superior nursing care.

Louisa May Alcott (Fig. 9–17) (1832–1888) was the daughter of Bronson Alcott, whose influence prompted the rise of the Trans-cendental Movement. Miss Alcott cooled feverish brows, soothed the fears of 12-year-old drummer boys and recorded her efforts in letters which she signed "Nurse Periwinkle." Later, her letters appeared in *Hospital Sketches*, published in 1863. Reflecting on her daily routine, she wrote:

Up at six, dress by gaslight, run through my ward and throw up the windows, though the men grumble and shiver. But the air is bad enough to breed a pestilence . . . till noon I trot, trot, trot,

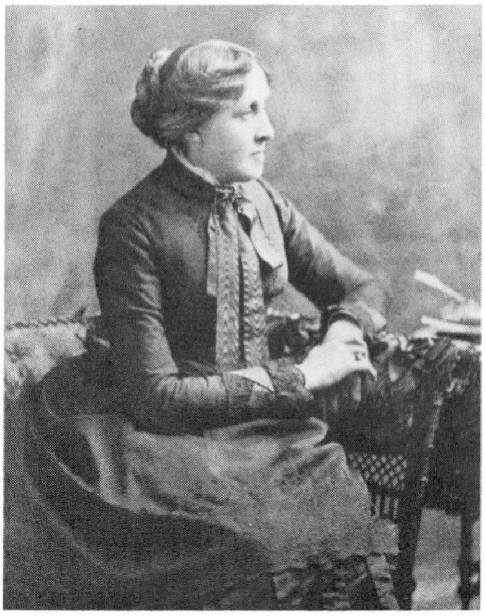

Figure 9–17. Louisa May Alcott in 1887.

giving out rations, cutting up food for helpless 'boys,' washing faces, teaching my attendants how beds are made or floors are swept, dressing wounds. . . . At twelve comes dinner for patients and afterward letter writing for them or reading aloud. . . . Supper at five sets everyone running who can run. . . . Evening amusements. . . . Then, for such as need them, the final doses for the night.

She reported that she "ministered to their minds by writing letters" to their families for them. She noted that many boys wore bags of camphor around their neck for protection against disease.

Her common sense and ability to protest against lack of organization in nursing service was displayed when she registered disapproval of the use of convalescents as attendants. She deplored not having enough help or the right kind:[20]

If any hospital director fancies this a good and economical arrangement allow one used up nurse to tell him it isn't, and beg him to spare the sisterhood who sometimes in their sympathy, forget that they are mortal, and run the risk of being made immortal, sooner than is agreeable to their partial friends.

Dr. Brockett's book[21] presents many nursing care studies of these heroic and good

---

[19]*Ibid.*, p. 121.

[20]Alcott, Louisa M.: *Hospital Sketches*. Boston, James Redpath, 1863, p. 74.
[21]*Op. cit.*, pp. 293–454.

nurses of the Civil War era. Several of the studies described the activities of Louisa May Alcott.

Of Georgeanna Woolsey's work, Dr. Brockett states[22] that she was one of the most efficient ladies where her constant cheerfulness, her ready wit, her never failing resources of contrivance and management in any emergency, made the severe labor seem light, and by keeping up the spirits of the entire party, prevented the scenes of suffering constantly presented from rendering them morbid and depressed.

Walt Whitman (Fig. 9–18) (1819–1892) has left a monumental record of the care of the sick during the Civil War in his collection of poems, *Drum-Taps,* and in *Specimen Days,* his diary, which contained vivid descriptions of his experiences as a hospital nurse in Washington. His younger brother George enlisted in the Thirteenth Regiment. When news reached Whitman that his brother had been

wounded, he rushed to Fredericksburg, Virginia, to be of assistance. His sensitive nature was so moved that he was unable to leave the sick. His major role was not so much to meet the physical needs as to meet the psychological ones. The emotional trauma suffered by these heroic soldiers could only be understood and appreciated by those who witnessed the tragedy.

He was a familiar figure wandering from ward to ward passing out books and other comforts, offering to listen to the boys and to write letters for them. He used his literary talents to expose the inefficiency and negligence that he noted as he observed the military procedures. His objective in these articles was to move the indifferent public. He played a dual role of war correspondent and nurse. His presentation of the sufferings of men and his efforts in their behalf are set forth in "The Dresser":

> Bearing the bandages, water and sponge,
> Straight and swift to my wounded I go,
> Where they lie on the ground after the battle
>   brought in,

---

[22] Brockett, L. P.: *Woman's Work in the Civil War: A Record of Heroism, Patriotism and Patience.* Boston, R. H. Curran Co., 1867, p. 327.

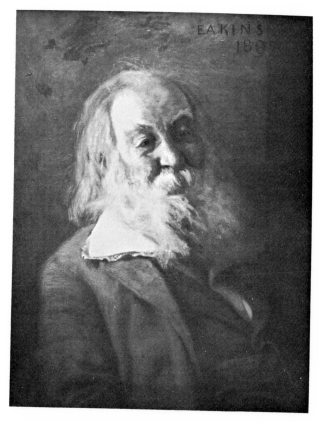

Figure 9–18. Walt Whitman by Thomas Eakins (1887). (Courtesy of the Pennsylvania Academy of the Fine Arts.)

Where their priceless blood reddens the grass,
   the ground,
Or to the rows of the hospital tent, or under
   the roof'd hospital,
To the long rows or cots up and down each
   side I return,
To each and all one after another I draw near,
   not one do I miss,
I onward go, I stop,
With hinged knees and steady hands to dress
   wounds,
I am firm with each, the pangs are sharp yet
   unavoidable,
One turns to me his appealing eyes — poor boy!
   I never knew you,
Yet I think I could not refuse this moment to
   die for you, if that would save you.

On the Confederate side, religious sisters and lay women gave heroic service. The Confederate Army did not appoint a director of nursing, but *President Jefferson Davis* bestowed the rank of *Captain* on a most deserving candidate, *Miss Sally Tompkins*. Miss Tompkins was a well-to-do young Southern lady who was active in the charitable works of her church. She had taken care of many sick persons so that after the battle of Bull Run when Judge Robertson had offered the use of his home as a hospital, she was placed in charge of it. When private hospitals were ordered closed, she begged President Davis to intercede for the soldiers and her hospital, and the Robertson hospital was not closed. She refused the customary remuneration but accepted food, medicines and other supplies in lieu of a salary.

The nursing care given by Miss Tompkins must have been of a superior quality because by the end of the war, her records indicated that only 73 patients died out of 1333 who had received care in the Robertson hospital.

Many refined, self-sacrificing ladies nursed the wounded day and night. Their heroic benevolence inspired others to join them. Among these women were *Miss Kate Cumming*, *Mrs. Ella Newson* and *Mrs. Gilmer*. Hospitals were named in honor of Mrs. Newsom and Mrs. Gilmer.

Kate Cumming's diary of her activities as a volunteer nurse with the Confederate Army has been preserved as an important primary source material of this epoch of history.[23]

---

[23]Cumming, Kate: *Kate: The Journal of a Confederate Nurse.* Richard Barksdale Harwell (ed.). Baton Rouge, Louisiana State University Press, 1959.

It was published in 1865. She states, "I had never been inside of a hospital and was wholly ignorant of what I should be called upon to do, but I knew that what one woman (Florence Nightingale) had done, another could."

Impressive are her accounts of the sick and wounded, their care, or lack of it, on battlefields and in hospitals. She relates problems concerning the quartermaster, transportation, food, shelter, fuel, lighting, clothing, communications and many tribulations. She describes amputations, hospital gangrene, contagion, smallpox and typhoid fever. In a sense of deep humility she bemoans with regret that "she failed to be more useful." Many of these cultured, dedicated women recognized the need for well educated nurses.

The mansion of *Robert E. Lee* was converted into a hospital, and here the wounded from the Civil War's first important battle, Bull Run, were brought. Now the mansion's beautiful estate is known as *Arlington National Cemetery*.

Temporary hospitals were organized in any available building. Other structures were hastily erected or tents were pitched. Public buildings were commandeered. At one time the Capitol in Washington was converted into a hospital; 400 wounded were nursed in the Senate and House and 300 in the rotunda. Hospital steamers are said to have originated during this war, and many were in service along the Ohio and the Mississippi. There were also hospital trains.

In many hospitals there were ward masters and orderlies who did as much of the nursing as they could. The women nurses dressed wounds, gave medicines and attended to diets. The hours of duty were long. There were many medical cases, fevers, dysentery and even smallpox, and many nurses died of disease contracted in the line of duty. (See Figure 9–19.)

Despite all efforts, many soldiers had insufficient care and many died from neglect. After some battles hundreds of wounded were laid in open sheds or temporary shelters without bedding, and there were only a few surgeons to look after them. The so-called "ambulances" were often only springless wagons.

During the Civil War, many of the medicines made from herbs were obtained from the *Shakers*, or the *United Society of Believers*

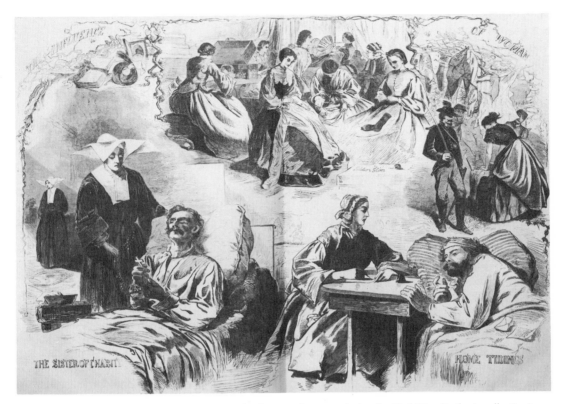

Figure 9–19. A montage of the activities and influence of women during the Civil War. (Author's collection.)

in Christ's Second Coming. They were the first group in the United States to grow herbs for the pharmaceutical market.[24] Their main industrial enterprise was the cultivation of herbs; they collected them, dried them or extracted the medicinal ingredients, and packed and shipped them.

The Shakers were meticulously clean and had an efficient system of preparing these medicines. In addition to the beautifully cared-for gardens, there was an herb house where the herbs were dried and packaged; another building was called the extract house where presses and boilers were located. Water, the well known universal solvent, was brought by clay pipes from mountain springs. This provided a pure water supply. Raffinesque,[25] the famous French-American botanist, said, "The best medical gardens in the United States are those established by the communities of Shakers or Modern Essenes."

---

[24]Andrews, Edward D., and Andrews, Faith: *Shaker Herbs and Herbalists.* Stockbridge, Mass., Berkshire Garden Center, 1959, p. 3.

[25]*Ibid.,* p. 4

THE RED CROSS SOCIETY

One of the dramatically significant movements of the nineteenth century was the development of the Red Cross society. It was originally an association of citizens, who undertook to render effective help in time of war or calamity. In the beginning it was meant only for war, but soon came to include all calamities that involved a considerable number of people.

For centuries there had been societies for helping the wounded in time of war, many of which had done efficient work. The Red Cross idea was far greater than anything that went before it, in that it placed the work on an *international* basis and suggested teamwork between nations, a thing almost unheard of before that time.

The plan originated in the mind of *Jean Henri Dunant,* a Swiss, and the work owes its effectiveness to the greatness of his ingenuity. Dunant said that Florence Nightingale had inspired him.

In 1859, while traveling in Italy, Dunant saw the field of Solferino on the day after the battle in which 300,000 were engaged.

He helped in caring for the wounded and was horrified by the needless suffering that he saw. He wrote a vivid description of it, began lecturing on the subject and interviewed kings, princes, generals and church officials. It was his vision and persistence that brought about this work of such incalculable value.

In 1863 Dunant formulated a plan by which he proposed to organize in every country an association for war relief. Each was to be an independent society, with a strong international bond of affiliation and a guaranteed neutrality of supplies and personnel. The result was that in October, 1863, an international conference was held at Geneva, Switzerland, where representatives of 16 nations agreed to a provisional program. This led to the formation of an international Red Cross society. The United States had sent no official delegate, as she was in the midst of the Civil War and harassed by her own problems.

In August 1864, a formal diplomatic congress was held, which signed what is known as the *Geneva Convention.* This stipulated that each nation that ratified the convention should have a national committee or society, civil in character and function, which alone should have the right to send a surgical corps to a war. Such organizations were at that time under way in 28 countries. The well known emblem of the society was also adopted.[26]

The convention was ratified at that time by 12 nations; by 1925 there were 52 national Red Cross organizations, and in 1945 a total of 67. Additions have been made to its program from time to time, and its provisions are now recognized as a part of international law.

In some countries similar societies found to be already in existence were affiliated or absorbed, keeping the original idea of co-operation. The idea of helping in diaster came early so that earthquakes, extensive floods or forest fires, famines and all catastrophes that needed more than local help were included. The present emphasis is on improvement of health, prevention of disease and relief in suffering.

In every country the society makes preparation beforehand for war or disaster; they

have at various centers great storehouses of every sort of material—tents, portable houses, furniture, tools, clothing and medical and surgical supplies. The Red Cross personnel are men and women who can leave their regular occupations; its organization provides means of getting together, on an hour's notice, a group of previously instructed workers. The efficiency of its organization has repeatedly been shown when governments were helpless because of official "red tape."

The First World War caused an unprecedented development of the Red Cross. In 1919 the great health authorities of the world formed a league that is a federation of the various national Red Cross societies. This league has expanded its program to include public health and has become interested in the control of tuberculosis and venereal diseases, and in child welfare.

Since these things involve an interest in the training of nurses, the *Division of Nursing* was promptly created by the League. Its directors have included Alice Fitzgerald and Katherine Olmsted of the United States of America, Mrs. Maynard Carter of England, and Yvonne Hentsch of Switzerland.

The *Florence Nightingale Medal* was established in 1912 by the International Red Cross Committee, to be given on alternate years to nurses "who have distinguished themselves in an exceptional manner by great devotion to their patients in time of war or peace." This medal has been given to organizations, graduate nurses, nurses' aides and to nurses who died in war.

In some European countries, the Red Cross had its own hospitals and trained its own nurses, the courses varying greatly in length and content. Some courses lasted three months, some three years in an accredited school of nursing. Some consisted of lectures to laymen and schoolchildren, or instruction in first aid. Red Cross hospitals sometimes cared for the sick poor or the army in peacetime.

The United States, the thirty-second country to enter the Red Cross, soon formed the *American Red Cross Society.* This was due largely to the tireless efforts of *Clara Barton,* a nurse who served during the Civil War and who, in 1870, undertook the work of the Red Cross in the Franco-Prussian War. In 1881 she organized in Washington a Red Cross Committee and so persuaded the

---

[26]During the Serbian War of 1876 the Turkish Government notified the powers that it would use the red crescent instead of the red cross as the insignia of its relief societies.

Government, that in 1882 it finally ratified the Geneva Convention and gave the committee official standing.

PUBLIC HEALTH

In the 1860's, New York City had a setting of filth and debris; pestilence ravaged the inhabitants. Garbage and refuse were thrown in the streets and the air was polluted by the slaughterhouses and leather tanneries. Communicable diseases, tuberculosis, small-pox, diphtheria, scarlet fever, yellow fever, cholera and dysentery, were rampant in the congested tenement house districts.

It took a group of distressed, public spirited citizens, who banded together into the Citizen's Association, to finally fight for sanitary and health reform. For years they submitted health bills into the legislature without success. In 1866 the Metropolitan Health Bill was passed and the Board of Health came into being.

An interesting highlight that provoked action was reported as follows:

"Why I believe I have got smallpox for I begin to itch all over," cried a New York State legislator as he listened to Dr. Stephen S. Smith explain the sanitary requirements of the Citizen's Association's metropolitan health bill. The date was February 13, 1865, and Smith described how wholesale clothing dealers had goods manufactured in tenement houses. City inspectors often found the clothing thrown over the beds of children with scarlet fever, measles, or smallpox—a condition which helped make the city vulnerable to epidemics.[27]

The health picture viewed by the Citizens' Association was discouraging, but persistence, plus the added impetus caused by the reappearance of dreaded cholera, which Europe faced in 1866, assisted in the passage of the necessary legislation. One of the first acts of the new Board of Health was to establish a bureau of records and vital statistics and an office of sanitary superintendence. When the United States faced another outbreak of cholera in 1866, isolation of the patients was enforced and disinfectants were used to cleanse the homes and surroundings of the patients. A central depot for distributing disinfectants was established and a special disinfecting corps was organized. This was a successful project and the new Board of Health was credited with preventing a more devastating outbreak of cholera.

A vigorous program aimed at a general "clean up" of the City of New York then ensued (Fig. 9–20). Unsanitary conditions of every nature became the target of the new Board of Health. Establishments that were

---

[27]McMahon, Margaret, and Erhardt, Carl: "Highlights of the First 100 Years." *Public Health Reports*, U.S. Department of Health, Education and Welfare, No. 1, *81*:87, 1966.

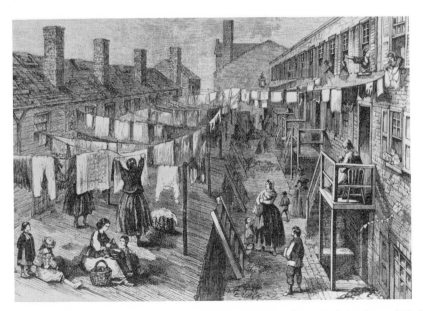

Figure 9–20. A congested tenement district in New York City. (Courtesy of New York Academy of Medicine and New York City Department of Health.)

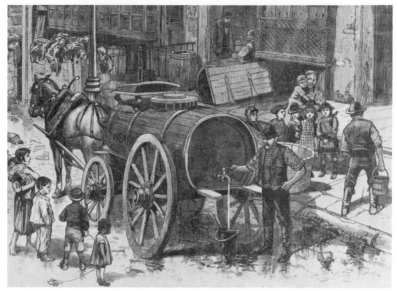

Figure 9–21. The disinfecting corps of the Health Department distributing disinfectants. (Courtesy of New York Academy of Medicine and New York City Department of Health.)

considered to be health menaces were required to relocate. Garbage and refuse disposal systems were enforced and cellars were personally cleaned out by the members of the Board of Health. Cellar apartments were ordered drained, renovated or vacated (Fig. 9–21).

Food markets were inspected as part of the initial plan for regulating and controlling the quality of produce. Finally, in 1869, a chemical laboratory was initiated to analyze the water supply of the city; it detected that well water was being contaminated with the drainage from privies. Typhoid fever was discovered to be transmitted in this way. The results of an analysis of cosmetics revealed that they contained injurious quantities of lead. Kerosene, which was used in the lamps of this period, was mixed with naphtha and caused many explosions that resulted in fires and serious burns. The Board of Health had achieved phenomenal success!

Practicing physicians were required to register cases of infectious disease with the Bureau of Records and Vital Statistics. By 1870 the registrar of this department devised the weekly statistical reports that have continued ever since. Birth, stillbirth, marriage and death certificates were examined with great care. The incredibly high infant mortality rate, particularly in the so-called

tenement districts, became apparent. Deaths of children under five years of age accounted for 48 per cent of the total mortality. Deaths of children under two years amounted to approximately 40 per cent of the total mortality.

A "summer corps" of physicians visited the tenement districts during July and August, treated the sick and distributed to mothers a pamphlet on infant care. The absence of, and urgent need for, nurses was obvious! In 1867, Elisha Harris, counsel to the Board of Health, predicted that nurses would become our "missionaries of health" and advise the public on health and sanitation.

Tuberculosis, called consumption or phthisis, was purported to be responsible for one fifth to one sixth of all deaths and this disease seemed to be associated with the underprivileged and minority groups. Poor food and unsanitary living conditions were considered to be the cause of tuberculosis.

An epidemic of smallpox struck New York City in the winter of 1874–75. It was the duty of the Health Department to provide a special corps of doctors to vaccinate the public (Fig. 9–22). Efforts were devised to prepare vaccine. Health education opportunities were recognized and pamphlets on child care, food handling, ventilation and prevention of dis-

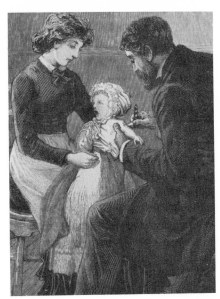

Figure 9–22. This newspaper drawing made in 1871 shows an early vaccination clinic where mothers brought their small children for smallpox vaccinations. (Courtesy of New York Academy of Medicine and New York City Department of Health.)

ease were available for distribution. Families were instructed in the need for cleanliness, disinfection and of isolating sick persons from other members of the family.

The smallpox epidemic, which resulted in a high mortality, prompted legislation to transfer the Smallpox Hospital on Blackwell's Island, under the control of the Commissioners of Charities and Corrections, to the control of the Health Department. It was renamed Riverside Hospital. Buildings were renovated and the nursing services of the Sisters of Charity were secured. The Board of Health eventually purchased a steamboat called the "Psyche" to transport patients to Riverside Hospital. Toward the end of the nineteenth century this hospital became too small for the demands made upon it, and a new and larger isolation hospital was constructed on North Brother Island. Again a larger steamboat was required, and the "Mayor Franklin Edson" was procured for hospital service. It has been reported that the after-cabin of the boat was divided in two parts to permit transportation of two types of contagious diseases without danger of mixed infection.

At a time of critical need in the history of the country there was response to the call for nurses from many dedicated and gifted persons.

The proper scientific and social ingredients had been added to the culture medium for the growth of nursing.

REFERENCE READINGS

Adams, G. W.: *Doctors in Blue:* The medical history of the Union Army in the Civil War. New York, Collier Books, 1961.

Alcott, Louisa May: *Hospital Sketches.* Boston, James Redpath, 1863. (New York, Sagamore Press, 1957.)

Alcott, Louisa M.: *Life, Letters and Journals.* Edited by Ednah D. Cheney. Boston, Roberts Brothers, 1889.

Austin, Anne L.: *The Woolsey Sisters of New York—1860–1900.* Philadelphia, American Philosophical Society, 1971.

Baker, Nina B.: *Cyclone in Calico.* Boston, Little, Brown & Co., 1952.

Blackwell, Elizabeth: *Pioneer Work in Opening the Medical Profession to Women.* London, 1895.

Boyden, Anna L.: *Echoes from Hospital and White House.* Boston, D. Lothrop and Company, 1884.

Brockett, L. P.: *The Camp, the Battle Field and the Hospital; or Lights and Shadows of the Great Rebellion.* Philadelphia, National Publishing Company, 1866.

Cook, Sir Edward: *The Life of Florence Nightingale.* Vols. I–II. London, Macmillan, Ltd., 1914.

Cope, Zachary: *Florence Nightingale and the Doctors.* Philadelphia, J. B. Lippincott Co., 1958.

Cumming, Kate: *The Journal of a Confederate Nurse.* Barksdale Harwell (ed.). Baton Rouge, Louisiana State University Press, 1959.

Dolan, Josephine A.: *The Grace of the Great Lady.* Chicago, Medical Heritage Society, 1971.

Hamlin, Cyrus: *My Life and Times.* Boston, Congregational Sunday School and Publishing Society, 1893.

Hobson, W.: *World Health and History.* Bristol, John Wright & Sons, Ltd., 1963.

Holland, Mary A.: *Our Army Nurses.* Boston, B. Wilkins & Co., 1895.

Leech, Margaret: *Reveille in Washington 1860–1865.* New York, Harper & Brothers, 1941.

Livermore, Mary A.: *My Story of the War.* Hartford, Conn. A. D. Worthington, 1890.

Lowenfels, Walter: *Walt Whitman's Civil War.* New York, Alfred A. Knopf, 1961.

Marshall, Helen E.: *Dorothea Dix: Forgotten Samaritan.* Chapel Hill, University of North Carolina Press, 1937.

Nightingale, Florence: *Notes on Hospitals*, 3rd ed. London, Longmans, 1867.

Nightingale, Florence: *Notes on Nursing*. London, Harrison & Sons, 1859. (Philadelphia, J. B. Lippincott Co., 1946.)

O'Malley, I. B.: *Florence Nightingale, 1820–1856*. London, Thornton Butterworth, 1931.

Parton, James, et al.: *Eminent Women of the Age*. Hartford, Conn., S. M. Betts Co., 1868.

Phelps, E. S.: *Our Famous Women*. Hartford, Conn., A. D. Worthington & Co., 1884.

Rathbone, William: *Sketch of the History and Progress of District Nursing from its Commencement in the Year 1859 to the Present Date*. New York, Macmillan, 1890.

Reed, William H.: *Hospital Life in the Army of the Potomac*. Boston, William V. Spencer, 1866.

Seymer, Lucy R.: *Florence Nightingale*. London, Faber & Faber, 1940.

Seymer, Lucy Ridgely: *Florence Nightingale's Nurses. The Nightingale Training School 1860–1960*. London, Pitman, 1960.

Seymer, Lucy R.: *Selected Writings of Florence Nightingale*. The Macmillan Co., 1954.

Strachey, Ray: *The Cause, A Short History of the Women's Movement in Great Britain*. London, G. Bell and Sons, 1928.

Tiffany, Frances: *Life of Dorothea Lynde Dix*. Boston, Houghton, Mifflin Company, 1890.

Wilson, Forrest: *Crusader in Crinoline: The Life of Harriet Beecher Stowe*. Philadelphia, J. B. Lippincott Co., 1941.

Woodham-Smith, Cecil: *Florence Nightingale, 1820–1910*. New York, McGraw-Hill Book Co., Inc., 1951.

Woolsey, Jane Stuart: *Hospital Days*. New York, Van Nostrand, 1868.

Wormeley, Katharine P.: *The Other Side of the War with the Army of the Potomac*. Boston, Ticknor, 1889.

CHAPTER 10

Relationship of Nursing to Society and Welfare Services in the Late Nineteenth Century

The late nineteenth century witnessed the development of programs in nursing and the fundamentals of the science of bacteriology.

THE NEED FOR NURSING EDUCATION

Florence Nightingale's work and the founding of her school at St. Thomas' were well known in America. It was not long before interested people grasped something of her vision that better nursing could be undertaken by educated women.

Doubtless the first attempt to train nurses on this continent was made by the Ursuline Sisters of Quebec, who, about 1640, taught the Indian women to care for their sick.

The family of Dr. Valentine Seaman, of New York, claims that he was the first person in the United States to found a school for nurses. His son says, "In 1798 Dr. Seaman introduced the first regular school for trained nurses, from which other schools have since been established." He enrolled about 24 pupils and gave them a course of lectures in anatomy, physiology, care of children and midwifery.

The events of the preceding 10 years—the Crimean War, the educational endeavors of Florence Nightingale and the Civil War—had focused attention on the necessity for nurses and on the importance of an educational system in which to prepare them. Interest was stimulated by doctors as well as enlightened citizens, and efforts to inaugurate a program for the preparation of nurses were made.

In 1869 at a meeting of the *American Medical Association*, Dr. S. D. Gross as chairman presented a report of the *Committee on the Training of Nurses*, which recommended that nursing be placed under the control of the medical profession. They proposed that there should be a school for the training of nurses in every large hospital, not only to supply demands of that hospital but also to care for families in their homes. The teaching was to be given by the medical staff as they were doing for the medical students. The county medical societies were to take the responsibility for the district schools. The recommendations of the committee were not adopted, fortunately.

The most popular woman's magazine of this period was *Godey's Lady's Book*, and in 1871, Mrs. Sarah Hale, its editor, wrote a significant editorial, which appeared in the February 1871 issue, entitled "Lady Nurses."[1]

Much has been lately said of the benefits that would follow if the calling of sick nurse were elevated to a profession which an educated lady might adopt without a sense of degradation, either on her own part or in the estimation of others. . . .

There can be no doubt that the duties of sick nurse, to be properly performed, require an education and training little, if at all, inferior to those possessed by members of the medical profession. . . . The manner in which a reform may

[1]Hale, Sarah: "Lady Nurses." *Godey's Lady's Book and Magazine*, 82:188–189, January to June, 1871.

be effected is easily pointed out. Every medical college should have a course of study and training especially adapted for ladies who desire to qualify themselves for the profession of nurse; and those who had gone through the course, and passed the requisite examination, should receive a degree and a diploma, which would at once establish their position in society. The graduate nurse would in general estimation be as much above the ordinary nurse of the present day as the professional surgeon of our times is above the barber-surgeon of the last century.

Mrs. Hale, in this brief thought-provoking editorial, identified the need for *professional nurses* to receive a well planned educational program with a specific body of knowledge that was different from, but in as great a depth as, that received by members of the medical profession. This knowledge was to be obtained in an educational rather than a service-centered institution with the attainment of an academic degree in addition to professional certification. Her words fell on deaf ears, and in 1873 a Dr. Aeneas Munro in *The Science and Art of Nursing the Sick* stressed the need for requiring that nurses be able to read and write and bemoaned the fact that so many could not do either.

In both England and America the need for trained nurses was so great that schools of nursing inevitably took root and grew. As in England, the pioneer nurses in America were unusual women who had vision, force, great courage and persistence. It was these few courageous women who laid the solid foundations on which we now stand.

At the time of the Civil War, there were said to be only 68 hospitals in the country; in 1872 a survey was made and 178 were found. From that time on, the number increased rapidly, unquestionably because of the improvement in nursing, and owing to the fact that doctors and patients found better and more convenient service in hospitals than in the average home. The process seemed slow, but in 30 years the picture had changed. In 1900 there were about 2000 hospitals in the United States. From that time on they multiplied at an incredible speed. Those already founded expanded their facilities.

THE INCEPTION OF SCHOOLS OF NURSING

The New England Hospital for Women and Children, staffed by women physicians, took its first step toward a school of nursing when Dr. Marie Zakrzewska came there in 1859. She suggested practical instruction in the hospital for women medical students, and that a school of nursing be established. The hospital charter was issued in 1863 and included a nursing school.

In the 1864 Annual Report of the New England Hospital for Women and Children, the adoption of the first bylaws on June 5, 1863 was recorded. It is interesting to read them carefully:

The objects of the Institution shall be
1st. To provide for women medical aid of competent physicians of their own sex.
2nd. To assist educated women in the practical study of medicine.
3rd. To train nurses for the care of the sick.[2]

In the early 1870's a committee was appointed to develop the plan for instituting a training school for nurses. It was described as:[3]

Education of Nurses

In order more fully to carry out our purpose of fitting women thoroughly for the profession of nursing, we have made the following arrangements:

Young women of suitable requirements and character will be admitted to the Hospital as school nurses, for one year. This year will be divided into four periods; three months will be given respectively to the practical study of nursing in the Medical, Surgical, and Maternity Wards, and night nursing. Here the pupil will aid the head nurse in all the care and work of the wards under the direction of the Attending and Resident Physicians and Medical Students.

In order to enable women entirely dependent upon their work for support to obtain a thorough training, the nurses will be paid for their work from one to four dollars per week after the first fortnight, according to the actual value of their service to the hospital.

A course of lectures will be given to nurses at the Hospital by the physicians connected with the Institution beginning January 21. . . . Certificates will be given to such nurses as have satisfactorily passed a year in practical training in the Hospital.

The inception of these programs of nursing education in hospitals revolved around practical experience obtained within the framework of the medical geography of the hospital, such as in the medical and surgical wards, as well as covering the service needs

---

[2]Munson, Helen W.: "Linda Richards." *American Journal of Nursing,* 48:552, 1948.
[3]*Ibid.,* p. 552.

of the hospital by providing coverage around the clock. They were considered employees rather than students because they were paid a meager salary.

On *September 1, 1872*, the *New England Hospital in Boston* (later transferred to Roxbury, Massachusetts) admitted a class of five students to the newly formed *Training School*. This school was administered under the direction of Susan Dimock, M.D. She had finished her medical education in Switzerland and had been to Kaiserswerth and knew its methods. Dr. Zakrzewska taught bedside nursing. The course was one year in length. No classwork was required, although lectures were given during the winter months. Books were not available for giving a background in nursing so that lectures without demonstrations comprised the educational aspects of the curriculum.

The course was a rigorous one. The hours of duty extended from 5:30 A.M. to 9:00 P.M. The living arrangements consisted of rooms between the hospital wards because the students had to take care of the patients night and day. Days off for illness had to be made up. At the end of the year on October 1, 1873, one student graduated.

When the second year began, a nurse was hired as a head nurse and instructor of the students of nursing, and a theoretical program was started. The length of the program was expanded to 16 months and by the time the school celebrated its fifth anniversary, it was an 18 month course. The so-called enrichment provided one month in the diet kitchen at the hospital and one month of district nursing in the community. There were now two head nurses, and a superintendent of the training school. In 1893, the program was lengthened to two years—in 1901, to three years.

Melinda Ann (Linda) Richards (1841–1930) was the one student who graduated on October 1, 1873, and has been called *"America's first trained nurse"* (Figs. 10–1 and 10–2).

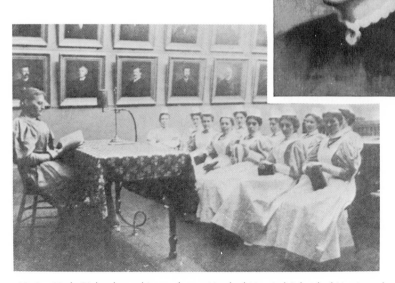

Figure 10–1. Linda Richards. (From a painting given to the New England Hospital for Women by its alumnae.)

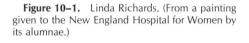

Figure 10–2. Linda Richards teaching a class at Hartford Hospital School of Nursing where she was matron from 1895 to 1897. (Courtesy of Hartford Hospital School of Nursing.)

Miss Richards had been a nurse in the Boston City Hospital. Going there with the idea of learning nursing, she had been greatly disappointed to find that the nurse's work and position were little more than that of a maid. She had been offered a position as head nurse there, but had refused it, claiming that she did not know enough and wanted more training. They had then directed her to the New England Hospital.

Miss Richards recorded her experiences, in which she mentioned that students did not wear a uniform; dark washable dresses were worn.[4] She related that "every second week" they had a free afternoon from two to five o'clock. They had no evenings out, no hours for study or recreation and no regular leave on Sunday. During the year's program only twelve lectures were given by the visiting staff of physicians and the only clinical instruction was given by the women interns when they ordered a treatment and the intern and student nurse together figured out the procedure. Medicines were kept in bottles that were numbered, not labeled, and there was no understanding of the medicine, its action or untoward symptoms to be observed. In addition to an absence of textbooks, no preentrance requirements were stated and no final examinations taken.

Miss Richards has given an account of the high maternal mortality rates due to epidemics of puerperal fever and of the astonishing duty of the patients in labor to make shrouds for the hospital. Many a patient must have wondered if she were making her own!

Her first assignment as a graduate was that of night superintendent at Bellevue. After a year there, she went to the Boston Training School as the new superintendent of the school. In addition to the position for which she was hired, she insisted upon giving actual patient care herself. Many days she worked day and night. She even requested a room in the hospital, in place of the comfortable room outside of the hospital, in order to watch the patients at night. Her reason was that it would be more convenient for her if she could be called at any hour of the day or night.

In 1877, Linda Richards visited England where she met Florence Nightingale and studied the methods at St. Thomas' Hospital.

Between 1885 and 1889, she was a medical missionary in Japan, establishing and directing the first training school for nurses there. In the following years, she assumed the position of superintendent of nurses at the New England Hospital for Women and Children, at Brooklyn Homeopathic Hospital, at Hartford Hospital and at the University of Pennsylvania Hospital. Her efforts were then directed to establishing schools in hospitals for the mentally ill. She died on April 16, 1930.

In 1879, *Mary Mahoney*, another important nurse, graduated from the training school of the New England Hospital for Women and Children. She was America's first Negro nurse to graduate from a school of nursing.

Mary Eliza Mahoney (Fig. 10–3) (1845–1926) enrolled on March 23, 1878 in the New England Hospital for Women and Children and completed her course of 16 months on August 1, 1879. Personal interviews were required in the selection of applicants. In addition to the previously described course of 12 months of nursing experience in medical, surgical, and maternal nursing and night duty, Mary Mahoney had four months that were needed "to prove the students' competency in all of these clinical areas" by sending them into the homes of the community for private duty under the direction of the school. There were three students who graduated with her out of the class of 40. Twenty-

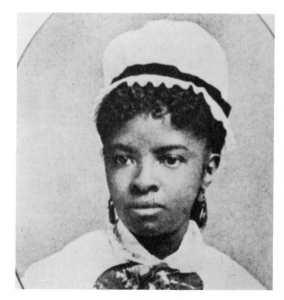

Figure 10–3. Mary Eliza Mahoney (1845–1926). (Author's collection.)

---

[4]Richards, Linda: *Reminiscences of Linda Richards.* Boston, Whitcomb and Barrows, 1911.

two were dropped by the school, which attests to the mental and nursing ability of Mary Mahoney and the fortitude with which she accepted a rigorous program. Her experience included being responsible for a ward and the care of the patients in that ward.

The hours of duty at this institution were from 6:00 A.M. to 9:00 P.M.

In *Pathfinders*,[5] Mrs. Adah Thoms has given a description of Mary Mahoney, who gave the address of welcome at the first convention of the National Association of Colored Graduate Nurses:

Miss Mahoney was small of stature, about five feet in height and weighed less than one hundred pounds . . . she was most interesting and possessed an unusual personality and a great deal of charm. . . . Although at this meeting Miss Mahoney seemed pleased to see and to know of the upward trend of the nursing profession, to hear her make comparisons between the years 1879 and 1909 would almost lead one to believe that the training of today was rather a hit-or-miss proposition. However, she was an inspiration to the entire group of nurses present. At the close of the convention she was made a life member of the Association, exempt from dues, and was elected chaplain. . . . Through her efforts on this occasion a demonstration for nurses was held at the New England Hospital. . . .

Miss Mahoney was a remarkable person. . . . She seldom missed a national nurses' meeting. Her last attendance was in Washington, when the Association met in August, 1921, as a guest of the Freedmen's Hospital Alumnae Association. This circumstance made it possible for the nurses to be received at the White House by President Warren G. Harding. The nurses carried a large basket of American Beauty roses which they presented to President and Mrs. Harding with the request that the National Association of Colored Graduate Nurses be placed on record as an organized body of two thousand trained women ready when needed for world service.

In her honor, the *Mary Mahoney Medal* was initiated in 1936 by the National Association of Colored Graduate Nurses. This medal is symbolic of the opportunities in nursing for those of all races, creeds and national origins.

The New England Hospital for Women and Children can boast of two other distinctions. It was the first institution in America to conduct a formal course for the training of nurses. It also had the distinction of graduating America's first trained nurse, Miss Linda Richards. The directors of this pioneer institution, which was founded by another minority, women in medicine, could well understand and be sympathetic with Miss Mahoney's desire to become a trained nurse. They, too, had experienced prejudice in their efforts to practice their profession. The opportunity they gave Mary Mahoney was extended to other Negroes up until 1951, when the school closed.[6]

The next year, 1873, was notable because in that year three of the important schools of the country—Bellevue in New York, the Connecticut Training School in New Haven, and the Boston Training School at Massachusetts General Hospital—were established. It is interesting that the New York and Boston schools were the result of the efforts of committees of laywomen and were opposed by doctors, and that the New Haven school was founded by doctors.

Bellevue Hospital Training School

In 1872 Louisa Lee Schuyler, who organized the New York State Charities Aid Association, enlisted the aid of certain members including Miss Abby H. Woolsey to visit *Bellevue Hospital*. They found a serious state of affairs. The nursing was done chiefly by women who were ex-convicts and collected fees from the patients for the crude and inefficient services that they rendered them; drunkenness and foul language were common; their food was poor and they slept on bundles of straw. The doctors of the house staff took temperatures, gave treatments and recorded the condition of patients. It was a repetition of the worst days in the hospitals of Old England. Dr. Gill Wylie, who was an intern there, said, "The nurses had the impossible task of attending to from twenty to thirty patients each. The night watchman was expected to assist in the care of patients. The wards looked well on the surface; but sepsis followed slight operations or injuries, and about 50 per cent of the amputations were fatal. One out of every eleven maternity cases died."

It was reported that in Bellevue Hospital there were 900 patients, "most of them in want, many in positive distress." The crowded conditions required that three patients sleep

[5]Thoms, Adah B.: *Pathfinders*. New York, Kay Printing House, 1929.

[6]Staupers, Mabel K.: *No Time for Prejudice*. New York, The Macmillan Co., 1961, p. 2.

on two beds, which were presumably strapped together, and five patients occupied three beds. There were no night nurses and only three night watchmen.

The report of these conditions stirred the women's nursing committee, which had asked in 1871 for a nurses' training school; the matter had been referred to the medical board, which did nothing about it. The committee felt that nursing *must* be improved, but most of the medical board disapproved of the women's interest in the matter. General James Bowen was the only commissioner who supported them, and a clergyman said publicly that it was not proper for ladies to visit a hospital of this sort.

Dr. Wylie offered to go abroad, at his own expense, to see what was being done there. He spent some time abroad and even conferred with Miss Nightingale, getting valuable advice from her. Meantime the committee, under the leadership of Miss Schuyler,[7] had succeeded in getting six wards set apart to use in making the experiment of a nurses' "training class." Funds were raised by subscription and a house was rented for the nurses' home.

---

[7]The National Institute of Sciences recognized Miss Schuyler as the founder of Bellevue's training school.

In May 1873, the *Bellevue Training School for Nurses* was founded (Fig. 10–4). The person who was selected to direct this new program was Sister Helen of the Sisterhood of All Saints. It was recorded that "all are lodged and boarded free of charge during the two years' course and are paid a small sum monthly while in the school, to defray their actual necessary expenses." In the beginning the course was one year in length. Miss Euphemia Van Rensselaer succeeded Sister Helen as the superintendent.

Linda Richards became night superintendent in October, 1874. At that time, Miss Richards started the practice of keeping records and of written orders. There was no classwork, and the lectures were irregular. She noted that, "The training did not compare favorably with that given at the New England Hospital, where far greater nicety in caring for patients was required."

The environment that nurtured the Bellevue Training School left much to be desired. There was a very high mortality rate because of blood poisoning or septicemia. The medical house staff dressed the wounds, going from patient to patient and spreading infection. Sponges for cleaning wounds were pieces of real sponge, one of which was used to cleanse wounds of many patients.

The incredibly high mortality rate caused

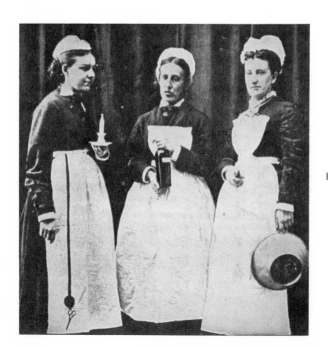

Figure 10–4. Three of the first nurses of the Bellevue Training School for Nurses.

by puerperal fever (two deaths out of every five deliveries), in the maternity service, prompted the Training School to offer to take charge of the entire maternity ward. The students of nursing had reported the unbelievable plight of the maternity patients. The obstetricians were violently opposed. A request for assistance to the State Charities Aid Association resulted in the assignment of the three maternity wards to Bellevue Training School in May, 1874. Linda Richards was asked to direct this project. Strong community backing was solicited and the Advisory Committee presented the following ultimatum to the Medical Board: "Gentlemen, we have learned the cause of mortality in the Lying-in wards of this hospital. We give you forty-eight hours to remove these women. If they are here at the end of this time, the whole story will be published in the Evening Post."

The President of the Board of Charity ordered the immediate removal of the 25 women who were waiting to be delivered, to the Charity Hospital on Blackwell's Island. Every patient survived. The maternity wards of Bellevue were closed; the story of Dr. Semmelweis had been repeated. The medical students and medical house staff had been guilty of transferring puerperal sepsis.

Connecticut Training School

In 1872 the New Haven Hospital appointed a committee of three doctors and a layman to report upon the practicability of training nurses. Dr. Gill Wylie's report upon European schools of nursing aided them in their investigation. The committee reported in April, 1873, that it was not expedient for the hospital itself to undertake such a work, but it recommended the establishment of a school as a separate organization with the hospital as its field.

The Connecticut Training School obtained its charter before Bellevue did, but was not opened until later. Dr. Francis Bacon, the husband of Georgeanna Woolsey, prepared a scheme of organization after studying the Nightingale plan of nurse education.

The school was founded, but there were no pupils, so they advertised for "probationers" through country newspapers, ladies' missionary societies and notices at railway stations and in post offices. All the early schools found it hard to convince young women that it was necessary to spend even six months' time in learning nursing. The Civil War, however, had done much to call attention to the need of training.

In October of 1873, the Connecticut Training School at the New Haven Hospital was established, with four pupils. Miss Bayard, a graduate of the school of the Woman's Hospital of Philadelphia, was in charge (Fig. 10-5).

Many serious and frustrating obstacles became apparent when the hospital steward and his wife exhibited animosity toward the new director and her students. The couple were terrified of losing their jobs and, therefore, they fought the new system. Miss Bayard resigned when fantastically incorrect and adverse newspaper publicity about the new school was printed.

A new director, Mrs. Allen, arrived and the distraught steward attempted to inflict harm whenever he could. She resigned May 13, 1874; however, there were courageous women who were willing and able to direct the school and guided it successfully. The desire of the teachers and students to save the lives of their patients prompted them to work longer hours than were expected and to request a ward for teaching purposes. The school contracted with the hospital to provide nursing service in exchange for educational services because it was critical for the students to see good patient care. This meant day and night coverage for instructor and students.

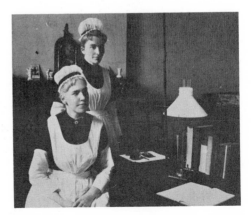

Figure 10–5. The office of the Connecticut Training School with the Superintendent and Assistant Superintendent of Nursing. (Courtesy of Yale Medical Library.)

They even tapped the meager school budget to purchase food and milk to supplement the patients' diets.

From the beginning, the aims of the nursing schools seemed to emphasize charitable service, with education incidental to this service.

The doctors liked the work of the nurses and were, from the first, enthusiastic about the school. (See Figures 10–6 and 10–7.)

Mrs. Georgeanna Bacon has written:

Our first four pupils arrived late in the evening, and in a dreary storm. . . . They and their superintendent found themselves at once plunged into hard work. The north ward was full of typhoid fever, ten cases, six men and four women, and wards 1 and 2 East and West were opened and filled during the first week. The committee's journal reads: 'Our nurses for the first five weeks did very hard work. The fever cases were severe, some of the patients entirely delirious. . . . The four nurses in turn sat up night after night and did duty during the day in the other wards, or diet kitchen, where the special diet for thirty was cooked and distributed to all parts of the hospital by the nurses who cooked it.' . . . No class of nurses has ever had such demand made upon its endurance as this pioneer class of pupils met and struggled through. All the typhoid fever cases recovered. . . . Everything was in a transition state. The nurses were crowded, as their numbers increased, into the three small rooms in the top floor, four in a room, – the clothes horse screens which divided their beds one from another were the first screens of the kind used in the hospital. . . . By the end of our second year we were able to send out our first graduates to private families.

Shortly after, the school was allowed to take eight students, and at the end of its second year the nurses were sent into private nursing. The payment for their services went to the Training School. Fortunately, this practice was discontinued in 1905, and by discontinuing it, the Connecticut Training School became eligible to register with the Regents in New York State.

In 1877, the school published the *New Haven Manual of Nursing*, a textbook created by a committee consisting of both nurses and doctors; it was a comprehensive text and soon found wide acceptance among the nursing schools, which by then were being organized all through the country.

A report of 1881 says: "The work was so hard many nurses broke down and were obliged to give up their profession. The members of the Training School Committee went on the wards and helped at this time. The Board of Managers feel the Hospital cannot go on successfully without the school, and the community cannot dispense with the services of the nurses here trained. If there were no school we should have to hire nurses and the lowest rate for which they could be

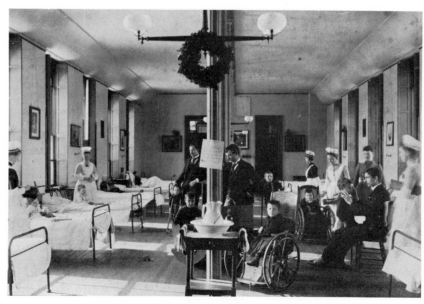

Fugure 10–6. A pediatric unit under the aegis of the Connecticut Training School (ca. 1878). Note that there are two faculty members supervising three students. (Courtesy of Yale Medical Library.)

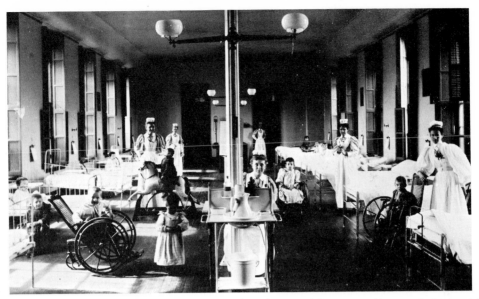

Figure 10–7. The same pediatric unit in Figure 10–6, about the turn of the century. Note one instructor at the right and five students. (Courtesy of Yale Medical Library.)

engaged for this harassing work would be $15 monthly."

An interesting comment appears in the 1881 yearly report: "It is perhaps well to state once for all, the school is thankful they are able to relieve suffering in the hospital, but the school does not exist primarily for this purpose but for the training of nurses for the public; the only school in this country or in Europe which is not supported by the hospital which it serves."

The public took kindly to the nurses, and there was an immediate demand for their services.

Boston Training School

In 1807 the *Massachusetts General Hospital* was started by a group of prominent doctors. It was a private enterprise, though designed for nonpaying patients, and a model hospital, noted for its cleanliness and good nursing. Mrs. G. L. Sturtevant, who was nurse there in 1862, tells us of the conditions of work:

The nurses were paid $7.50 a month, head nurses $12. There were no maids; the nurses washed the dishes and did the cleaning. The night watchers left the ward at 5 A.M., making a verbal report to the head nurse. The day nurses went on duty at that hour, had breakfast at six, and remained on until 9:30 P.M., taking an occasional hour off if they could get it. They slept in small rooms between the wards, two nurses in a folding bed. In the daytime the room was used for doctors' consultations or for dressings and minor operations.

The committee that was formed to present the matter of a Boston Training School to the Massachusetts General Hospital consisted of a group of men and women of intellect and social prominence. The hospital trustees and staff did not approve of a school for nurses, but the standing of the committee was such that they were compelled to consider it.

It was finally agreed that the hospital should allow the school to open as an experiment. Subscriptions were secured for the expenses of the school, and pupils were sought. Six young women were accepted, and on November 1, 1873, the *Boston Training School* was opened.

The committee had asked Florence Nightingale and Thomas Rathbone to find them a superintendent of nurses but had no encouragement. They finally selected Linda Richards, as being "the most desirable person to be had in America." She found the school still on trial and rather discredited by the staff. She saw that the nurses were working much as their untrained predecessors had done;

there were no maids, and, therefore, nurses were occupied doing dish-washing and dining-room work, washing poultice cloths and taking turns at doing night duty and being head nurse. Cotton was expensive, so all soiled dressings and poultice cloths, of which there were many, had to be washed (in the patients' bathtub) and ironed by the nurses.

Miss Richards reorganized the work, got classes under way and developed the school. "Her major job was to prove to the staff that trained nurses were better than untrained ones. One means she sometimes used to demonstrate this was to care for the sickest patients herself. Gradually the staff realized their value and began to refer to 'our school' with pride." By the end of her first year Miss Richards had convinced the doctors that the new régime was a success, and the school was accepted by the trustees. Miss Richards remained for two and one-half years, and when she left to study training school work in England the school was on a permanent basis. For some decades *Training School for Nurses* was the accepted term, and students of nursing were called *pupils*.

In analyzing the development of the new program at Massachusetts General Hospital,[8] it is noted that: in 1874, a thermometer was requested for the use of nurses in taking care of patients and a month of night watching was added to the program; in 1875, cooking became an essential addition, there being no cooks in hospitals; in 1876, pupils were permitted in the operating room; in 1889, a class on "insanity" and one on "bacteriology" were added; in 1891, pupils were responsible for cleaning and sterilizing instruments for Saturday operations; by 1896, pupils were required to assist with operations on Saturday. (The reason for students in the operating room only on Saturday is not given.) Gradually, a graduate nurse was placed in charge of the operating amphitheater, pupil nurses assisted at operations and, finally, assumed the responsibility of administering the ether. By 1895, *Miss Annabella McCrae* became a full-time instructor in the teaching of nursing procedures. In 1896, pupil nurses received instruction in the administration of hypodermic injections.

In 1896, The Boston Training School ceased to be an independent school and was made an integral part of the Massachusetts General Hospital.

St. Catharine's Training School

In 1874, nursing education in Canada was initiated when The St. Catharine's Training School and Nurses' Home came into being. The name was changed later to *The Mack Training School for Nurses* in connection with St. Catharine's General Hospital in honor of the founder, Dr. Theophilus Mack.

Parts of the correspondence between Miss Lavinia Dock and Dr. Howard Dittrick of Cleveland appear in the history of Mack Training School for Nurses.[9]

Miss Nightingale's new plan of training was begun in St. Thomas' Hospital in 1860, and only four or five years after that, Dr. Mack, having comprehended her work and its meaning—determined to have a hospital with a home for nurses on Miss Nightingale's plan, with a trained nurse at its head. This is where he outdistanced all others on the American continent.

Today, when this system is universal, we do not realize its immensely revolutionary character in Miss Nightingale's day. It was unknown in English hospitals, although British matrons held dignified and respected positions. It heralded, in fact, a phase of the "woman movement" although this was not foremost with Miss Nightingale.

Dr. Mack and his intelligent community, familiar with Miss Nightingale's work in the Crimea and in the English hospital world, adhered to her principles, and determined as early as 1864 to establish and follow them loyally. Beginning in a small way, in that year—they developed their purpose so well that in 1873 they sent Miss Money to England to bring out a staff of nurses trained in the "Nightingale System," and she returned with three from Guy's Hospital, and several probationers.

The final success was the result of the efforts of Dr. Mack, who in 1874 sent to England for nurses and founded a school that has always been worthy of the name and produced some able nurses. Its establishment made trained nursing in Canada practically simultaneous with that in the United States.

---

[8]Sleeper, Ruth: "The two inseparables—nursing service and nursing education." *The American Journal of Nursing*, 48:678–681, 1948.

[9]Seventy-fifth Anniversary (1874–1949) of the Mack Training School for Nurses. St. Catharine's General Hospital, p. 3.

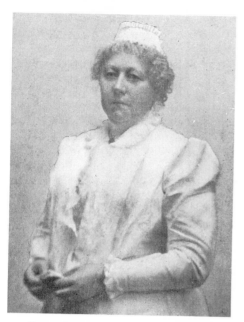

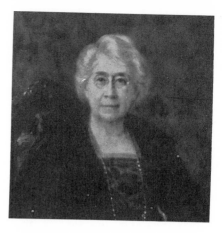

Figure 10–10. Mary Anges Snively. (Courtesy of *The Trained Nurse and Hospital Review*.)

Figure 10–8. Nora Gertrude Livingston.

The *Montreal General Hospital* was founded in 1821, and in 1875 the Board applied to Miss Nightingale for help in establishing a school. She sent them five nurses, but these were not successful. Finally, under *Nora Gertrude Livingston* (Fig. 10–8), a graduate of the New York Hospital, a superior school was established, which gave the first preliminary course and was the first three-year school in America. Flora M. Shaw (Fig. 10–9), one of its

graduates, established in 1920 the University School at McGill University.

The *Toronto General Hospital*, established about 1830, had a similar history. In 1877 an attempt was made to establish a nursing school, but it did not really flourish until 1884 when it was taken over by *Mary Agnes Snively* (Fig. 10–10), one of the founders of the Canadian Nurses' Association and a graduate of Bellevue, New York. During her 26 years of service, Miss Snively elevated the standards of the Toronto General Hospital school.

The establishment of good nursing education had been accomplished, and with the early schools of nursing came the dawn of modern nursing.

It was most unfortunate that hospitals saw an economic advantage in the establishment of schools of nursing. A few recognized the duty of providing skilled nurses for the community, but most of them stated frankly that their schools were organized "to provide better nursing *for the hospital*." Also it was promptly discovered that students in training were not only more easily disciplined and controlled but were cheaper and more satisfactory than hired nurses.

In consequence, during the 1880's, and even more in the 1890's, many schools were started in small private and special hospitals where it was impossible to give adequate training or experience. The independent schools disappeared as hospitals began to control the "training" of nursing.

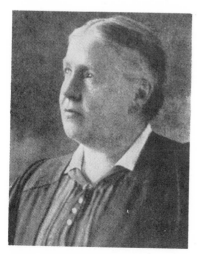

Figure 10–9. Flora Madeline Shaw. (Courtesy of *The Trained Nurse and Hospital Review*.)

PROBLEMS OF EARLY SCHOOLS

Society had accepted the social and financial obligation to educate teachers for elementary and secondary schools, but society did not recognize the obligation or benefit of financing programs to prepare nurses and thereby upgrade patient care. The early schools had great difficulty surviving as independent schools.

The early schools of nursing faced many problems; one of the most difficult was whether to supply nursing service or to educate students of nursing. This led to a fusion of the two aims. The necessity of obtaining financial aid was also a serious problem. Drives to encourage wealthy residents of the community to donate funds stimulated the schools to promise in return that they would permit students to care for members of the donors' families in their homes in times of illness.

Senior students were the ones who were sent into this community private duty nursing. Sometimes in periods of financial crises, all members of the senior class were on private duty and the least experienced students were giving nursing care to the hospitalized patients. The fees obtained from caring for these patients in their homes went into the school treasury.

An interesting hand-written note from the office of the Editor-in-Chief of the *American Journal of Nursing* and signed by Miss Sophia F. Palmer on August 12, 1904, was sent to the Superintendent of Nurses of the Connecticut Training School. Miss Palmer states: "The objection to sending nurses out [into homes] is that it deprives the nurse of a part of her legitimate education whether the money is used for the hospital or the training school. . . . Either the hospital or the community should carry the burden of the cost of the school. . . ." Miss Palmer sarcastically stated that this "is a great reflection upon the city and the members of the Board of Directors of the hospital."

In many schools, students upon admission were immediately assigned to the wards as workers (employees) and, when placed on the hospital payroll, were paid a stipend. Students were not sustained by the kind of self-respect that is accorded members of a profession. It has been stated that "heavy demands of the wards made it impossible for all students to attend their weekly lecture [class]." Certain students were assigned to take full complete notes and later had to read them to those who were unable to attend the class.

The two-year programs consisted of a first year that provided experience in patient care and a second year of ward administration. Also, these students were responsible for the instruction of new students. Their roles might be summarized as comforters of patients, housekeepers, financial providers (private duty), trainers of themselves and teachers of younger students.

Divisions of Nursing

Three divisions of nursing, hospital work, private duty and visiting or district nursing, were recognized.

Hospital nursing positions at first were only those of superintendent of nurses and perhaps an assistant, and operating and night supervisors; these were the only graduates employed. Usually the head nurses were students. Doctors gave lectures and the superintendent of nurses gave most of the classes, in both sciences and nursing arts. Gradually the better schools added instructors, graduate head nurses and graduates for general duty.

As the increasing number of schools produced a body of trained nurses, there was a marked demand for them to do *private duty* in private homes. People did not go to hospitals for medical illnesses, rarely for obstetrics and not always for surgery. Even major operations were often done in private homes. Typhoid, lasting a month or more, was prevalent for about one third of the year; pneumonia had a high death rate. The vast majority of graduate nurses did private duty. People began to understand what a trained nurse was and gave her their confidence. Twenty-four-hour duty was the rule for years.

Duties of Nurses

An item of equipment that has become commonplace is the clinical thermometer, and yet it was scarce and not readily available to nurses in the latter part of the nineteenth century. The doctor carried the thermometer and on occasion he, not the nurse, took the temperature. A nurse's assignment involved making and applying turpentine stupes to relieve abdominal distention and to encourage peristaltic action. Mustard plasters and poultices made of ginger or onions or flax-seed assisted in drawing out the "laudable pus" from an infection. Carbolic acid gargles were given to patients and, of course, the pre-paring and giving of numerous enemas, cleansing as well as nutritive, occupied much of her time and effort. Since intravenous in-fusions were unknown during this period, nutritional supplementation was achieved by the rectal administration of egg nog with brandy or chicken broth. Cupping and the application of leeches were also her duty.

Answering a patient's questions about his condition or planning a program of teaching him about his health needs was not permitted. Nurses were instructed to answer very briskly "I don't know—ask your doctor." The need of additional education caused many nurses to take postgraduate courses. These courses were supplements to the experience they had received. Several offered instruction as well as work experience, but frequently they were inaugurated to provide low cost service to hospitals without schools.

Because of ignorance of the cause of many diseases, of surgical intervention, and of the spread of disease, as well as the absence of important pharmaceutical preparations such as antibiotics, many patients were hospitalized for long periods of time. The physical, emo-tional, spiritual, recreational and nutritional aspects of nursing care were crucial to the patient's comfort and well-being. It is a well-known fact that patients came to the hospital for nursing care because the attainment of a cure was dubious. Many patients, families and doctors have recorded that it was nursing care alone that brought the patient back to health. Many interesting beds were designed and even an invalid lift assisted in at least making the long hours more comfortable (Figs. 10–11, 10–12 and 10–13).

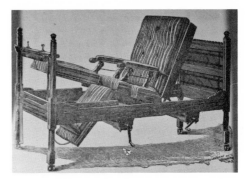

Figure 10–12. An adjustable chain bed (ca. 1880). (Author's collection.)

NURSING LEADERSHIP

In *A Century of Nursing*, written in 1876, Abby Woolsey stressed the desirability of ele-vating nursing to an educated and honorable profession. She pleaded for quality in educa-tional programs, expressing the feeling that nursing schools should be practically normal schools (the predecessor of the state teachers' colleges). A Committee of the Bellevue Train-ing School mapped plans for a "College of Nursing"; this did not become a reality.

John Eaton, Commissioner of Education, in a public address conveyed the impression that the training of nurses should be an edu-cational endeavor and must be planned on educational lines. His address was published

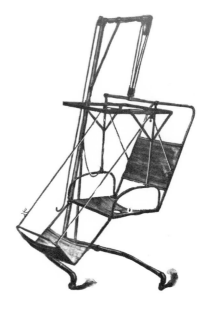

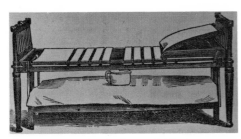

Figure 10–11. The Crosby invalid bed (ca. 1877). (Author's collection.)

Figure 10–13. An invalid lift (ca. 1880).

under the title, "Training Schools for Nurses," by the Bureau of Education, Washington, in 1879.

In addition to the founding of these early schools of nursing in the last quarter of the century, there were some dynamic leaders in nursing education and teaching tools such as textbooks were published.

Isabel Hampton Robb (1860–1910) was a most outstanding leader in nursing and in the education of students of nursing. Born in Welland, Ontario, Canada, after attending St. Catherine's Collegiate Institute for several years, she accepted a teaching position. She decided to enter the field of nursing and in 1881 was admitted to *Bellevue Training School* as a student nurse (Fig. 10–14) and graduated in 1883. She was a remarkably constructive thinker and had the rare ability both to create and make practical application of new ideas.

In 1886, she became *Superintendent of Nurses at Illinois Training School in Chicago.* The school contracted with Cook County Hospital for clinical experience for the students. The ability of Miss Isabel Hampton as an organizer began to be noted in this position. She put into practice a graded system of theory. Through her good judgment, she terminated the practice of students' doing private duty as part of their education.

In 1889, Miss Hampton journeyed to Baltimore to organize a new school at *Johns Hopkins Hospital.* Here her fertile mind gave birth to new ideas, and many innovations were attempted. She became "Principal" instead of "Superintendent"; she established policies for a twelve-hour day, which included time allowance for meals, definite recreation, rest and study periods, and a limit on the day's work. Her aim was quality nursing care that combined a happy balance of intellectual and manual skills. She had the ability and persistence to achieve it. Of her leadership qualities, Miss Nutting has commented:[10]

Planning, initiating, directing, and controlling, —such activities provided for her an element in which she lived and moved with the greatest ease and freedom. She was in every sense of the word a leader, by nature, by capacity, by personal attributes and qualities, by choice, and probably to some extent by inheritance and training; a follower she never was.

Realizing the need for textbooks, Miss Hampton wrote *Nursing—Its Principles and Practice for Hospital and Private Use.*

Another challenging assignment was given to her. During the World's Fair in Chicago in 1893, the International Congress of Charities, Correction and Philanthropy was to be held, and a section for nursing was included. Miss Hampton needed the thinking and advice of Florence Nightingale, as well as nurse edu-

---

[10] Nutting, M. A.: "Isabel Hampton Robb—her work in organization and education." *American Journal of Nursing,* *10*:19, October 1910.

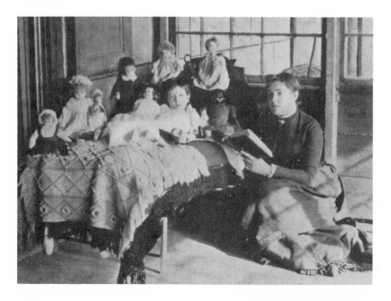

Figure 10–14. Isabel Hampton as a student nurse caring for a little girl surrounded by her dolls. (Author's collection.)

cators in this country. Miss Nightingale shared her thoughts generously through correspondence, and a firm friendship blossomed between these two dynamic leaders.

During the Congress, the nurse educators were called together by Miss Hampton and the *Society of Superintendents of Training Schools for Nurses* evolved. She became the first president.

Miss Hampton's attractiveness, combined with poise and a charming manner, have been written of by many admirers. Dr. Hunter Robb became her chief admirer and in June of 1894, Isabel Hampton married Dr. Robb. She resigned from active nursing, but remained an ardent supporter in the fight for better preparation for nurses, especially nurse educators, and of a better quality of care for patients (Fig. 10–15).

Her revolutionary but sound ideas were presented in 1895 at the annual convention of the American Society of Superintendents of Training Schools for Nurses. She advocated a *three-year course* and an *eight-hour day!* This was at a time when many students were working twice that number of hours. Another suggestion was to terminate the practice of giving stipends each month and with the money saved, she suggested establishing

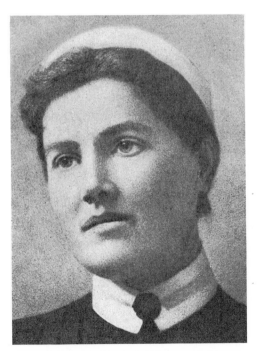

Figure 10–15. Isabel Hampton Robb. (Author's collection.)

libraries. This would change the status from employee to student.

Mrs. Robb felt that an organization was needed for *all nurses*, not just for nursing school administrators. In 1896, she became the first president of the newly formed *Nurses Associated Alumnae of the United States and Canada*, which was a nation-wide union of alumnae associations. In unity there could be strength.

Unlike Florence Nightingale, Isabel Hampton Robb believed that the status as well as preparation of practitioners of nursing would be benefited by licensing examinations and registration. A form of legal control would protect patients from incompetent nurses as well as elevate the standards for the nurse, as it did for both the physician and the lawyer. Her efforts played a large part in the development of the courses established in 1898 at Teachers' College.

Isabel Hampton Robb's brilliant career was ended abruptly in 1910 when she was killed in a tragic accident.

A trust fund was established to perpetuate the memory of this brilliant leader. The *Isabel Hampton Robb scholarships* have permitted many nurses to receive a more enriched background; hopefully, this has been used to elevate the quality of nursing care, as well as that of nursing education.

Mary Adelaide Nutting (Fig. 10–16) (1858–1948) was born in Quebec and later attended private schools in Montreal, Boston and Ottawa, receiving special instruction in music and art. She was a member of the first class to graduate from Johns Hopkins and became principal of this school when Mrs. Robb resigned. Her concepts of nursing education seemed to parallel those of Mrs. Robb, and Miss Nutting carried out many of the reforms Mrs. Robb had initiated.

In 1907 Miss Nutting was appointed to the faculty of Teachers' College, Columbia University, and became the first professor of nursing in the world, a position that she held until her retirement in 1925. Out of gratitude for her outstanding leadership, The Adelaide Nutting Historical Nursing Collection was dedicated to her memory and has been exhibited at Teachers' College.

Among her many achievements were: raising the standards of basic nursing education, assisting in the establishment of nursing organizations, preserving the past in the four-volume *History of Nursing* written in collabora-

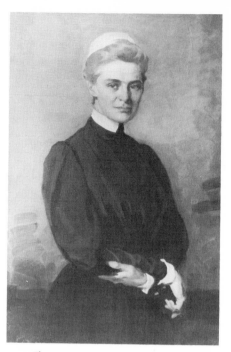

Figure 10–16. Mary Adelaide Nutting. (Author's collection.)

tion with *Lavinia Dock*, encouraging provision for financial support for schools of nursing and, thus, permitting separation of schools of nursing from hospital ownership and control, developing programs at Teachers' College for nurses in teaching, public health, supervision and administration, and coordinating nursing services during World War I. Other contributions included a brochure entitled *A Sound Economic Basis for Schools of Nursing,*[11] and, in 1912, *The Educational Status of Nursing.*[12]

Miss Nutting received an honorary Master of Arts degree from Yale in 1921. The Liberty Service Medal was awarded to her for her humanitarian and patriotic services. The National League of Nursing Education designed the Adelaide Nutting Medal for Leadership in Nursing Education, presenting the first medal to Miss Nutting in 1944.

---

[11] Nutting, M. A.: *A Sound Economic Basis for Schools of Nursing.* New York, G. P. Putnam's Sons, 1926.
[12] Nutting, M. A.: *Educational Status of Nursing.* Bulletin No. 7, U.S. Bureau of Education, 1912.

UNIFORMS

Nurses' uniforms were not designed or worn by lay nurses until the latter part of the nineteenth century. *Euphemia Van Rensselaer* (Fig. 10–17) has been credited with recognizing the need for a uniform and designing one.

Miss Van Rensselaer was born in 1840 of an illustrious family. Her mother was Elizabeth King, the daughter of Governor King of New York and the niece of Charles King, President of Columbia University; her grandfather, Rufus King, had been one of the early American statesmen and was ambassador to Great Britain on two occasions. Miss Van Rensselaer's father was Brigadier-General Van Rensselaer whose death from typhoid fever prompted her to become a trained nurse.

The niece[13] of Miss Van Rensselaer relates the story in this way:

The story I heard from my Mother was that Euphemia Van Rensselaer volunteered for service at Bellevue when the two Miss Schuylers—granddaughters of the General—organized the States Charities Aid Association. Up to that time the only nurses were the old women collected by the Hospital. The Misses Schuyler, inspired by Florence

---

[13] Personal correspondence with Mrs. Christopher Wyatt (Euphemia Van Rensselaer Wyatt).

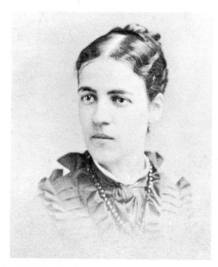

Figure 10–17. Euphemia Van Rensselaer (Sister Marie Dolores) in 1878. (Courtesy of Mrs. Christopher Wyatt.)

Nightingale were determined to relieve this impossible situation and procured volunteers. In 1876 it was determined to have uniforms but this did not suit the volunteers. It was then that my Aunt set the example by taking home some material and having a uniform made for herself. When Miss Van Rensselaer was seen duly clad the others decided to follow suit. She later became an Anglican nun in Clewer, England and then when her brother, who was a clergyman in the Episcopalian Church came over to Rome, she followed him and joined the Sisters of Charity. She was sent to Nassau to found a Mission and on her return organized Seton Hospital for tuberculosis which was taken over later by the City. She then organized the Grace Institute—a trade school for women—and ended her life in a Day Nursery in her brother's parish—St. Francis Xavier's—the Jesuit Church at 16th Street and Sixth Avenue. She died about 1912 in the New York Foundling Asylum.

Euphemia Van Rensselaer designed the blue and white uniform, apron and cap of the Bellevue Training School.

The nurse's cap has always been and still is distinctive. It probably originated when all women wore caps indoors; this would account for the lace frills on the cap that Florence Nightingale designed for her school in 1860. At one time the cap that entirely covered the hair was thought correct, and the "dusting cap" pattern was much used. Since these were ugly, the style gave way to one which covered the knot of hair that was usually on top of the head. Caps either were not washable (book muslin or organdy) or had elaborate frills that required special laundering. About 1910, simply made, easily laundered caps began to be used. The use of black bands for graduates or seniors shows the military influence, an attempt to indicate rank. The present customs in this matter are so varied they are meaningless.

NURSE AUTHORS

In the early years of nursing, practically all textbooks used by nurses were written by doctors. Miss Nightingale's *Notes on Nursing* (1859) probably did much to make nurses feel that they were capable of writing their own textbooks and knew best how to present the art of nursing.

With the exception of the texts, Bellevue Training School's *Handbook of Nursing* (1878) and Connecticut Training School's *Handbook*

on Nursing (1879), which were the joint work of doctors and nurses and used for thirty years, the first nursing textbook in America was written by Mrs. Clara Weeks-Shaw, a graduate of the New York Hospital.

Clara S. Weeks's *A Textbook of Nursing* (1885) made the distinction between true nursing care and the mere execution of the doctors' orders.

Diana C. Kimber has been credited with writing the *first textbook on anatomy for nurses* in 1893. She was born in Oxfordshire, England. She came to New York and entered Bellevue Training School in 1884 after receiving an excellent liberal education both in England and in Germany. The teaching field attracted her and, feeling the need for a textbook on anatomy, she undertook the assignment of writing one. It was the *first scientific book written by a nurse for nurses.* She returned to England in 1898, entering an Anglican nursing sisterhood. From this spiritual environment, she went forth to care for the sick poor in their homes, carrying out her high ideals of service.

Minnie Goodnow (Fig. 10–18), well known author, educator, war nurse, and administrator, was one of the pioneers in the field of textbook writing. She wrote the first textbook on chemistry for nurses in the United States in 1911, the well known *Nursing History* in 1916[14] and the first *Physics for Nurses* in 1919. Miss Goodnow saw active service overseas during World War I and had a colorful background as an administrator for over forty years. She died in 1952.

Bertha Harmer was a graduate of Toronto General Hospital. She received the degrees of B.S. and M.A. from Columbia University and was instructor of St. Luke's Hospital, New York City. Assisting in organizing the Yale School of Nursing, Miss Harmer was one of its professors. For some years she was in charge of the Graduate School of Nursing at McGill University, Montreal. She wrote a textbook entitled *Principles and Practice of Nursing.* She died in 1934.

Lavinia Dock's *Textbook on Materia Medica for Nurses,* published in 1890, was another milestone. Miss Dock graduated from Bellevue Hospital in 1886. She held executive positions in Bellevue, Johns Hopkins and the Illinois Training School, and worked long

---

[14]This textbook is successor to Miss Goodnow's many editions of *Nursing History.*

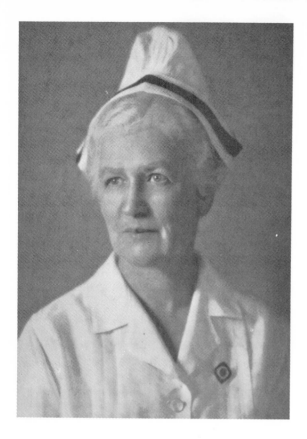

Figure 10–18. Minnie Goodnow.

at the Henry Street Settlement. She was for several years Secretary of the International Council of Nurses and one of its chief promoters.

The first general history of nursing, with the exception of two pamphlets, was written by Americans, M. Adelaide Nutting and Lavinia L. Dock. Its four volumes have constituted a standard reference. The school at Johns Hopkins University, Baltimore, was the first to put the history of nursing into its curriculum.

Lavinia L. Dock (1858–1956) was one of the great women in nursing history, contributed to the improvement of the status of women and was active in many movements contributing to social welfare.

SOCIAL SERVICE

The closing years of the nineteenth century saw a resurgence of *humanitarianism.* Many individuals and groups endeavored to relieve the physical and social sufferings of others.

Leprosy continued to plague many people, and devoted care for its victims was still needed.

In 1873 *Father Damien* de Veuster (1840–1889), a young Belgian priest, requested to be sent as a missionary to Molokai in the Hawaiian Islands. Singlehanded he cheered his heartsick victims, built homes for them, nursed them and buried them. Thus began the magnificent story of courage, devotion and sacrifice that remained an inspiration to his patients and followers.

In 1894, the State of Louisiana realized the need for a place to care for the many victims of leprosy. Money was raised, an abandoned sugar plantation was purchased and a physician, Dr. L. A. Wailes, volunteered to take care of the lepers. When he quickly realized that more assistance was needed, he resigned. In 1896 *The Sisters of Charity of St. Vincent de Paul* received the petition for help from the Board of Directors of the "Louisiana Leper Home" and the nuns offered to send some members of their community. Sister Beatrice, a trained nurse from

Boston, joined four other nuns and took over the settlement. The Sisters worked for many years under incredible hardships to make the institution a suitable place in which to live and work. Patients received a home and nursing care. Their excellent work was done in a spirit of devotion. In 1917, Congress passed a law authorizing the purchase of this institution and named it the *National Leprosarium*. Because of World War I, this transfer was not completed until 1921. Since then, the U.S. Public Health Service has been responsible for this project. The Sisters of Charity have remained an integral part of the staff.

In "Nurses at Carville" three primary areas have been identified in the care of the patient with leprosy (Hansen's disease)—the importance of a strong nurse-patient relationship, the accurate recording of observations, assessments and facts, and the "nurse's role as an educator on health problems related to leprosy."[15]

Sister Mary Anne Hain, director of nursing at the Carville, Louisiana, Public Health Service Hospital, was the recipient of the 1971 Federal Nursing Service Award given annually by the Association of Military Surgeons of the United States to a nurse member for outstanding accomplishments in the advancement of professional nursing.

William Booth (1829–1912) was an ardent religious leader who was fired with enthusiasm to rescue poor souls who were living in the slums of London. He knew that hunger, dirt and misery needed to be removed before spiritual assistance could be rendered.

In 1878, he organized and became the first general of the *Salvation Army*. He taught Christian principles and practiced Christian living by giving food, clothing and shelter to the poor, as well as aiding them in finding suitable, useful work. His labors extended to other lands. The gracious assistance given by his army to the United States' soldiers during World Wars I and II can never be forgotten.

William Booth's book, *In Darkest England and the Way Out* (1890), reflects his belief that to restore a man to humanity is to restore him to God.

The *Settlement House Movement* was started at Toynbee Hall in London by Oxford University students who studied community problems and aided in alleviating them.

Jane Addams (1860–1935) graduated from college in 1881. One night two years later, she wandered through London's East End and for the first time saw the slums of a big city. She was determined to do what she could to relieve the problems of city slums. (See Figure 10–19.) In Chicago in 1889, she and Ellen Gates Starr purchased a big old house and opened the doors to the neighborhood; this was the beginning of *Hull House*. Help of any sort was available to neighbors. This was the spirit of social service. Jane Addams was a leader in the fight for suffrage for women. She, with Nicholas Murray Butler, was the recipient of the 1931 Nobel Peace Prize.

The *Young Men's Christian Association* (Y.M.C.A.) was started to develop the spiritual, social, physical and intellectual well-being of men. It was organized in 1844 in London and in 1851 in America. Physical training has become an important part of the program.

During the Civil War, several branches of the Young Men's Christian Association joined to form the United States Christian Commission for the welfare of soldiers in camps and hospitals. In the First World War, they cared for prisoners as well as providing recreation for the soldiers. In the Second World War, they cooperated with other agencies to form the United Service Organization (U.S.O.) which planned recreational programs for the armed forces.

The *Young Women's Christian Association* (Y.W.C.A.) was founded to assist women and

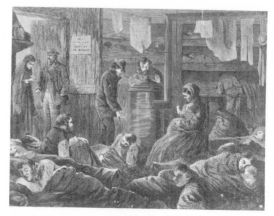

Figure 10–19. Underground lodging for the poor in New York. (Author's collection.)

[15]Hughes, Sister Ann Elizabeth; Bertonneau, Sister Dorothea; and Enna, Carl D.: "Nurses at Carville." *The American Journal of Nursing*, Vol. 68, No. 12, December 1968.

girls spiritually, socially, intellectually and physically. In 1855, Lady Kinnaird in London encouraged a group of women to provide homes for women workers. In 1866, there was a Young Women's Christian Association in Boston. Local associations spread until it became the vast organization it is. The Young Women's Christian Association units in this country have been a source of housing for women in every large city.

The next humanitarian project was the establishment of the *Grenfell Mission. Sir Wilfred Grenfell* (1865–1940) was an English medical missionary who went to Labrador in 1892 (Fig. 10–20). He built a chain of hospital centers and nursing stations, established cooperative stores and built schools, libraries and orphanages. In 1912, the International Grenfell Association consolidated the work of the American, Canadian and English branches that supported his mission. Sir Wilfred supervised the work of his staff and gave assistance by cruising along the coast in the hospital steamer, Strathcona II.

Patients were reached by dogsled in the winter and by boat in the summer. Thus, another amazing project had been developed for the welfare of mankind.

NURSING IN THE SPANISH-AMERICAN WAR

The year was 1898, and American patriotism was being fanned to fever pitch by the slogan "Remember the 'Maine.' " The United States battleship "Maine" had been sunk mysteriously on the fifteenth of February in Havana harbor. This was one of the many incidents that finally incited President McKinley to ask Congress for authority to intervene in Cuba's struggle to be free from Spanish control and domination. He was authorized to permit enlistment of volunteers.

There was no organized army nurse corps although training schools were in existence and trained nurses were available; furthermore, there was no system by which nurses could be provided for war service. Congress appropriated the necessary funds and gave the Surgeon General the authority to employ nurses under contract.

The Nurses Associated Alumnae of the United States and Canada (now the American Nurses' Association) had been formed for such a short time, and although this was an organization representing the trained nurses of both countries, it was not recognized as the spokesman for nursing nor was it prepared to undertake the task of listing qualifications or recruiting nurses for this war service.

A physician, *Dr. Anita Newcomb McGee,* was the person who assumed the task. Through her prompting, the Surgeon General asked the Daughters of the American Revolution to carry out the procurement of nurses. The Surgeon General felt that nurses would not

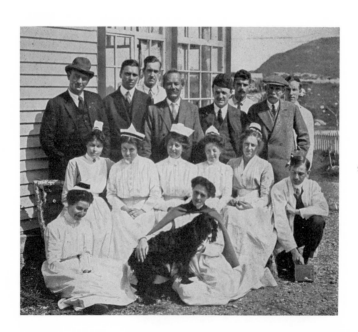

Figure 10–20. Dr. Grenfell (center) and his staff at St. Anthony's Hospital, Labrador, 1914.

be needed because military surgeons were opposed to their presence in military hospitals. The gentle but firm insistence of Dr. McGee won out, and as she was vice president of the Daughters of the American Revolution the offer to recruit was accepted. Dr. McGee established standards of admission to the service as well as a valuable system of keeping records. Credentials were evaluated, statements being obtained from schools from which the applicant graduated, as well as a certificate of good reputation.

Nurses were recruited; they were needed desperately, not so much because of war casualties but because of the typhoid fever that afflicted many of the soldiers in camp. Other communicable diseases that threatened the troops in Cuba were yellow fever, malaria and dysentery.

When Dr. McGee was appointed Acting Assistant Surgeon General, she was responsible for the Army Nurse Division. At this time she terminated the assistance of the Daughters of the American Revolution. The efforts of Dr. McGee and the excellence of the work of the nurses in this war led to the establishment of a permanent Army Nurse Corps. Commenting on the achievements of the nurses in general an officer was quoted as saying, "When you were coming, we did not know what we would do with you. Now we do not know what we would have done without you."

Many members of the Associated Alumnae and many women prominent in the nursing world served in the war. (Among these were Mary Gladwin, Eugenie Hibbard, Esther Hasson and Anna Maxwell.) A total of nearly 1600 graduate nurses served.

These army nurses invariably won the esteem and recognition of the officers and men. Their supporters included the surgeons who had originally been most prejudiced against them. The continued employment of women as army nurses was undoubtedly due to the skill and devotion that they showed at the time of the Spanish-American War.

During the Spanish-American War, a military physician, *Major Walter Reed,* was appointed chief of a committee to study the cause and spread of typhoid fever in the army camps. After much searching, it was determined that flies, aided by unclean practices in general, were the most obvious source of contamination.

At the end of the war, it was apparent that disease had taken a heavier toll of lives than the bullets of the enemy. Yellow fever had been a particularly virulent and fatal enemy. Burning sulfur candles as a means of prevention of this disease did not appear to be successful. When a person died, all his personal effects, called "fomites," were burned. This could include even the burning of his home. This was still no solution to the problem. The United States government sent physicians to *Cuba* with the assignment of finding some method of control of this malady, which had been endemic in Havana for more than 200 years. The physicians were *Drs. James Carroll, Aristides Agramonte, Jesse W. Lazear and Walter Reed.*

Dr. Carlos Finlay, a Havana physician, had been striving for 19 years to convince his medical colleagues that yellow fever was caused by a common house mosquito. Major Walter Reed and Dr. Agramonte consulted Dr. Finlay who shared his theories about yellow fever and even gave them a supply of mosquito larvae of the suspected species. Human volunteers were needed.

Heroic Americans volunteered, and the first ones were doctors. Some survived, but others died, martyrs to the cause of science. The experiments proved that yellow fever was transmitted by the bite of the mosquito now called *Aëdes aegypti.*

One of the unsung heroines of this scientific project was a nurse, *Clara Louise Maass* (1876–1901), who lost her life in the yellow fever experiments in Cuba and was accorded full military honors.

Miss Maass entered the Newark German Hospital Training School for Nurses (Lutheran Memorial Hospital, Newark, New Jersey) in 1893 and graduated in 1895. She was one of the first to volunteer to care for the sick and wounded soldiers in army camps in this country and in Cuba. She responded to the call for nurses in the government hospitals in the Philippines and was stationed at Manila. Her patients were critically ill from typhoid fever, smallpox, and yellow fever. She was distressed that there was no method of prevention or cure for these diseases.

In 1901, Clara Maass returned to Cuba and was employed by the sanitary department of Havana. She was assigned to a hospital that was an inoculation station for the yellow fever experimentation. She volunteered and succumbed to the treacherous affliction. The epitaph on her monument

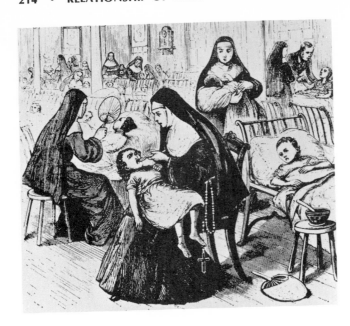

Figure 10–21. The Sisters of Charity at St. Vincent's Infant Asylum in New Orleans, Louisiana caring for victims of yellow fever.

reads: "Greater love hath no man than this, that a man lay down his life for his friends."

A devastating epidemic of yellow fever had occurred in many of the southern states. Many people packed their families and possessions and attempted to flee to safety. A lack of physicians helped add to the devastation of the population. Many nurses, such as the Sisters of Charity, to the best of their ability aided the sick (Fig. 10–21).

PUBLIC HEALTH PROBLEMS

Two community problems of vital importance were those of contagious disease and environmental sanitation. Many civic improvement groups attempted to solve these problems. *The Association for Improving the Condition of the Poor*, as well as the *State Charities Aid Association*, emphasized the dangers in tenement dwellings because of overcrowding, poor ventilation, inadequate water supply and absence of decent privies. As a result, the sanitary police force was increased and, by 1887, the New York Health Department was required by law to inspect tenement dwellings twice a year.

Public dispensaries were available for medical care of the poor (Figs. 10–22 and 10–23). The need for well prepared nurses to teach and care for people in homes, outpatient facilities and clinics, as well as assist in a dynamic program of prevention of disease, was obvious.

In the 1870's and the first part of the twentieth century, *tuberculosis* was among the leading causes of death. The microorganism, the tubercle bacillus, that caused the disease was identified about 1882 by Dr. Robert Koch. It was determined that this infection was spread from person to person, as well as by drinking milk from diseased cattle. A tuberculosis control program was initiated; it included hospital facilities to isolate and care for victims of this disease, tuberculin tests for cattle, regular inspection of milk and meat supplies and mandatory reporting of cases.

Patients were admitted to such psychologically depressing institutions as the *Hospital for Incurables* (Fig. 10–24). The importance of healthful surroundings was pointed out by Dr. Edward L. Trudeau, who was stricken with tuberculosis in 1872 while nursing his brother. He had been taught as a medical student that tuberculosis "was a noncontagious, generally incurable and inherited disease, due to inherited constitutional peculiarities, perverted humours and various types of inflammation."

Trudeau, fearing an early death, retired to the Adirondack Mountains. He was surprised to discover a lack of suitable living

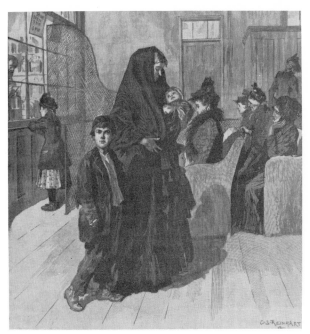

Figure 10–22. A public dispensary in the 1890's. (Courtesy of New York Academy of Medicine and New York City Department of Health.)

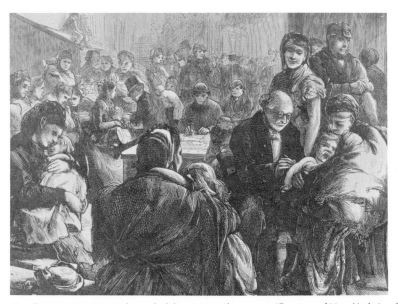

Figure 10–23. Smallpox vaccination at the end of the nineteenth century. (Courtesy of New York Academy of Medicine and New York City Department of Health.)

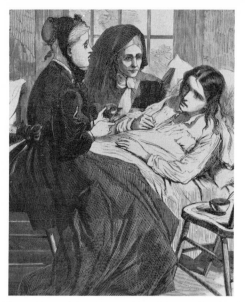

Figure 10–24. A patient and her visitors at the Hospital for Incurables on Blackwell's Island. (Courtesy of New York Academy of Medicine and New York City Department of Health.)

arrangements for patients of moderate means. In 1885 he established the Adirondack Cottage Sanatorium, which became known as the Trudeau Sanatorium. The importance of rest, sunshine, fresh air and nutrition was emphasized.

The widespread acceptance of the inevitability of tuberculosis, often referred to

as the white plague or galloping consumption (Fig. 10–25), is reflected in several of the operas of the period, such as Verdi's *La Traviata* and Puccini's *La Bohème*. The association of this disease with celebrities of the century is presented in Waksman's book[15] and a special chapter is devoted to tuberculosis in literature and the arts. Among the victims of tuberculosis were Keats, Shelley, Robert Louis Stevenson, Goethe, Schiller, Washington Irving, Elizabeth Barrett Browning, Chopin and Chekhov.

Opium or opium derivatives were taken to soothe the effects of the disease. It has been reported that Coleridge wrote "Kubla Khan" after taking large quantities of opium.

Edgar Allen Poe described the effects of tuberculosis from which he had first-hand observation in his family, as did Ralph Waldo Emerson and the Brontës.[16] There are also textbook presentations of the disease in *Nicholas Nickleby, David Copperfield* and *Wuthering Heights*.

There was clearly a need for the practical application of the components of good nursing care for tuberculosis patients and their families.

---

[15]Waksman, Selman A.: *The Conquest of Tuberculosis.* Berkeley and Los Angeles, University of California Press, 1964.

---

[16]Hobson, W.: *World Health and History.* Bristol, John Wright & Sons Ltd., 1963. See Chapter X, The white plague.

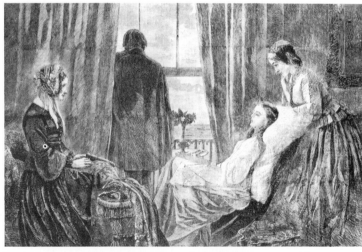

Figure 10–25. This picture entitled "Fading Away" reflects the devastation and frustration of the effects of tuberculosis, not only on the teen-ager but also on the family. (Author's collection.)

PUBLIC HEALTH NURSING

In Liverpool, England, in 1859, after a lengthy illness, the wife of *William Rathbone* died. Mrs. Rathbone had all the comforts that wealth and affection could provide. In his grief, Mr. Rathbone pondered the predicament of the poor families bereft of money and comfortable surroundings who might be faced with long-term sickness. Mrs. Mary Robinson, the nurse who had been such a comfort to his wife and the Rathbone family, was asked to try an experiment for three months. She was to give nursing care and comfort to poor patients and was given the necessary appliances for usual bedside care as well as medicines and nourishing foods. Included in her assignment was the responsibility to teach families to improve their standard of living.

The conditions Mrs. Robinson found were worse than anything she could have imagined, and in despair she returned after one month to Mr. Rathbone to resign from her assignment. After much persuasion on his part, she returned and continued in her project.

Mr. Rathbone believed in the value of personal service in relieving the needs of the poor. He convinced the Liverpool Relief Society to adopt a system of dividing towns into districts and districts into sections. To each district a committee of "Friendly Visitors" was assigned. Initial inquiries were conducted by paid agents before the case was turned over to the care of the friendly visitor of that section, to be handled with tact and kindness. Mr. Rathbone's book, *Social Organization of Effort in Works of Benevolence and Public Charity by a Man of Business*, presented his beliefs and suggestions for social welfare.

He was convinced of the need and value of district nursing. He felt that many persons with long-term illnesses would not be admitted to a general hospital, that many patients preferred to stay at home with their loved ones, that there were not enough hospitals available to meet the demands made upon them and that the cost was far less when the patient stayed at home. These were urgent reasons for action in the development of district nursing.

Mr. Rathbone consulted Miss Nightingale who encouraged him to organize a training school for nurses in the Liverpool Royal Infirmary. There would be the dual benefit of improving the nursing care within the hospital and of providing nurses for the sick of the community. Mr. Rathbone had constructed a home for nurses, and he presented it to the Royal Infirmary; this solved a housing problem. In 1862, the *Training School and Home for Nurses of the Royal Infirmary* began the program of providing nurses for the hospital, private duty and district nurses.

By 1865, in the town of Derby in England, a trained nurse was placed as a "Lady Superintendent" in charge of all district nursing units to supervise the quality of the nursing care they gave.

An interesting project developed in relation to *Mrs. Ranyard's Bible and Domestic Mission*, which she had organized in 1857. The Bible women visited the poor to read to them and pray with them (Fig. 10–26). These eager women recognized the need for being prepared to minister to ever-present physical needs as well as the spiritual. Finally, in 1868, the nurses' branch of the mission was established in London. After proper preparation as a Bible woman, three months' training followed in the medical and surgical wards of the hospital, plus a month's training in obstetrics. No classes seem to have been given; mere presence in the hospital setting seemed all the preparation that was available. Caring for patients with contagious diseases was not permitted because of the danger of spreading infection.

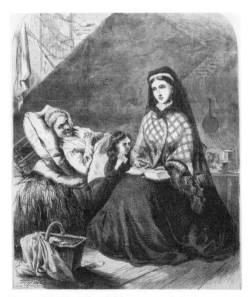

Figure 10–26. The Bible woman bringing a spiritual message, alms and compassion. (Author's collection.)

In 1874, a committee was established in London called *The National Association for Providing Trained Nurses for the Sick Poor*. The objective of this group was to improve the quantity and quality of nursing care. The committee developed a logical plan for solving this problem by determining what nurses were available. what preparation was needed and how other groups had handled this problem.

Miss Lees, a pupil of Florence Nightingale, was placed in charge of investigation. About 700 to 800 letters were sent to clergymen and medical officers in London. Data revealed great need for nurses, but personal interviews showed that district nurses had poor preparation, if any. The cases presented the ways by which nurses carried infection from one house to another.

The conclusions of this committee were: There was need for more district nurses. Hospital nurses' training schools should provide preparation for care of the sick in their homes. Under the prevailing system there was too much emphasis on distribution of alms, which was not nursing, and too little on giving nursing care. Nurses needed to be given guidance, direction and supervision. There was too little consultation between nurses and doctors in planning for patient care. There was much too little teaching given to the patient and his family.

After reviewing their conclusions, the following proposals were drawn up: (1) An independent training school should be established in close proximity to a hospital similar to Miss Nightingale's school and its relationship to St. Thomas' Hospital, but under the control of the trustees of the school. (2) Close to the hospital would be a district home where four to six nurses could live with a superintendent (supervisor). After the year's training in the hospital, a three months' apprenticeship would be given in district nursing. (3) Payment should be obtained for this service, provided a patient could afford to pay. This would permit many patients to receive care who were in need of as well as deserving of this service—poverty-stricken families—but who were unable to procure it. (4) An alternate plan was presented in case the previous suggestions were not acceptable or feasible. A superintendent could be appointed to manage a less elaborate but essentially identical program without developing the special training school.

This remarkable report was published in 1875 and received favorable attention by the public. The fourth suggestion was adopted, and Miss Lees was appointed Superintendent. Many gentlewomen were recruited because it was Miss Lees' belief that this type of nursing required the highest type of women, who were well educated, to demonstrate the actual nursing care that involved teaching opportunities. This organized effort was called *The Metropolitan and National Nursing Association for Providing Trained Nurses for the Sick Poor.*

The uniform adopted and worn by the Metropolitan Nurses was a dress of brown trimmed with dark blue linen, with large apron and oversleeves of the same material to be worn when on duty. The outdoor uniform consisted of a large dark blue cloak, blue alpaca in summer. A black straw bonnet, trimmed with black silk and piped with pale blue silk, lined with white muslin with a stiffly crimped muslin border and wide white muslin strings, completed the uniform. At that time, bonnets were worn when on duty. A leather bag was pinned to the uniform and contained pin cushion, scissors and dressing forceps. Each nurse carried a small leather handbag, containing disinfectants, hand towel, soap and surgical dressings.

The training of these nurses was the important function of this Association. Miss Lees selected applicants with care, and they remained in the Central Office for one month under observation as they accompanied a more experienced nurse on calls. If these women were considered suitable, they went into the hospital for one year and then returned for a six months' course in district nursing under the guidance of the superintendent (supervisor), who went with her on each new case, teaching her how to care for each patient. This appears to have been a good use of the apprenticeship system.

Special classes were given in anatomy, physiology, hygiene, diseases of women and ways of peptonizing foods. Examinations had to be passed after the completion of the classes.

This experiment proved successful. Better educational methods, added to greater individual intellectual capacity, were two points raised by Miss Lees (then Mrs. Dacre Craven) in her address given at the World's Fair in Chicago.

District nurses should feel themselves beyond

and before all things, the servants of the sick poor. They instruct—but practically and by example. District nursing means, the care of the sick poor in their own homes, where there are no proper appliances, and where the nurse can rarely see the doctor,—in some cases, not at all. She must know how to put the room of each patient into such good sanitary condition that the patient may have a fair chance of recovery, and how to extemporize hospital appliances where these are required. She must be so well trained in nursing duties as not only to know how to observe and report correctly on every case under her charge, but to allow no change to pass unnoticed; and to be able to apply, provisionally, suitable treatment, until the medical man shall have arrived. She must know how to purify the foul air of the room without making a draught; to dust without making a dust; to ice drinks without ice; to filter water without a filter; to bake without an oven . . . She must be content to be servant and teacher by turns. . . . A district nurse must have a real love for the poor and a real desire to lessen the misery she may see among them; and such tact as well as skill that she will do what is best for her patients even against their will. No district nurse should ever give alms or relief of any kind, beyond the highest of all—that of nursing service. . . . A nurse's business is to nurse—but she has also to teach the poor those sanitary laws which are household words with the well-to-do.[17]

Thus important groundwork for the development of community nursing had been laid. Another opportunity was presented when *Queen Victoria* celebrated the fiftieth anniversary of her reign as Queen. Of the 76,000 pounds raised by the women of England, 70,000 pounds were used to establish the Institute for the Training and Supervising of District Nurses. Properly qualified nursing associations already in existence were given an opportunity to affiliate. This consolidation would upgrade and standardize the community nursing service. A form for affiliation was devised.

In 1889, the *Queen Victoria Jubilee Institute for Nurses* was founded by royal charter. This Institute was connected with the historically famous St. Katherine's Hospital, founded by Queen Matilda in 1148. This group of nurses was called "Jubilee Institute Nurses" but became known as the *"Queen's Nurses."*

In addition to the plan for preparation of these nurses, which resembled the one

developed by Miss Lees, there was special training available for those who would work in the rural areas. This program ranged from four to eighteen months according to the background of the individual and was given at the "Maternity Charity and District Nurses' Home." This type of preparation provided trained nurses and midwives.

In America, after the War of 1812 that left wives and children without a breadwinner and after the devastation and death wrought by the epidemics of yellow fever, a *Ladies' Benevolent Society* was organized for the relief of persons suffering from anguish, sickness and poverty. Cases were investigated, relief was given in proportion to needs and work was provided for the unemployed.

By 1832, Dr. Joseph Warrington had organized the society of *Lying-in Charity for Attending Indigent Women in Their Homes.* This group instructed prudent women as nurses.

By 1877, the *Woman's Board of the New York City Mission* recognized as great a need for nurses to go into the homes of the poor to care for physical needs as their missionary members cared for spiritual needs. (See Figure 10–27.) These nurses received their training at Bellevue.

The *Visiting Nurse Society of Philadelphia* employed nurses to care for the sick in their homes in 1886. The service was extended to persons of moderate means who paid, as well as to the poor to whom the care was given free. A uniform was adopted in 1887, and in 1891 Miss Linda Richards assumed charge of the Philadelphia Visiting Nurse Society.

In 1886, the *Instructive District Nursing Association* was founded in Boston, Massachusetts. Teaching was an important aspect of the home care of the sick and the principles of hygiene and sanitation as well as health subjects and aspects of illness were taught. The Instructive District Nursing Association was the first to recognize the educational opportunities in visiting nursing.

Annie Brainard[18] has said:

It was a fortunate thing that the first District Nursing Association in America should have laid such stress on the educational side of the work, and as proof that their attitude was accepted by America as the right and proper one, we may

---

[17]Proceedings of the International Congress of Nurses, 1893.

[18]Brainard, Annie M.: *The Evolution of Public Health Nursing.* Philadelphia, W. B. Saunders Co., 1922, p. 208.

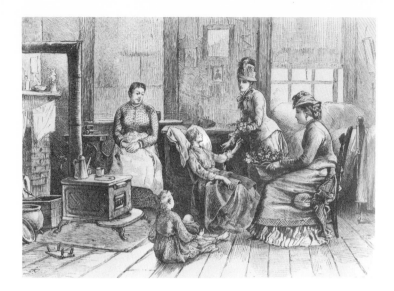

Figure 10–27. Members of The Flower Mission visiting the sick. (Author's collection.)

cite the words of Isabel Hampton (the late Mrs. Robb) who five years later in an address to the International Congress of Nurses (1893) said: "In District Nursing we are confronted with conditions which require the highest order of work, but the actual nursing of the patient is the least part of what her work and influence should be among the class which the nurse will meet with. To this branch of nursing no more appropriate name can be given than 'Instructive Nursing,' for educational in the best sense of the word it should be."

In 1889, the *Chicago Visiting Nursing Association* was another early agency. A white Maltese cross was sewn on the sleeve of the uniform of each nurse member of this agency. Miss Edna Foley, a graduate of Hartford Hospital, was one of the early superintendents of this public health nursing agency in Chicago. She was the author of the *Visiting Nurse Manual* and president of the National Organization for Public Health Nursing from 1920–1921.

Another pioneering endeavor was the course in public health nursing given by the *University of Michigan* to provide instruction for students who were engaged in field work with the Detroit Department of Health as well as those with the Visiting Nurse Service.

Lillian D. Wald (1867–1940), who graduated from the New York Hospital Training School for Nurses in 1891, was shocked by the neglect of a woman in a back tenement who was critically ill in unbelievably distressing surroundings. Miss Wald conceived

the idea of establishing a neighborhood nursing service for the sick poor of the lower East Side in New York City.

She was fortunate in interesting two prominent and wealthy lay persons, Mrs. Solomon Loeb and Jacob H. Schiff, and she had the encouragement and support of her classmate in nursing, *Mary Brewster.* The world-famous *Henry Street Settlement* was opened in 1893 on the top floor of a tenement on the lower East Side (Fig. 10–28).

Duffus[19] entitled his biography of Lillian Wald *Neighbor and Crusader,* and this is well named, for neighborliness was her motivating thought and approach as she carried on her intensive crusade of assistance to the less fortunate. Her concept was that the visit should be like that of a really interested friend, rather than that of an impersonal, paid visitor.

The experiment was a success, and at the close of the second year this organization moved into a house on Henry Street purchased by Mr. Schiff. Here there was added to the already existing personnel both nurses and social workers. In due time there was an organized program of social and educational activities in addition to the nursing service. It became a *generalized social settlement project* (Fig. 10–29).

As nursing in general and community

[19]Duffus, R. L.: *Lillian Wald, Neighbor and Crusader.* New York, The Macmillan Co., 1938.

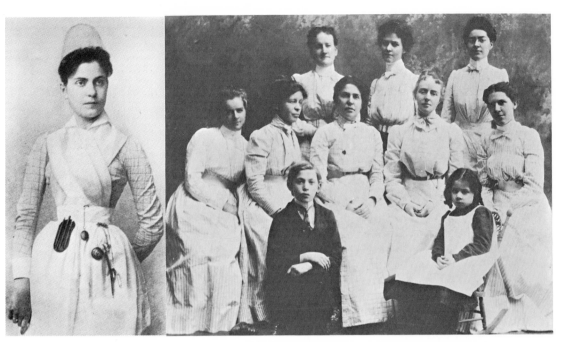

Figure 10–28. *Left:* Lillian Wald in her student uniform. In the early years of the Visiting Nurse Service the nurses wore the uniform of the school from which they were graduated. *Right:* Lillian Wald and her staff. She is seated in the middle of the second row with Lavinia Dock to her right. (Courtesy of the Visiting Nurse Service of New York.)

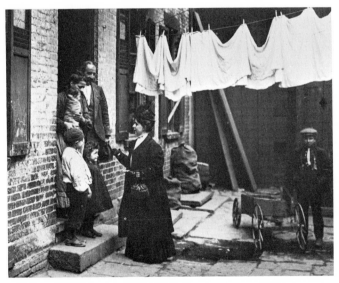

Figure 10–29. A nurse from the New York City Department of Health instructing tenement dwellers about health and sanitation in 1895. (Courtesy of New York City Department of Health.)

nursing in particular enlarged its concept of duties and opportunities, more nurses with special assignments and preparation were needed. Nurses were specializing in maternity, in infant welfare and in tuberculosis work. Gradually, there came to be an overlapping of functions, with several nurses working in the same household at the same time; this was a most disturbing situation for everyone, including the perplexed family. Eventually, there was a plan developed for all nursing to be of a general nature with supervisors who had specialized preparation and who acted as resource persons for nurses who needed special instruction in the care of patients.

There were *public health nurses* in Canada from about 1885. The work became highly developed under the Victorian Order and was for some years considered superior to almost any other in the world.

The Victorian Order nurses go into the simple homes in the little fishing villages in Nova Scotia and Cape Breton; into the workingman's cottages in the larger towns; into the tenements in the cruel slums of our larger cities; into the schools, the milk stations, the homes where tuberculosis holds its victims; into the little hospitals, away up in the mining towns or out on the beautiful prairies; out into the ranches in the ever lovely foothill region, where they become the country nurses; or into the tiny hospitals in the mountains, and away out to the Pacific coast branches. The Victorian Order nurse seems to fit into her particular corner as if she had been there all her life and it was good to be there. The committees, with hardly an exception, work as though their existence depended on the results, throwing all their energies into the service and loving their work.

Practically all public health nursing in Canada has been conducted by the *Victorian Order of Nurses for Canada*. Founded in 1897 by Lady Aberdeen, its name came from the fact that that year was Queen Victoria's Diamond Jubilee.

The Order's work has been threefold: public health nursing, chiefly in cities; the Lady Minto Cottage Hospital Fund for small hospitals in outlying and thinly populated districts; the Lady Grey Country District Nursing Scheme for visiting nurse care in Canada's many sparsely settled places, including work among the Indians. The order has always had much lay interest and support.

Elizabeth Smellie (Fig. 10–30), member of the original V. O. N. committee, was for many years head of the order, and organized

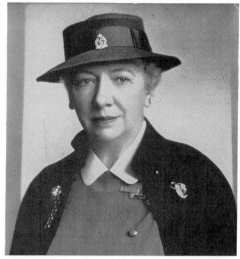

Figure 10–30. Lieut. Col. E. L. Smellie, formerly Matron-in-Chief, Royal Canadian Army Medical Corps. (Courtesy of *The Canadian Nurse.*)

the Canadian Women's Army Corps during World War II, similar to the U.S. WAC.

INFANT WELFARE

Marked progress had been noted in interest in the welfare of infants and contributions toward their care (Fig. 10–31). The *Crèche*, a type of day nursery for the care of poor babies, was established through the efforts of the Mayor of Paris in 1844.

During the later years of the nineteenth century, it was realized that one of the major reasons for such a high infant mortality rate was the milk used in the feeding of infants. It was essential to obtain a pure supply of cow's milk. (See Figure 10–32.)

In 1889, two milk distribution centers were constructed, one in New York City and one in Germany. The objective was to provide clean milk for only poor sick babies. This project was of relatively little value because after the child became well the supply of impure milk was again used, and sickness returned.

BACTERIOLOGY, PREVENTIVE MEDICINE AND ASEPTIC SURGERY

It was *Louis Pasteur* (1822–1895), the great French chemist, who finally disposed of the

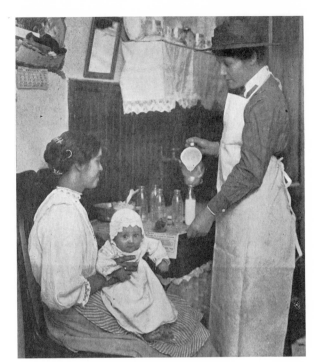

Figure 10–31. The baby welfare nurse. (Brainard, Annie M.: *The Evolution of Public Health Nursing,* 1922.)

long-accepted theory of spontaneous generation or abiogenesis. It is interesting that this great scientist and benefactor of medicine and society was trained as a chemist, not a physician.

In 1860, he began to study the air. Drawing air through a tube containing a plug of cotton, he noticed that the cotton often became black with dust, and inspection of the dust under the microscope revealed bacteria. Presence of airborne bacteria was confirmed. He found that living ferments abounded on many objects and in water. He experimented with heating flasks of broth, expelling the air in the process, and demonstrated that no growths of bacteria appeared.

The wine industry sought the aid of Pasteur because of the spoilage of wine. He investigated it and discovered yeast plants and tiny microscopic substances, bacteria, contaminating the wine. He held that fermentation resulted from airborne growths on the ripened fruit. Pasteur instructed the manufacturers to heat the wine to a certain tem-

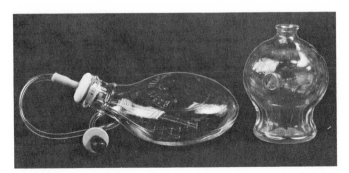

Figure 10–32. Two nursing bottles of the late nineteenth century. The cut glass one at the right still has a place for the finger or a cork to regulate the air. The bottle at the left gives less opportunity for transmission of organisms into the milk. A toddler could pull this one around on the floor. (Courtesy of Miss Kate Hyder.)

perature to kill the ferments without injuring the flavor of the wine. This process of heating liquids and rapidly cooling them has been applied to other liquids, and this familiar method is referred to as pasteurization.

The silk industry profited by Pasteur when he determined that parasites caused the disease that was threatening the silk-spinning moth larvae, *Bombyx mori*. His next project came when he was asked by the French Government to inspect the farm animals that were dying in the pastures. Pasteur discovered that the disease was *anthrax* and that it was caused by bacteria. He devised a vaccine that, when inoculated into animals, protected them against the disease.

Pasteur's last and perhaps his greatest accomplishment was his study of *rabies* in 1880. His efforts resulted in the development of a method of vaccinating dogs[20] and, thus, immunizing them against rabies. The fact that the cause of the disease had not been established was a serious disadvantage; however, he produced the well known *Pasteur treatment for rabies*. This was used on a young boy, Joseph Meister, after he had received many serious bites from a rabid dog. The treatment was a success and was reported in *A Method of Preventing Rabies After a Bite*. Now the popularity of the *madstone* (Fig. 10–33) in the treatment of dog bites dwindled. The madstone was a calculus, which on rare occasions formed in the stomach of the deer. Being rare, it was treasured by the owner and heavily insured. The madstone was dipped in warm milk and

---

[20] It has since been realized that many other animals can transmit rabies.

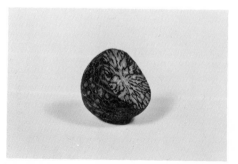

Figure 10–33. This madstone was found in an eighteenth century medicine chest and was the property of a physician. (Author's collection.)

then placed on the person's body, where the bite occurred. This object supposedly had the ability to draw out the evil aspects of this affliction.

One success after another crowned the efforts of Louis Pasteur, a real benefactor of society.

Joseph Lister (1827–1912) was the first to apply Pasteur's phenomenal discoveries to the field of surgery. The conditions existing in the hospitals at this time were indescribable. Surgical patients and those admitted with injuries as well as obstetric patients were exposed to severe infections, such as blood poisoning (septicemia), erysipelas, puerperal fever, lockjaw (tetanus), and "hospital gangrene."

Lister's particular field was surgery, and he was shocked and horrified at the contagious nature of infection associated with open wounds and with the appallingly high death rate that followed. He dedicated himself to the duty of investigating and thus correcting methods of surgery, as well as dissipating the obnoxious odor of the wards, a situation which was partly due to poor ventilation.

He pondered the swiftness of the surgeon who operated amid the screams of his unanesthetized patient; then he watched for the inevitable signs of infection that seemed localized in the hospital wards. With the availability of anesthesia, many more surgical operations were performed; the amount of infection increased, and the surgeons talked freely about the formation of "laudable pus." Lister felt that it must be due to the surgeon, his instruments, his assistants and his methods of carrying out technique. He had studied the work of Pasteur and immediately applied the germ theory of disease to his surgical procedures. He looked for some method of keeping germs out of wounds and decided upon the use of carbolic acid. In 1865, Lister used carbolic acid (phenol) successfully in treating a compound fracture. He used it to disinfect his instruments, to saturate the surgical dressing and to spray the solution into the air above the incision during the operation. His success increased as his methods and techniques were improved.

Infections and the dangers of infections were drastically reduced as a result of his contributions, and Lister received many honors for his heroic efforts. Among them, he was raised to the peerage; from then on he was called Lord Lister. In 1903 he saw the Lister

Institute of Preventive Medicine become a reality.

Surgical aseptic technique has replaced Lord Lister's technique, and hospitals have been transformed from the places of stench, horror and death.

Robert Koch (1843–1910) was the brilliant German physician who proved that every infectious disease was caused by a specific microorganism. Thus was laid the foundation for the science of bacteriology. Koch was possessed of an intense scientific curiosity. He proposed four "postulates" by which a specific organism can be proved to cause a certain disease: (1) Obtain a specific organism from blood or tissue of a diseased person. (2) Make a pure culture of this organism. (3) Produce the disease condition in another person or animal by inoculation with material from the pure culture. (4) Procure the same specific organism from the now-diseased second person or animal.

His contributions included: a method for growing or culturing microorganisms, a system of staining microbes with different colored dyes to be seen under the microscope and photographed, and detection and identification of the specific causative organisms of several diseases, such as the anthrax bacillus and the tubercle bacillus. In addition to identifying the bacillus of Asiatic cholera, Koch proved the spread of this disease by way of water, food and clothing.

Now the solution to the perplexing and mysterious aspect of disease (formerly explained as evil influences, demons, the night air) was that all carried these invisible causative organisms called microbes.

As spontaneously as fire ignites dry timber, one scientific investigation led to another; all were productive. Many specific organisms were identified and there was hope that vaccines or medications for treatment and prevention of disease would be forthcoming.

In 1872, Cohn, who first classified bacteria as plants, published the first modern classification of bacteria.

In 1874, Armauer Hansen of Bergen, Norway, isolated the lepra bacillus. Leprosy is now called *Hansen's disease* after him.

The discoveries of bacteria continued in rapid succession throughout the rest of the nineteenth century.

Ernst von Behring (1854–1917) was a Prussian doctor who spent some time, in the latter part of the nineteenth century, at Koch's Institute for Infectious Diseases. His studies there resulted in the introduction of a new principle—that of using serum from immunized animals in the prevention of diseases. In 1892, with Dr. Kitasato, he produced diphtheria antitoxin, and later that year he prepared tetanus antitoxin.

On Christmas night in 1891, von Behring successfully treated, by using diphtheria antitoxin, a child suffering from diphtheria in Bergmann's Clinic in Berlin.

Another theory that needed to be exploded was the still popular humoral theory. It was examined scientifically by the great German pathologist, *Rudolf Virchow* (1821–1902), who proposed in 1855 that the basic unit of life was the cell, that cells change in response to internal as well as external stimulus or irritation. Changes in cellular structure result in pathological conditions.

The field of *psychiatry* has benefited by the efforts of *Daniel Hack Tuke* (1827–1895), as well as members of several generations of Tukes; it seems to have been a family undertaking. His great-grandfather, William, was a devout member of the Society of Friends, more commonly known as Quakers, and was opposed to brutality in any aspect. This abhorrence was carried into the care of the mentally ill from the time he visited several hospitals, including Bedlam, and observed the inhumane treatment given to these unfortunate creatures who were not treated as sick individuals (Fig. 10–34).

Through the efforts of William Tuke and his son and daughter-in-law, money was raised to establish a home where these patients could be treated as human beings. The home, called "The Retreat," seemed well named because it was a place of security, a haven during a stormy period of life. An additional advantage was that good care was provided inexpensively. The construction of the building was unique because in place of barred windows, it had window frames made of steel that looked like wood. The building itself had a homey, comfortable appearance in a setting of trees. The interior atmosphere was as conducive to convalescence as the exterior.

William's grandson continued the fight for better care of the mentally ill. In 1854, he described the disgraceful conditions of the York Insane Asylum and Bedlam. The directors seemed to have labored under the impression that these patients were devoid of

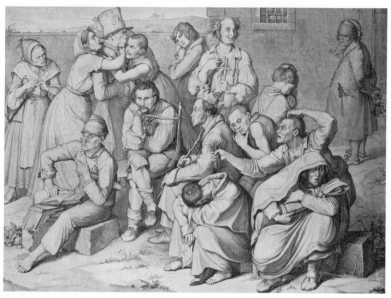

Figure 10–34. The Madhouse, by Wilhelm Kaulbach. (Courtesy of Philadelphia Museum of Art.)

feelings because some of them were chained in a sitting position; others were placed in a squatting position; some of them were clothed; many others nude; all of them were cold, even to the point of freezing; and the lack of sanitary facilities made the total environment unbearable. Solitary confinement of the patient in a chamber of horrors with occasional floggings was used. Fear technique was used for disciplinary measures. (See Figures 10–35 through 10–38.)

William Tuke's great-grandson Daniel also continued the fight for this cause. He became a physician and eventually one of England's most celebrated psychiatrists. He gave courses in psychology, maintained a private practice and was chief psychiatrist at the York Retreat. Tuberculosis interrupted his work, and he had to seek a climate more conducive to cure.

Among his writings are *A Manual of Psychological Medicine, History of the Insane in the British Isles, The Influence of the Mind upon the*

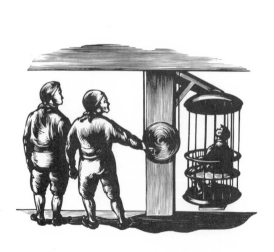

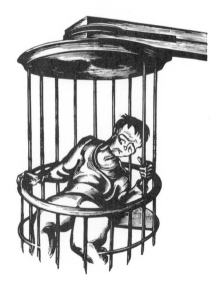

Figure 10–35. A whirling cage—an early device for calming psychiatric patients. (Courtesy of Smith Kline & French Laboratories.)

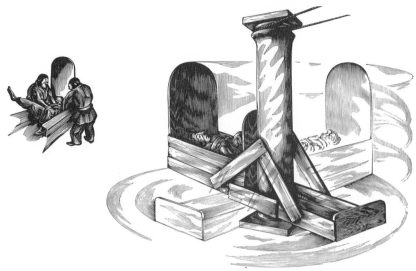

Figuse 10–36. The revolving bed—an early device for calming patients with mental illness. (Courtesy of Smith Kline & French Laboratories.)

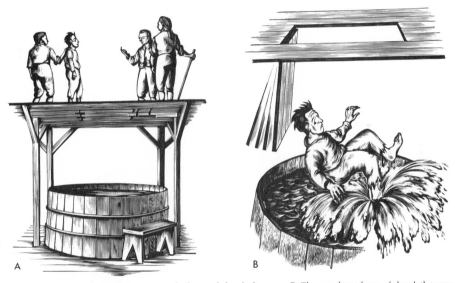

Figure 10–37. *A,* Enticing the patient to an early form of shock therapy. *B,* The resultant form of shock therapy. (Courtesy of Smith Kline & French Laboratories.)

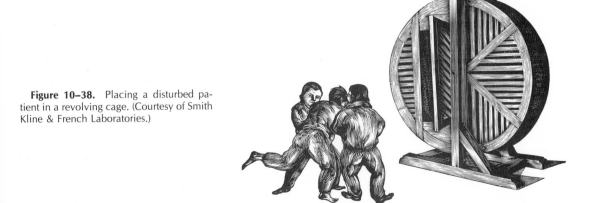

Figure 10–38. Placing a disturbed patient in a revolving cage. (Courtesy of Smith Kline & French Laboratories.)

Body in Health and Disease and his famous compilation, *Dictionary of Psychological Medicine.*

DISCOVERY OF RADIUM AND X-RAY

Two discoveries occurred at the close of the nineteenth century that were of tremendous significance to many aspects of society including the medical field.

The first was made by the German physicist, *Wilhelm Roentgen* (1845–1922), who discovered the *x-ray* in 1895. In his capacity as a professor of physics and mathematics, he had been fascinated by the studies on radiation and stumbled upon his great gift to society. In searching to find the invisible light in his laboratory, he connected an induction coil to a Crookes tube. It threw out light and glowed with a phosphorescence when electricity was passed between two electrodes inside the tube. In order to eliminate any visible rays, Roentgen completely covered the tube with black paper and excluded all light from the room. On the table across from the tube, Roentgen placed a screen covered with a chemical preparation that emitted a fluorescent glow. There was no visible light anywhere and yet something had to come from the tube — his invisible ray — that caused the screen to give off a greenish glow. These rays penetrated many things, including human flesh, but the bones remained opaque. His photograph of this was scarcely believable even to him.

His news was eagerly received, and honors, including the Nobel Prize in Physics in 1901 and an honorary degree of Doctor of Medicine, were accorded Roentgen.

The application of x-ray to the field of medicine was at first only in a meager diagnostic aspect. Later, this was expanded greatly, and its therapeutic uses have been realized.

The second disclosure was that of *radium* by *Pierre and Marie Sklodowska Curie*. The realization came about in a most unusual way. Marie, in selecting a problem for her doctoral dissertation, chose to pursue further some research that had been carried out by the French physicist Henri Becquerel. He had worked with uranium salts and noted the presence of rays of undetermined origin.

As her experimental work progressed, Pierre joined her in this exciting study. Their efforts were reported in 1898 in a paper discussing a new radioactive substance contained in pitchblende, the ore that was the source of the uranium. The extracted substance, radium, has been found to possess the ability to destroy some types of malignant cells and tissues. The Curies shared the Nobel Prize in physics in 1903 for their accomplishment. Madame Curie received it again for chemistry in 1911; in 1906, her husband was struck and killed by a careless motorist.

To society they both made a monumental contribution whose benefits have still not been fully realized.

EDUCATIONAL PROGRESS IN MEDICINE

There was an obvious need for a unifying force to weld the members of the health allied groups. An opportunity to discuss common problems, to share evidence of progress, to set standards for acceptable practice, to upgrade the educational background of the practitioner, all played a part in the establishment of local and then *national organizations.*

In 1832, the British Medical Association was formed; in 1841, the Pharmaceutical Society of Great Britain was established; in 1847, the American Medical Association was founded and in 1852, the American Pharmaceutical Association was developed.

One of the first items of business of the newly formed American Medical Association was a resolution asking for the separation of licensing functions from teaching institutions.

Beginning in 1883, the *Journal of the American Medical Association* was published for the dissemination of information to its members. The process of intellectual upgrading in the health sciences was underway.

The fruition of the plans to establish these organizations was a triumph, but overall development came slowly. The improvement of the educational preparation of practitioners was not easy or immediate.

There was a striking variation in the educational background and preparation of practitioners in medicine in the nineteenth century.

An example of the lack of uniformity in educational preparation is detected when one reads some of the biographies of the period. An educated gentleman left Massachusetts to avail himself of a homesteading opportunity. In 1871, he went to Kansas, after being wounded in the Civil War. Needing pharmaceutical supplies, he wrote to a supply firm for the necessary medicines. Probably because of the tone of the letter, he was mistaken for a doctor, and his supplies were addressed to "Dr. Waugh." When they arrived at the small town railway office, the clerk noticed the address, paying particular attention to the gentleman's title and immediately "Dr. Waugh" began to practice medicine, although under marked and voluble protest. When Kansas required doctors to be licensed, this gentleman, without instruction, formal or otherwise, was reputed to be the only one to pass the medical examinations in three counties.

The course of study in medical education ranged from no preparation in basic education or medicine to good preparation. The profession was going through a period of trial and error. There were good as well as poor forms of apprenticeships, opportunities in proprietary schools and, at last, the beginning of schools under the sponsorship of universities. It is interesting to observe that in 1848 the need for practical demonstration for students of medicine was realized and recorded as was the necessity for clinical teaching.

In reviewing the accomplishments of the *Association of American Medical Colleges*, which was organized in 1890, one notes only a recommendation of a minimum standard of high school graduation as a prerequisite for the study of medicine! Yet, conversely, Johns Hopkins University in 1893 made a bachelor's degree a prerequisite for admission to its medical school. This wide diversity in the background of doctors compelled the leaders in medicine to consider the establishment of some required standard of preliminary education.

An outstanding *medical center* came into existence in Baltimore when Johns Hopkins University opened in 1876, Johns Hopkins Hospital was founded in 1889 and Johns Hopkins School of Medicine was established in 1893. A distinguished faculty was obtained; among them was Dr. William Welch, professor of pathology; Dr. William Osler, professor of clinical medicine; Dr. William Halsted, professor of surgery; and Dr. Howard Kelly, professor of gynecology and obstetrics.

The new school of medicine was a graduate school; the faculty felt that a sound liberal foundation was essential before the student attempted professional study.

Sir William Osler (1849–1919) was a Canadian who received his degree in medicine from McGill Medical School in Montreal. He spent two years studying medical practices abroad.

Dr. Osler practiced medicine and taught at the Philadelphia General Hospital. He revolutionized the teaching of medicine by initiating bedside study as well as textbook study (Fig. 10–39). He was reputed to be a most inspiring clinical instructor. He lectured at

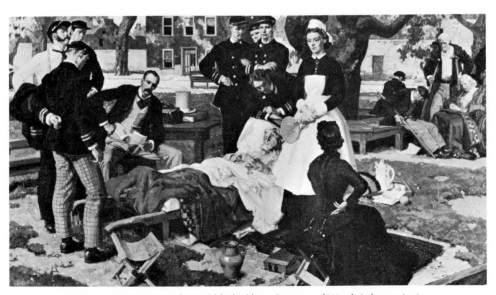

Figure 10–39. Dr. Osler at Old Blockley. (Courtesy of Wyeth Laboratories.)

autopsies, which became so meaningful to the students that the postmortem house became too small to accommodate the numbers who wanted to attend.

In 1888 Dr. Osler, an eminent professor of clinical medicine, was appointed physician-in-chief of Johns Hopkins Hospital. In 1891 he wrote his famous textbook, *Principles and Practice of Medicine*. It was because of Dr. Osler's efforts and inspiration that the Rockefeller Institute for Medical Research came into being in 1904. When his career ended, he was Regius Professor of Medicine at Oxford University.

William S. Halsted (1852–1922), in addition to being professor of surgery, was in charge of the surgical service at Johns Hopkins Hospital. He applied the principles of Lister's doctrine to his aseptic techniques of surgery. Many innovations in surgical procedures were due to his use of rubber gloves. Love rather than Lister was the motivating force behind the inception of rubber gloves as part of the operating room equipment. Scrubbing for surgery meant scrubbing and using the chemical solution of mercuric chloride. This proved injurious especially for the delicate hands of the operating room scrub nurse which were becoming precious to Dr. Halsted. In 1890, before Miss Caroline Hampton became Mrs. Halsted, Dr. Halsted consulted the Goodyear Rubber Company about the problem. Loose-fitting rubber gloves, easily boiled and most protective, were produced. Another first had been achieved.

In this century many devices, including the hypodermic syringe, the cystoscope, laryngoscope and bronchoscope, were invented. These instruments were useful for diagnostic as well as therapeutic purposes. Many bacteria had been identified, and three ways of destroying bacteria — by heat, chemicals and vaccines — were determined. The closing years of the nineteenth century were filled with important discoveries and developments in bacteriology and parasitology. Among the most outstanding events were the demonstrations of Sir Ronald Ross of the malarial parasite in the mosquito, the use of serum against snake venom by Albert Calmette, the explanation of the side-chain theory by Paul Ehrlich, the use of ultraviolet light by Niels Finsen and the discovery of the transmission of yellow fever in the mosquito by Reed, Carroll, Lazera and Agramonte in 1899.

The progress in biological and physical sciences and medicine in this century had been beyond belief.

Thomas Eakins (1844–1916), a famous American painter, has left two paintings that present the remarkable progress made in the scientific basis of patient care in the last quarter of the nineteenth century.

The first painting, the *Gross Clinic* (Fig. 10–40) (1875), presents grand rounds with Dr. Gross explaining to medical students the surgical operation that is being performed. He appears to be completely oblivious to the feelings of the patient and to the agonizing horror of the patient's mother who sits at the right of Dr. Gross.

The second picture, the *Agnew Clinic* (Fig. 10–41) (1898), presents Dr. Agnew presiding at grand rounds. The setting for both pictures is presumably a surgical clinical amphitheater, the audience presumably medical students, but the scene has definitely changed in the years from 1875 to 1898. The concepts presented as a result of the scientific investigations of Pasteur, Koch and Lister have made the surgeons aware of the necessity of shedding their street clothes and replacing them with white operating gowns; the instruments appear to be bathed in carbolic acid solution; the patient is covered; the anesthetist is giving ether (note the can of ether in his hand and the ether cone over the patient's nose and mouth); thus, the advantageous use of ether by Dr. Morton has been noted, and since schools of nursing had been opened a nurse appears in the operating room but not as an assistant to the surgeons.

Her name was *Mary V. Clymer* and her diary-type notebook was discovered in November of 1961.

School records reveal that at her graduation in 1889 she was awarded the Nightingale medal. Her instruction included cooking and her recipes record her ability to concoct such things as jellied soups, beef tea and arrowroot. The ingredients for poultices and good liniments are also presented. "A good nurse," she relates, "must be kind, firm, gentle, and possessing a good deal of magnetism. Never be curious. Be watchful but not officious. Unnecessary noise with tongue or coal scuttle is to be avoided."

The full impact of the necessity of surgical aseptic technique had not been comprehended or was not being practiced.

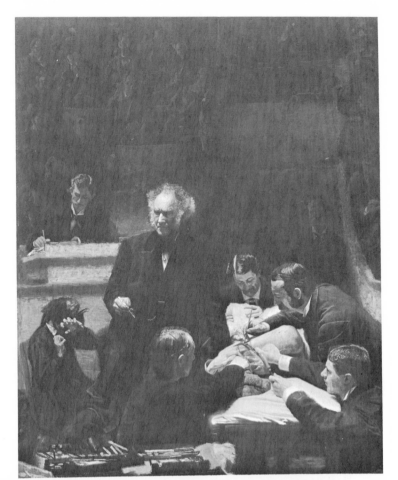

Figure 10–40. The Gross Clinic, by Thomas Eakins (1875). (Courtesy of Jefferson Medical College, Philadelphia, Pa.)

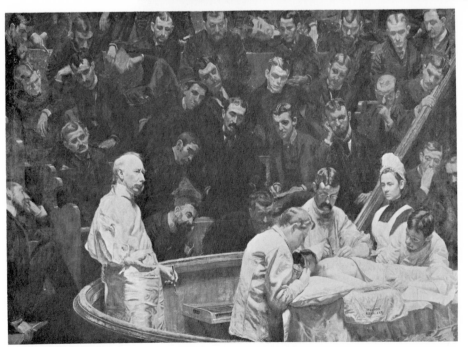

Figure 10–41. The Agnew Clinic, by Thomas Eakins (1898). (Courtesy of Philadelphia Museum of Art.)

REFERENCE READINGS

Bernheim, Bertram: *The Story of Johns Hopkins.* Surrey, England, Windmill Press, 1949.

Burton, Katherine: *Sorrow Built a Bridge.* New York, Longmans, Green & Co., 1937.

Christy, Teresa E.: *Cornerstone for Nursing Education.* New York, Teachers' College Press, 1969.

Colvin, Sarah T.: *A Rebel in Thought.* New York, Island Press, 1944.

Cooper, Page: *The Bellevue Story.* New York, Thomas Y. Crowell, 1948.

Cushing, Harvey: *The Life of Sir William Osler.* New York, Oxford University Press, 1925.

Duffus, R. L.: *Lillian Wald, Neighbor and Crusader.* New York, The Macmillan Co., 1938.

Faxon, Nathaniel W.: *The Hospital in Contemporary Life.* Cambridge, Mass., Harvard University Press, 1949.

Flexner, James T.: *Doctors on Horseback.* New York, Viking Press, 1937.

Giles, Dorothy: *A Candle in Her Hand.* New York, G. P. Putnam's Sons, 1950.

Hampton, Isabel A., et al.: *Nursing of the Sick — 1893.* New York, McGraw-Hill Book Co., Inc., 1949.

Hanaford, Phoebe: *Daughters of America, or Women of the Century.* Augusta, Me., True & Co., 1882.

Kittredge, George L.: *Witchcraft in Old and New England.* Cambridge, Mass., Harvard University Press, 1929.

Marshall, Helen E.: *Mary Adelaide Nutting.* Baltimore, Johns Hopkins University Press, 1972.

Osler, Sir William: *Aequanimitas.* Philadelphia, Blakiston Co., 1932.

Parsons, Sara E.: *History of the Massachusetts General Hospital Training School for Nurses.* Boston, M. Barrows, 1922.

Pugh, Garrett F., and Fisher, A. J. B.: *Ethics and Health in Late Victorian Society.* London, Arundel, 1970.

Richards, Linda A.: *Reminiscences of Linda Richards.* Boston, M. Barrows, 1911.

Staupers, Mabel K.: *No Time for Prejudice.* New York, The Macmillan Co., 1961.

Thoms, Adah B.: *Pathfinders.* New York, Kay Printing House, 1929.

Vallery-Radot, Pasteur: *Louis Pasteur.* New York, Alfred A. Knopf, 1958.

Waksman, Selman A.: *The Conquest of Tuberculosis.* Berkeley and Los Angeles, University of California Press, 1964.

Wald, Lillian: *House on Henry Street.* New York, Henry Holt, 1915.

Wald, Lillian: *Windows on Henry Street.* Boston, Little, Brown & Co., 1934.

Walker, Kenneth: *Joseph Lister.* London, Hutchinson & Co., 1956.

Weeks-Shaw, Clara S.: *A Text-Book of Nursing.* New York, D. Appleton & Co., 1897.

CHAPTER 11

Nursing and the Scientific, Technological and Societal Changes of the Early Twentieth Century

A reflection of the setting in which nursing prospered in this century reveals the exploration of outer space, as well as the penetration of every area of the earth and of man, the development of new sciences, the expansion of old ones, and a fusion of many sciences—literally, an explosion of knowledge and technology. It has been said that much which was unknown has become known and much which was invisible has become visible.

The twentieth century has also witnessed a phenomenal improvement in the general standard of living, lengthening of the span of life, the identification of the causes of many diseases, the ability to conquer most bacterial diseases and the provision for a scientific plan of care for the patient and his family. In this century, the center of medical care has been the hospital; the prevention and rehabilitative as well as the curative aspects of patient care have received increasing attention. The influence of wars, the marked progress in transportation and communication, the remarkable inventions, along with scientific achievements, have had an influence on keeping individuals healthy, on initiating changing patterns of the care of the sick, on the expansion of the field of medicine in general and on the refinement of nursing in particular. (See Figure 11–1.)

The past years have presented the transition from candlelight to satellite, from the horse and buggy era to the jet age, from the laying on of hands to impersonal electronic monitoring. The struggle for freedom and independence of new nations, the trauma of international tensions and threat to survival itself have all played a part in writing the current history of society.

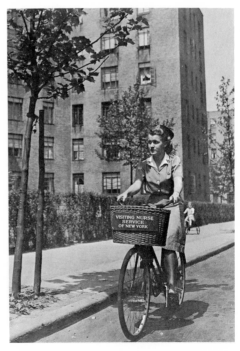

Figure 11–1. In 1944 during the gasoline shortage of World War II, nurses rode bicycles in the Bronx and Queens in New York. (Courtesy of the Visiting Nurse Service of New York.)

233

PROGRESS IN TRANSPORTATION, COMMUNICATION AND OTHER TECHNOLOGICAL AREAS

The *automobile* has been responsible for many occupational opportunities as well as bringing medical assistance to a patient much more quickly than ever before. Car accessories, gas stations, tourist facilities, construction of roads, motor busses—all have changed American life. Travel opportunities broadened knowledge and provided recreational diversions, but they also encouraged contact with new diseases and increased the accident rate.

Helicopters have proved of immeasurable value because of their high degree of maneuverability. Many patients are flown great distances and reach medical centers more quickly (Fig. 11–2).

Another practical use of the helicopter as a miniature hospital that flies through the air has been tried out in West Germany. The name for this unique vehicle is the Clinocopter. Its purpose is to go to the scene of traffic accidents to save lives that might otherwise be lost because of improper care and delay in ambulances' reaching the patient. A professional team, a surgeon, assistant and nurse, accompanies the Clinocopter. The equipment necessary for emergency surgery, down to a complete x-ray unit, has been installed.

In the area of *communications*, use of the *telephone* has become widespread, as have motion pictures, radio, and television. The benefits of television in the educational field have been realized through the use of closed circuit television as a teaching aid.

In July, 1962, *Telstar* was launched. Scientists were thus able to demonstrate the transmission of international television as well as voice messages and telephone conversations from continent to continent by way of a satellite orbiting the earth. The effects of this form of communication have been far-reaching. Telstar as a system of international communication can provide much in the way of recreation and education in art, music and drama that formerly only wealthy people could afford. It offers an excellent medium for health teaching and instructional programs of medical significance as well as the obvious and important news coverage.

During the twentieth century there were many offshoots from the main stem of biological and physical sciences, and there occurred a marked expansion in older, better established ones.

One of the most significant contributions in scientific advances occurred in 1905 when Albert Einstein proposed his theory of relativity. Much evidence accumulated about the electrical nature of living systems and gradually the relationship of human beings with electrical fields was noted.

The science of *bacteriology* has increased in scope and depth. The *electron microscope* has

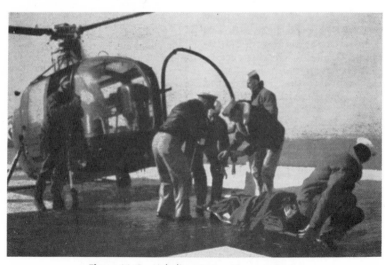

Figure 11–2. A helicopter awaiting a patient.

made it possible to study *viruses* and many causative organisms in greater detail than had previously been possible. Many valuable vaccines have been developed in this century. Associated sciences, such as *parasitology*, have evolved. An examination of the structure of the cell has become as important to the biologist as the atom has to the physicist and chemist.

Thus the study of *cellular biology* and *cytology* developed. The scientific bases of *pathology* in studying diseased tissues have aided in more accurate diagnostic tests and research for more efficient ways of treating patients. Developments in chemistry, including the introduction of biochemistry, seem little related to the alchemy of centuries past.

When atoms were split or smashed artificially by means of a cyclotron, the *atomic age* was ushered in. There are many useful purposes for atomic energy, such as radioactive isotopes for medical research. *Radioactive isotopes,* or those elements which have become radioactive when consumed as "atomic cocktails," are lethal to diseased tissue. In medical experimentation bacteria are "tagged" with a radioactive element such as phosphorus or iodine in an attempt to detect how the bacteria bring about disease in the human body. The action of a drug may be traced within the body in a similar manner. The use of nuclear reactors, cobalt machines, x-rays combined with motion pictures, and computers to plot programs for administration of lethal rays to diseased tissues are medical facts. Many doctors have a background in nuclear physics. The atom in medicine has become a potent force in patient care. There are technical atomic energy research centers such as Oak Ridge, Tennessee as well as medical atomic energy research centers such as the one at Brookhaven on Long Island.

Chemical progress has benefited society in many ways—in the pharmaceutical industry, in the field of foods and nutrition as well as in the cosmetic field. *George Washington Carver* (*ca.* 1864–1943) employed his theories in "chemical gymnastics." An example is his changing the peanut into a multiplicity of useful preparations.

Biochemists have added much to our knowledge of the chemistry of digestion; studies in *nutrition* have advanced the knowledge of this subject in this century. By using a fluoroscopic screen, Dr. Walter B. Cannon studied the digestive organs of cats who had eaten radiopaque meals. In addition he studied the effects of emotions on digestion and increased the knowledge of food utilization, transmission of nerve impulses and actions of the endocrine glands.

Vitamins, those necessary ingredients discovered in small amounts in certain foods, have been synthesized chemically so that vitamin deficiency diseases are now being eliminated from the roster of illnesses.

In 1910 when Dr. Paul Ehrlich (1854–1915) and his Japanese assistant Dr. Sahachiro Hata proclaimed the benefits of Salvarsan (606) as the magic "chemical bullet" for the treatment of syphilis, *chemotherapy* became a vital factor in medical science.

Many drugs have been synthesized in the chemical laboratories and chemotherapy has become one of the major aspects of patient care. In 1936 sulfanilamide, the first of the many sulfa miracle drugs, was available for the treatment of bacterial infections. *Sir Alexander Fleming* (1881–1955) of St. Mary's Hospital in London was responsible for providing an important contribution, that of *penicillin,* in 1939. The expansion and scientific progress in the field of pharmacology in the twentieth century has been phenomenal.

Tuberculosis had been a dreaded disease during the nineteenth century. The work of *Laennec* provided an instrument for listening to the chest; the combined efforts of many had stressed that the disease was contagious; *Robert Koch* had detected the causative organism; *Wilhelm Roentgen* had discovered a method of detecting evidence of tuberculosis in the body; and, because of the development of tests, bovine tuberculosis could be controlled in cattle.

The tubercle bacillus had been proved to cause destructive lesions in many parts of the body in addition to pulmonary tuberculosis—in the brain (meningitis), skin (lupus), glands of the neck (scrofula), bones, joints and spine (Pott's disease), and kidneys and intestines.

Tuberculosis (all forms) was the second leading cause of death in 1900, causing 194.4 deaths per 100,000 in that year or 11.3 per cent of the total. By 1959 the death rate from this disease had fallen to 6.7 per 100,000; it was no longer in the top ten death-dealing diseases for it accounted for only 1 per cent of all deaths. It has been calculated that the death rate from tuberculosis has declined by 98 per cent.

New treatments have drastically reduced tuberculosis as a major health problem today.

There was a second industrial revolution in the twentieth century, which brought new machinery and new methods into many agricultural as well as industrial areas. This was helpful from the viewpoint of work simplification, but it was exceptional from the viewpoint of the better produce, which markedly reduced the chance of transmission of disease. In the dairy industry, in addition to testing the cattle, farmers have introduced milking machines that milk the cows under sanitary conditions, thus eliminating milk handlers. The milk is sent under proper refrigeration to plants where it is pasteurized.

There has been a rapid growth of cities because of the increase of factories, mechanization of farming and the advancement in methods of travel and transportation. Improvements have been made in purifying water supplies, in meat inspection laws, in sanitary garbage collection and disposal, in sewerage systems for the sanitary disposal of human excreta, in street cleaning departments, in housing laws, in the increasing numbers and health supervision of public parks and recreation centers, in industrial hygiene and safety measures and in atmospheric sanitation.

MECHANICAL REFRIGERATION

In 1851, Dr. John Gorrie was granted the first patent for a cool-air machine. In treating patients who had high fevers, Dr. Gorrie believed firmly that if the room temperature could be lowered, his treatments would have a greater degree of success. In desperation, he relinquished his medical practice and devoted his full time to the problem of cooling air, and of freezing water artificially or ice-making. This achievement led to air conditioning. In 1914 his statue was placed in Statuary Hall of the Capitol at Washington, D. C., in recognition of his pioneering efforts.

Dr. Gorrie laid the foundation for the ultimate development of refrigeration, which has been so essential in shipping and storing fruits, vegetables, meats and dairy products. Cleaner, more healthful produce is available, permitting a more varied and balanced diet for more people.

Packaging of frozen foods has provided an opportunity for a well balanced diet through all seasons of the year. Cryotherapy, the use of cold in medical treatments, surgery, hypothermic equipment and anesthesia, has been developed in this century (Fig. 11–3).

IMPROVEMENTS IN HOSPITALS

It should prove rewarding to contemplate the role of hospitals at the turn of the century and their influence in conjunction with certain physicians and nurses in weaving the fabric of tradition with which the profession of nursing has had to cope. (See Figures 11–4 and 11–5.)

In 1883 the State Charities Aid Association of New York published a book entitled *Hand Book for Hospitals*. It had been prepared to assist public spirited citizens in understanding proper organization and management of hospitals. The citizens were requested to consider the purpose for which the hospital was built, and to remember the need of good care for everyone; in considering a plan of care, the importance of the family and family ties of patients should receive careful attention. Hospital administration should exercise control in demanding that all things purchased for the welfare of patients and staff be of good quality. It was proposed that even the ice, which was purchased in a period before refrigeration, should not be cut from ponds or streams which receive drainage or seepage from foul sources making it unfit for use.

In discussing interior details including appliances the advantages of *air beds*, which might be seen at the General Hospital in New Haven, and *water beds*, which were in use at Hartford Hospital, received attention. Many step-saving techniques and devices were described. A dining room for every ward was recommended with only the really sick and those patients who would be offensive to other patients being served in bed. The social and psychological rewards in achieving a turning point toward recovery were noted in a cheerful, attractive setting amid sociability and good food.

The Committee's concern extended to the realm of the nurse and it requested suitable living arrangements for her physical and mental health. In fact, they state: "the efficiency of the nurse is so important for her

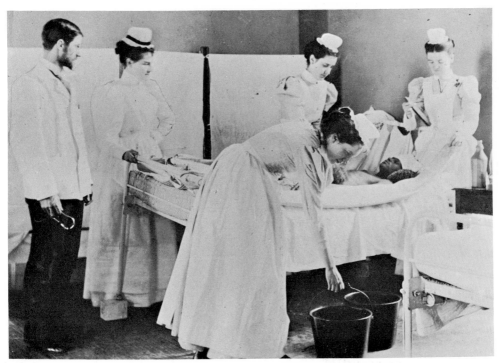

Figure 11–3. Three students of nursing prepare to give a patient who has typhoid fever a slush bath to reduce his temperature (1905). The foot of the bed has been elevated by shock blocks. (Courtesy of Hartford Hospital School of Nursing.)

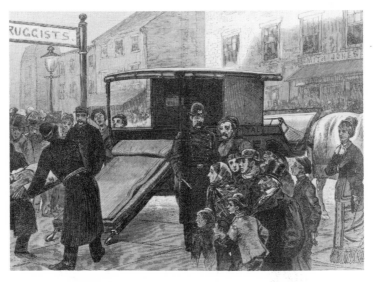

Figure 11–4. A New York City Ambulance in 1879.
(Author's collection.)

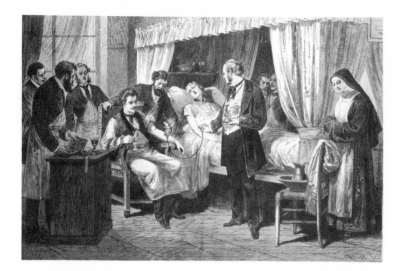

Figure 11–5. A blood transfusion at the Hospital de La Pitie in Paris in 1874. Blood from the donor is caught in the funnel and enters the recipient's circulatory system. Physicians and medical students observe the treatment. (Author's collection.)

charge (the patient) that her health and comfort should be considered for this reason as well as for her own sake."[1]

Two types of patients received special attention with an earnest plea for better care for both—maternity patients and the mentally ill. The plight of the pregnant woman, including the constant danger of puerperal fever, and the cruelty in the plan for care of the "insane" person were clearly delineated. The need for well planned care including diversional therapy for the mentally ill patient was presented by Dr. Mary Putnam Jacobi in her comment: "Rightly understood it means the creation around each patient of a new world, built up out of his own awakened and directed activities."[2]

In concluding the book, the State Charities Aid Society begged the reader to reflect again upon the objective "for which the hospital building, its corps of nurses, and its superintendence exist." They reiterated, "Let no one forget that this primary object is the curing of the sick. A hospital is not founded solely to provide a field of experiments and break in raw young medical men to practice."[3] It was felt to be the moral obligation of the citizens of communities to provide a healthful setting so that the sick poor could return home as well as possible

and as soon as possible. They were charged to become active in considering human rights.

This book produced a heated reaction on the part of physicians who felt a rebuttal of the arguments should be published in the hope of stifling many of the proposals. The person who rose to rally physicians and their influential friends was Dr. Charles Francis Withington.

From their inception, hospitals had been programmed to provide relief during times of sickness for those who had been unable to provide for themselves. Many philanthropists had insured the delivery of such care for the poor through generous endowments with stipulations for use of these funds.

Dr. Withington pleaded the cause of medical leaders to permit hospitals to be used for clinical instruction for medical education. He acknowledged that money and instructions left in trust, with the lapse of time and change of circumstances, mandated a reconsideration with a modification, if not a redirection, of the use of such funds which might not have been the intention of the donor.[4] He further stated that there are few endowed institutions which are carried on precisely as their originators supposed they would be. It was his feeling that if these generous people were alive today and apprised of all the facts in the case, they would exercise the same judgment and generosity

[1]State Charities Aid Association. *Hand Book for Hospitals.* New York, G. P. Putnam's Sons, 1883, p. 88.
[2]*Ibid.,* p. 188.
[3]*Ibid.,* p. 235.

[4]Withington, Charles Francis: *The Relation of Hospitals to Medical Education.* Boston, Cupples, Upham, 1886.

which characterized their lives and they would endorse the action made necessary by changed conditions.

Dr. Withington felt that there was incumbent upon intelligent and conscientious administrators of endowed institutions a moral obligation to conform to the needs of medical students for clinical experience. His book was written to ease the conscience of the hospital administration and placate the public, who might protest this trend of ignoring the obligation of providing for the comfort and well-being of individuals, and of permitting patients to be used for the purpose of advancing medical science.

The first section of the book addressed itself to the "peculiar obligation" of hospitals in regard to medical education resting on the possession of clinical material with the right to use it. He recognized the need of medical educators for patients and the impossibility of obtaining the consent of well-to-do persons who pay for their medical attention to allow themselves to be used for purposes of clinical instruction. It was his feeling that free patients, in consideration of the benefits they are receiving, should give such compensation as they have it in their power to make, which was the opportunity for clinical instruction.[5] He referred to the presence of "various appliances" which the hospitals could provide such as post-mortem examinations and opportunities to perform surgical operations.

The second section of Dr. Withington's book presented "the possible conflict between the interests of medical science and those of the individual patient and his indefeasible rights."[6] He agreed that occasionally it was "at the expense of the individual that truths of the greatest general utility have been learned." But he assured the public that in this country this is less likely to happen, but "even with us it may be well to draw up . . . a Bill of Rights which shall secure patients against any injustice from the votaries of science. The occupants of hospital wards are something more than merely so much clinical material during their lives and so much pathological material after their death."[7]

After stating the above, Dr. Withington questioned the extent to which a patient may rightfully be made the subject of experimentation. Experimentation in treatments and medications may become essential and a physician may feel the need to test for himself and the good of science some new and hitherto untried remedy. He states, "there is here the puzzling ethical fact that he would be unwilling, were the patient one of his own family, to subject him to the risk of the proposed novelty."[8] He continues, "it may be proper for him in the interests of medical science to establish its usefulness" or its lack of value; therefore, appropriate cases have to be obtained. He did inveigh against human experimentation for its own sake and without patient knowledge and encouraged the use of volunteers for such programs of experimentation. Patient consent was not discussed, although he said that physicians had no right to make any man the unwilling victim of such an experiment. "A temptation kindred to the above is the recommendation of hopeless surgical operations," and he felt that surgeons "had no right to take advantage of the patient's extremity to recommend a procedure which can have no other advantage than to enhance the operator's reputation for boldness."[9]

Another source of tribulation for a poor patient was that of overfrequent physical examinations which were injurious to many patients. A patient who was critically ill with pneumonia had to be subjected to the frequent exposure of the chest and the auscultation and percussion of students who wanted to learn about the pneumonic process. No mention was made of the exhaustion of the patient and the interruption of his rest; this should have been objected to by the nurse in charge of the patient. And one pondered where was the nurse when he presented the value of students checking the exact amount of pleuritic effusion or the precise size of a hypertrophied heart without compromising the patient's safety and then relating that "it is our duty to learn them, for there is no conflict between the interests of science and the individual." Dr. Withington seems to contradict himself.

The only instance in which the presence of a nurse was mentioned was the statement that doctors should not examine a female patient without a nurse in the room. He admitted that the greatest objection of women

[5]*Ibid.*, p. 9.
[6]*Ibid.*, p. 14.
[7]*Ibid.*, p. 15.

[8]*Ibid.*, p. 16.
[9]*Ibid.*, p. 17.

coming to a hospital was the unnecessary exposure to which they were subjected and the unnecessary pelvic examinations performed by students. He blithely proposed that "there is no violation of modesty when there is no consciousness of exposure. An operation may be performed upon a woman before a whole amphitheatre of students and provided she is unconscious . . . of her surroundings and never learns . . . of the circumstances, there has been no violation of her modesty."[10]

In treating the subject of pelvic examinations, he assumed that the patient's concern was due to the presence of the many and inexperienced students who were probing her body rather than because of the danger of transferring infection. He pontificated that patients who suffered from puerperal fever should not be admitted to or retained in a general hospital but implied that they should be sent to an isolation hospital or pest house.

The last section of the book referred to the factors which increased the educational value of hospitals. These revolved around the prestige of a medical school affiliating with a hospital and attracting intelligent young medical men as house officers. The "preparation of young men, through the educational influence of hospitals, for the practice of their profession . . . by no means exhausts the educational capacity of the hospital." He made the disconcerting statement that "The most useful handmaid of medicine is nursing,"[11] adding that "in many cases, notably in the acute fevers, the labor of the nurse is undoubtedly more important than that of the physician. For the reduction of medicine from a science to an art good nursing is absolutely indispensable."

Dr. Withington reported that many well-known physicians who had experience with both systems, agreed that the character of the nursing care was vastly better where training schools existed than prior to their inception. There were several reasons for favorable response on the part of doctors toward nurses who were as well prepared as training schools permitted them to be; the hospital stay was decreased for the patient, thereby enabling a greater number of patients to be treated in a year. The nurse who was doing private duty in the home provided "enormous relief to the practitioner (of

medicine) who no longer is obliged to attend personally to pass a catheter, make a hypodermic injection or renew a surgical dressing. Much time thus saved from the drudgery of his profession can be devoted to scientific improvement."[12] He did recognize that significant information about the patient or symptoms or other phenomena of disease which might not be noted by the doctor in the short time of his visit could be noted and recorded or reported by a well-prepared nurse.

The benefit of hospitals having a training school was emphasized and it was felt that "to the hospitals themselves this would involve little, if any additional expense." He opined that the "cost of maintenance of the nurses is increased only as women of high social grade require a little more privacy in their domiciliary accommodation than those who are less refined. But on the other hand, as apprentices to a craft, they are willing to work for a less compensation than women who are gaining no instruction."[13] He encouraged those who were willing to consider the merits of a training school not be discouraged by the cost of a building to house student nurses but rather to realize the monetary return from the use of the rooms vacated by students which would be available for the sick patients who pay for service rendered. He admitted that "money received from paying patients, who are usually ready to take such rooms, will pay the expense of the nurses' dormitory. . . . There is no question but that an equal outlay of money will secure as good nursing service to a hospital under a training school system as the same money would purchase in the labor market."[14]

In turning to the contemplation of training schools, Dr. Withington presented his arguments for the benefit of medical groups first and then that of hospitals. He indicated that there were two systems of nurse education, the first of which being the independent one where a committee obtained a charter and selected a superintendent of the training school. Under this system a contract with the hospital management agreed to supply the nursing for some or all of the wards while the hospital furnished a money payment for compensation for work done or maintenance of nurses or both. He makes

---

[10]*Ibid.*, p. 20.
[11]*Ibid.*, p. 29.

[12]*Ibid.*, p. 30
[13]*Ibid.*, pp. 30 and 31.
[14]*Ibid.*, p. 31.

no mention of students of nursing securing an education. According to the second method, "the hospital management itself, for the sake of securing good nursing for its wards and of supplying the community with well-trained nurses," for private duty, "undertakes the same work, but of course there is no contract between the two parties, and the one executive head of the hospital administers also the training school."[15]

He then sums up the presentation by focusing on where nursing should be located and under whose control it should be placed. "Independent training school managers may in their zeal for the education of their pupils, make such a distribution of the latter, that the hospital administration shall suffer. The balance of advantage to all interests, therefore, seems to be with the method which makes the training school a department of the hospital and under its administrative control. Then the hospital staff at whose immediate disposal this most important instrument (nursing) lies, can in case of failure or incompetency look, as in all other cases of difficulty, to the one executive head to have the matter righted."[16] It is important to realize that he was not pleading that medical education become a department of the hospital and under its control nor in case of medical incompetency that this important "instrument" (medicine) be chastised by the hospital administrator.

The preceding data from what must have been a controversial book presents factual evidence of some of the reasons for the trials which nursing has faced in this century.

A book entitled *Nurses and Nursing* was purported to be written by a "nurse" named Lisbeth D. Price in 1892. She was not a graduate of a school of nursing and admitted that compiler was a more appropriate term than writer of the book in question. An obstetrician wrote the introduction, stressing the need for the book and the capability of the author. The purpose was to "lay down the laws for the conduct and direction of nurses, and their responsibilities towards physicians, patients, and themselves." He indicated that capable, well-educated nurses are *almost* as essential as the educated physician.

In her preface, Miss Price's opening re-

mark was that "a strong line of demarcation should be drawn between that which a nurse should know and that which she should not know, that the theoretical portion of her studies must of necessity be more or less superficial." The reason for her literary contribution, she states, was that the textbooks which she had seen, "though in the main seemed good, are prone to enter into certain subjects too deeply"—while the practical side of nursing has been too superficial.

The initial chapter of her book bore the title, "The Limitations of the Duties of the Nurse." She commenced:

There are few professions—perhaps it may be said with truth, that there is *no* profession—which has its limitations marked with such rigid distinctions, as that of nursing.

She then elaborates:

There are many reasons . . . for these strong limitations. The chief one is this: the profession of nursing is dependent upon the medical profession; from it, in fact, it has emanated.[17]

Her lack of knowledge of her historic heritage is obvious. Another incredible observation was recorded: "The 'doctor's duty to the nurse' is a perversion of fact that looks distorted, even in writing; no such relation exists. The nurse to the doctor should be a human automaton, that listens to him attentively, and obeys him implicitly, nothing more. . . ."

Thus ends a trilogy of works that depict the efforts of a public spirited group of citizens seriously interested in the welfare of all human beings including nurses; a medical educator speaking for his colleagues and his students and trying subtly to mold the nurse's role and her educational program to the desires of medicine; and lastly a "nurse" who appears to have been flattered into permitting herself to assume the role of chastiser of her own colleagues. Through her eyes one sees her self-effacing demand for the role of the nurse as a passive servant to the doctor.

There has not been a great overall increase in the total number of hospitals since the turn of the century but rather in the size of hospitals. The total space of hospitals, which was once utilized only by patients' beds, is now

---

[15] *Ibid.*, p. 33.
[16] *Ibid.*, p. 34.

[17] Price, Lisbeth D.: *Nurses and Nursing.* Philadelphia, George W. Jacobs and Co., 1892, p. 1.

shared with diagnostic testing areas or therapeutic equipment needed for patient service.

The architecture of the newer buildings has been planned with greater understanding of the needs of the patient as well as those who care for him. Still greater progress in this area is needed. Many hospitals have progressive units, ranging from *intensive care* of a patient when he is critically ill to a do-it-yourself plan in which a minimal amount of care is required. The ancient custom of *"rooming-in"* with the sick loved one has been revived in some hospitals. In order to reduce expense, a motel system of patient care is another innovation in the medical setting.

Color is used more effectively in hospitals today than it has been in the last two centuries; the therapeutic value of music is beginning to be understood. Safety aspects are noted as is the use of many modern inventions to make care easier for both patients and nurses.

The construction of beds has been another area of marked change; the iron bed, which had to be lifted frequently by nurses to elevate the foot or head, has been replaced by electric beds (Fig. 11–6). Certain variations of beds provide greater comfort and ease in

assisting a patient or permitting him to do things for himself.

The feats of the physicists and engineers have been phenomenal. The theoretical principles behind many of their inventions are being applied to techniques and equipment used in the care of the sick.

The progress in the advancements of those scientific endeavors that have changed medical care have been so great that not all could possibly be described. In 1901, *Karl Landsteiner* described his phenomenal research with blood grouping, which led to a knowledge of blood testing and made possible blood transfusions. Willem Einthoven invented the string galvanometer, which provided the impetus needed to develop electrocardiography.

The year 1921 witnessed the announcement by Drs. Banting and Best of the isolation of *insulin* as the active ingredient in the pancreas needed for the metabolic activity of diabetic patients. Endocrinology became an important and recognized field. Surgery of the chest was another milestone in the progress of medicine.

The victims of an incurable disease, *pernicious anemia*, were aided by the research of

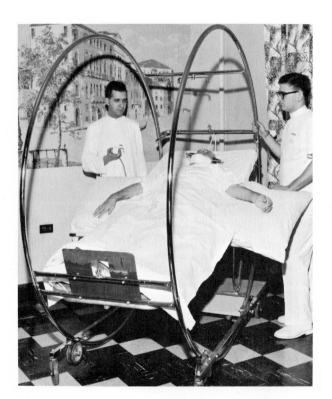

Figure 11–6. Alexian Brothers giving care to a patient in a CircOlectric Bed. (Courtesy of Alexian Brothers Hospital, Chicago.)

Drs. Minot and Murphy in Boston, who recommended that raw liver be included in the diet. Now pharmaceutical companies prepare liver for injection and another once fatal illness can be controlled.

In the early 1930's an artificial respirator called an "iron lung" was invented that was instrumental in keeping many patients alive, especially those who were paralyzed by poliomyelitis. These have been reduced in size and are now battery-powered.

The wonder drugs such as the *sulfa drugs—sulfanilamide, sulfapyridine* and *sulfathiazol—* were developed. These were beneficial in combatting such infections as those caused by streptococcus and staphylococcus. Methods of preserving the qualities of blood for therapeutic purposes were introduced. *Blood banks* were established for preserving human blood plasma and serum, which were used in transfusions. *Shock therapy* was used in psychiatry; *corneal transplants* were successful; additional information in relation to the blood, such as the knowledge of the *Rh factor,* was forthcoming.

In the decade between 1940 and 1950, World War II presented to medicine many new problems that involved a knowledge of *atomic medicine* as well as war injuries and an expansion in the field of *tropical medicine.* In addition to blood banks, many other banks, such as those for bone and tissue, became a reality. Powerful drugs such as atabrine (as a substitute for quinine), antihistamines for relieving allergic conditions, cortisone and ACTH, and of course the radioactive isotopes were processed. Supersonic and ultrasonic vibrations were used in medicine at this time.

In 1944 *Dr. Helen Taussig,* a pediatrician, carried out a research project on the plight of blue babies and emphasized the need for corrective surgery. This resulted in heart surgery, which was successfully achieved by *Dr. Alfred Blalock* of Johns Hopkins.

Cancer detection tests such as the vaginal smear test by *Dr. Papanicolaou* became available by 1948. The field of rehabilitation received a new status because of the efforts of *Dr. Howard Rusk* whose philosophy and teaching have been a boon to mankind.

During the years since 1950, *space medicine* has evolved as an offshoot of the growing field of astronautics. In 1955, *Dr. Jonas Salk* produced a vaccine for the prevention of poliomyelitis. Mass inoculation of children

and adults with Salk vaccine and Sabin oral vaccine have been responsible for the virtual disappearance of poliomyelitis. The oral poliomyelitis vaccine has been a favorable replacement for the inoculations.

Many surgical operations, such as open-heart surgery and artificial tissue transplants, have been carried out in this period. Scientific equipment, such as the artificial heart and artificial kidney apparatus, has been devised.

The use of electric monitoring, automatic thermometers, dialysis equipment, inhalation therapy, and data processing and computers have all become innovations in patient care. The lifesaving battery-operated pacemakers are now being supplied by nuclear power. This enables the pacemakers to operate longer than the earlier ones.

The remarkably unselfish and heroic efforts of many medical missionaries have been observed and their valiant work recorded. The contributions of *Dr. Albert Schweitzer* and *Dr. Tom Dooley* in their efforts as ambassadors of good will will not go unremembered.

The position of women in medicine has become more secure in this century.

A famous woman doctor was *S. Josephine Baker* (1873–1945).[18] The growing field of *public health* interested Dr. Baker and in 1901 she joined the New York City Department of Health. She recognized the need for a program of health education to try to prevent needless suffering and misery. She became Assistant Commisssioner of Health and engaged in an expanding program dedicated to the health and welfare of children. She was responsible for the creation of the New York City Division of Child Hygiene and directed this program.

Her goal in establishing this important section was "to prevent children from dying by preventing them from becoming ill." Educational programs absorbed her interest and emphasized the need for well prepared nurses whose role in teaching was recognized.

When she first started her crusade in the interest of infant welfare, she blamed much of the high infant mortality from gastrointestinal diseases on the city milk supply. She believed that the raw milk sold in the local grocery stores was a "diluted germ culture." Her suggestion was the establishment of baby health stations where bottled pas-

[18]Baker, S. Josephine: *Fighting For Life.* New York, The Macmillan Company, 1939.

teurized milk, sold more cheaply than the raw milk, was accompanied by educational material on child care. The taxpayers would not approve this plan but it won the financial support of a wealthy lady who maintained 30 of these baby stations. Their success prompted the adoption of the station plan by the municipal authorities.

Dr. Baker was instrumental in establishing the *United States Children's Bureau* in 1912. Her interest in growing professionally was evidenced when she became the first woman to earn the degree of Doctor of Public Health. Dr. Baker was also the first woman physician to be accepted for a position with the Federal Government.

Dr. Baker was a founder and one of the early presidents of the American Child Hygiene Association. All of her professional life was devoted to the service of providing for children a healthier, happier world in which to grow. Child health programs began to evolve.

WHITE HOUSE CONFERENCES ON CHILDREN AND YOUTH

The White House Conferences have been devoted to the interests of children and youth.

1909 — The First White House Conference was centered around the care of dependent children. As a result of this conference:

1912: Congress established the United States Children's Bureau.
1915–1919: The Children's Bureau helped states create divisions of Maternal and Child Health. All of the activities of the Children's Bureau have been directed toward three worthwhile objectives: "(1) to insure to the children of the nation the right to be born as normal healthy babies and to develop into vigorous young persons ready to take their places in the adult world; (2) the remedying of conditions in our society which are obstacles to normal child health and development, and (3) the prevention of these harmful conditions."

The Children's Bureau has been concerned with employed children. When the Bureau was established by Congress, there was specified in the Act the need for investigation of "dangerous occupations, accidents, and diseases of children; employment and legislation affecting children in the several states and territories."

1919 — The Second White House Conference emphasized child welfare standards. Concern was expressed for the high maternal and infant death rates partially due to too rapid industrialization. Results of this conference included:

1921: Sheppard-Towner Act (Maternal Child Act) passed.
1924: Child Labor Law amendment was proposed.
1928–1931: Committee on Cost of Medical Care was appointed.

1930 — The Third White House Conference stressed child health and protection. This conference resulted in:

1930: Children's Charter was enacted.
1935: Social Security Act was passed.
1935–1936: The National Health Survey was attempted.

1940 — The Fourth White House Conference selected as the theme, "Children in a Democracy." Continued study on responsibility of Federal, state and local government for maternity and child care was approved. Religion was emphasized. Grants-in-aid for research and for upgrading health professions were proposed.

Results of this conference were:

1942: Emergency Maternity and Infant Care Act was passed.
1946–1947: Hill Burton Act (hospital construction) was adopted.
1948: The Nation's Health — A report to the President was prepared.

1950 — The Fifth White House Conference accepted the challenge of a healthy personality. This was the first of many conferences that encouraged all disciplines to work together on the problems. Youth was also represented. Two major problems discussed were delinquency and mental retardation.

1960 — The Sixth White House Conference for Children and Youth used the same techniques as in 1950 for multidiscipline conferences, but there were 7000 attending and the results were not as easy to summarize. The "migrant minor," the American Indian problem, the physically handicapped, the illegitimate child and the Black child were discussed. Results were:

1960: President asked Governors to set up physical fitness programs in each state.
A permanent White House Conference committee was established to improve implementation

on local level of recommendations of the 1960 conference.

Eventually well-child clinics were set up. In the 1950's babies were tested to detect phenylketonuria (PKU) and state laws required PKU testing for all newborns. In the 1960's legislation was enacted for reporting of "the battered-child syndrome" in the hope of preventing child abuse.

At the beginning of this century, the circumstances surrounding the transmission and continuance of such diseases as typhoid fever, cholera, summer diarrheas and food poisoning were beginning to be studied. The control of milk-borne, water-borne, and food-borne diseases was claiming attention. Eventually adequate measures for obtaining sanitary water supplies and sewage disposal systems were put into practice.

New laboratory techniques received impetus from the eager health workers in departments of health. In 1907, an outbreak of typhoid fever in New York City was traced to a contaminated water supply. In the same year "Typhoid Mary" was located by Major George A. Soper of the U. S. Army. She was taken into custody by the New York City Health Department. Laboratory tests impelled the adoption of registration and supervision of typhoid carriers. By 1917 food-handlers were examined to detect possible typhoid carriers.

Bureaus of health education were established, followed by bureaus of infectious diseases; many bureaus of preventable diseases included divisions of industrial hygiene.

The identification of the causative organisms of many communicable diseases, together with the knowledge of the spread of disease and the institution of programs of immunization, led to civic action. Homes and family members were quarantined and the homes were placarded to warn all neighbors and friends of the presence of such diseases (Fig. 11–7).

The Federal Government attempted to control, inspect and supervise the quality of foods as early as 1879. At that time, a bill had been submitted to Congress to prohibit the adulteration of substances to be used as food and drink.

An American novelist and socialist *Upton Sinclair* (1878–1968) was instrumental in bringing about certain health reforms. His novel, *The Jungle*, published in 1906, described the shockingly filthy conditions in

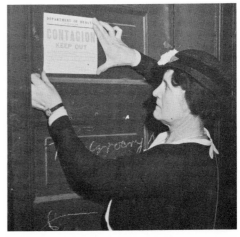

Figure 11–7. A home being placarded. (Courtesy of New York City Department of Health.)

the Chicago slaughterhouses, and instilled horror in the minds of the public and then action. President Theodore Roosevelt received scores of letters demanding federal action to raise standards in the meat industry. *The Jungle* symbolized the consumer cause and put the federal government firmly into the consumer protection business. It was not until 1906 that President Roosevelt signed the bill that enforced the proposal to prohibit the manufacture and sale of adulterated and misbranded foods. This law was to be administered by the Department of Agriculture. In 1938, President Franklin D. Roosevelt signed a bill which created the *Federal Food, Drug, and Cosmetic Act*. The Food and Drug Administration was transferred from the Department of Agriculture by the Reorganization Act and was placed under the control of the Federal Security Agency with a Commissioner of Food and Drugs.

The influence of public spirited citizens has continued in the fight for better health. The ecology movement was greatly influenced by Rachel Carson's *Silent Spring* (1962), as well as by the multifaceted activities of Ralph Nader, whose early efforts in *Unsafe at Any Speed* (1965) aroused Congress to study and take action against the automotive industry for manufacturing unsafe automobiles. In 1962, President John F. Kennedy enunciated what has been called the consumer bill of rights: the right to be informed, the right to choose, the right to safety and the right to be heard.

The Public Health Service was established by an act of 1798, authorizing marine hospitals for the care of American merchant seamen. In 1902, Congress renamed the Marine Hospital Service the Public Health and Marine Hospital Service under the direction of a surgeon-general. By 1912 this title was changed to the *United States Public Health Service* (U.S.P.H.S.). The duties of this branch of the Federal service rapidly became more complex. In 1918, it added the Division of Venereal Diseases, and in 1929 a narcotics division, which was renamed the Division of Mental Hygiene. It was responsible for hospital facilities at Lexington, Kentucky, and Fort Worth, Texas, for the care and treatment of those addicted to narcotics. The passage of the Federal Social Security Act of 1935 had important, far-reaching effects. The passage of the National Cancer Act of 1937 brought into existence the National Cancer Institute. Rapidly the responsibilities of the U.S.P.H.S. were increased. In 1946 the Hospital Survey and Construction (Hill-Burton) Act was passed, and in 1948 the National Heart Institute was founded. The National Institute of Allergy and Infectious Diseases and the National Institute of Dental Research were formed by reorganizing several existing units. *The National Institutes of Health* were developed. Since 1950 the National Institutes of Arthritis and Metabolic Diseases as well as the National Institute of Neurological Diseases and Blindness have been added.

In 1952, the U.S.P.H.S. established, on the grounds of the National Institutes of Health in Bethesda, Maryland, a research hospital center of 500 beds called the *National Clinical Center*.

THE DEPARTMENT OF HEALTH, EDUCATION AND WELFARE

In 1946, the Federal Security Agency was involved in further reorganization, which included the transfer of the Children's Bureau from the Department of Labor, the Food and Drug Administration from the Department of Agriculture, and the National Office of Vital Statistics from the Bureau of the Census of the Department of Commerce. In 1953, the Federal Security Agency was changed by an act of Congress to the Department of Health, Education and Welfare. In addition to the administrative offices, the following have become an integral part of the Department of Health, Education and Welfare: the Public Health Service, the Office of Education, the Social Security Administration, the Food and Drug Administration, the Office of Vocational Rehabilitation and St. Elizabeth's Hospital.

VOLUNTARY HEALTH AGENCIES

Many voluntary health agencies have exerted a tremendous influence on the preservation of health as well as prevention of disease through this century. Research efforts have been aided by their financial assistance. Some of the better known ones are the National Tuberculosis and Respiratory Disease Association, the American Cancer Society, the American Heart Association, the National Foundation for Infantile Paralysis and the National Association for Mental Health.

PUBLIC HEALTH EDUCATION

The University of Michigan awarded the first degree in public health in 1910. Two years later a program of study had been developed at the Massachusetts Institute of Technology. The University of Pennsylvania receives the credit for establishing the first school of public health. In 1941, the *Association of Schools of Public Health* was formed, whose Committee on Professional Education led to the development in 1946 of a system of accreditation of programs granting degrees in public health.

In 1949 the *American Board of Preventive Medicine and Public Health* was established. The sponsors of this new organization were the American Medical Association, the American Public Health Association, the Association of Schools of Public Health, the Canadian Public Health Association, and the Southern Medical Association. Carefully selected field residency programs have been developed in order to improve the educational backgrounds of those whose duty it is to protect and preserve the health of the public.

WORLD HEALTH ORGANIZATION

International health work has been carried on for many years. As early as 1902, the Pan-

American Sanitary Bureau was established; by 1907 the International Office of Public Health came into being; and by 1921 the Health Organization of the League of Nations was developed. In 1923, a consolidation occurred with the International Office of Public Health being absorbed into the Health Organization of the League of Nations.

In 1946, a constitution for a *World Health Organization* (W.H.O.) was accepted by 61 nations. The duties of the Health Organization of the League of Nations and the United Nations Relief and Rehabilitation Administration (UNRRA) were absorbed by this new World Health Organization. The Pan-American Sanitary Bureau became the regional headquarters for W.H.O. for the Americas; the international headquarters are in Geneva, Switzerland. The main objective has been to assist all peoples in the attainment of the highest possible level of health.

The World Health Organization as a specialized agency of the United Nations has been the world's directing and coordinating authority in international public health. It acts as an educational channel whereby health workers may receive the latest scientific and medical information and get assistance in applying this knowledge to their own countries.

Just as the children of the United States have the United States Children's Bureau, the children of the world have an agency specially dedicated to their interest and needs, the *United Nations International Children's Emergency Fund (UNICEF)*. Large sums of money have been spent on food, clothing and medicines for victims of catastrophic emergencies as well as for children of underdeveloped countries. Programs for the eradication of specific diseases have been instituted.

CHANGE IN MEDICAL EDUCATION

In 1848, a year after its organization, the *American Medical Association* stressed the need for clinical teaching to include demonstrations for proper education of medical students. Doctors had been more interested in practicing medicine than in the educational preparation of practitioners of medicine. When the *Association of American Medical Colleges* was organized in 1890, they recommended a minimum background of high school graduation as a prerequisite for medi-

cine. When *Johns Hopkins School of Medicine* opened in 1893, however, a bachelor's degree was required of applicants for admission to the Medical School, which was a four-year medical school program. These two diametrically opposed courses of action prompted the need for a required standard.

It has been recorded that the failure of the schools of medicine to keep abreast of scientific progress led to the establishment of *state medical boards* during the closing years of the nineteenth and early years of the twentieth century. These boards were empowered to examine all candidates and to license those who were successful in meeting the standards set by this Board of Examiners in Medicine. For some years they were hampered by lack of financial backing and by too many political controls.

In 1904 The American Medical Association established a *Council on Medical Education* to investigate the problems of medical education that had been identified as lack of educational standards, lack of prepared faculty and meager resources.

Carnegie Foundation was asked to make a survey of medical education. This foundation was eminently qualified to do this because it had completed studies in law and theology and was prepared to study medicine as well. A forceful scholar, *Abraham Flexner*, undertook the survey. His report, often referred to as "The Flexner Report," was published in 1910 in the book, *Medical Education in the United States and Canada*. His report was a highly explosive document that shocked and aroused the public to action.

The Flexner Report emphasized the need for fulltime faculty. They should be experienced teachers skilled in a medical specialty. Formerly, practicing physicians devoted their free time to their teaching responsibilities and medical students frequently received little clinical instruction.

The changes that were instituted because of the Flexner Report were remarkable. The devastating criticism provoked an immediate revolution in medical education. The proprietary diploma schools of medicine disappeared and university medical schools were reestablished. Many of the weaker schools closed, partly because of social pressures and inability to attract students. Many schools gained in strength through university affiliation, and nearly all schools were able to secure financial backing through private endowment or state support. The apprentice gave way to the university student of medical science. The faculty became university professors whose time was devoted entirely to instruction and research.

The admission requirements for medical schools changed and were enforced for all candidates for the profession of medicine. By 1914, high school graduation was required; by 1916 this changed to a requirement of one year of college, and by 1918 to two years of college. The necessary base of broad liberal education was becoming essential before the professional superstructure of medicine was added.

Flexner's criticisms stimulated a more dynamic intellectual climate. There was a dramatic metamorphosis of the physician from an artisan to a scientist. The medical teaching was patient-centered rather than procedure-centered. The physician accepted newly discovered facts. The numbers of medical researchers and clinical investigators increased, and they contributed incredible discoveries.

In 1962 medical educators carried out some self-evaluation and the trend seems to be a shortening of the total program with greater emphasis on humanities.

The span of life has been increased as a result of research in medical science, public health and sanitation, improvements in the living conditions of the less fortunate and the elimination of contagious and infectious diseases.

The Flexner Beacon has lighted up a half century of medical progress. It shines brightly today, for this study revolutionized the whole basis for the education of doctors in the U.S. and in the decades that followed American medicine shot far ahead of the rest of the world.

SCIENCE OF LIFE

The science of life, with its roots deeply implanted in ancient Greece, has blossomed during these last 50 years of expansion of scientific discoveries and delineation of scientific knowledge. There has been less hostility and more genuine acceptance of new concepts and theories and scientific revelations.

The field of genetics has changed the understanding of man. A substance referred to as DNA has been found to be present in all cells and determines the chemical nature of cells—their structure and functions—thus, the inherited characteristics as well as the control of bodily activities.

The American physiologist Walter B. Cannon coined the term *"homeostasis"* to refer to the system of self-regulation by which living organisms maintain a constant norm. Because of the inadequacy of this concept, the term *homeokinesis* has supplanted it. This implies broader, more dynamic interactions which strive to maintain life's structure.

Until recently, the degree of magnification was restricted by the ability of the human eye to observe enlarged images. Another obstacle to high magnification was the amount of light that was available. The *electron microscope* has overcome both deterrents because beams of electrons in a vacuum chamber now replace ordinary light. The image received by a photographic plate registering on a fluorescent screen is infinitely more sensitive than the human eye. Extremely minute structures such as viruses have been observed by the electron microscope.

As Dr. Howard Rusk has so aptly challenged, "years have been added to life—but life must be added to these years."

CHAPTER 12

Nursing as an Emerging Social Force in Health Care in the Twentieth Century

Developments in Nursing and Social Sciences

At the turn of the century, there was a marked expansion in the number of schools of nursing, and it seemed that this trend would continue. The quality of many schools was due to the vision of leaders of nursing who were attuned to social progress as well as needs of society. The role of the nurse had been molded by the social concept of woman's role in society. Again, nurse leaders were adamant for the rights of women and and were found among the marchers in the suffragettes' pilgrimages. An article in the *New York Herald Tribune*[1] describes an immortal triumvirate of suffragettes who led the march from New York City to Albany to demand the right of women to vote; one of these leaders was "Little Doc Dock" (Lavinia L. Dock) a member of the staff of the Henry Street Settlement.

In this male-dominated society in which the status of the physician was superior, the role of the nurse became a subservient, dependent one.

ORGANIZATIONS FOR NURSES

During the nineteenth century, it was realized that in unity there was strength. This concept had been followed by industrial, social and political groups in forming unions, parties and societies for workers. Members of other professional fields had associations for their members that brought individuals together for united action.

Group consciousness had permeated the professional boundaries of nursing, resulting in the formation of official organizations. The first evidence was the founding of the *Royal British Nurses' Association* in 1887 by *Mrs. Bedford Fenwick* (Fig. 12–1). In America, the

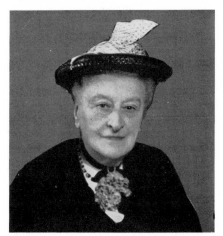

Figure 12–1. Mrs. Bedford Fenwick. In the Greco-Turkish war, 1897, she was in charge of a military hospital.

---

[1]Bugbee, Emma: "Suffragettes' 1912 Pilgrimage," *New York Herald Tribune*, Sunday, March 28, 1965.

first signs of union appeared in the organization of alumnae associations. These groups fostered the idea of cooperation but centered it around the school and hospital of the alumnae groups. Later, opportunities of a broader scope were recognized.

American Society of Superintendents of Training Schools

In 1893 at the World's Fair in Chicago eighteen superintendents of training schools gathered together and held an important meeting. The person who sparked the initial movement at this international gathering was Mrs. Bedford Fenwick of London who encouraged the inclusion of nursing at the Hospital and Medical Congress. Dr. John S. Billings, chairman of the Congress, agreed and a sub-section on nursing was provided. The chairman was Miss Isabel A. Hampton, Superintendent of Nurses at Johns Hopkins Hospital.

This resulted in the formation of the *American Society of Superintendents of Training Schools*, which aimed to promote fellowship among the members, to establish and maintain a universal standard of training, and to further the best interests of the nursing profession. In order to qualify for membership, it was mandatory that each person be a graduate in good standing of a training school connected with a general hospital giving not less than a two-year course of instruction and that each hold the position of superintendent of a training school connected with a recognized general hospital. These requirements were not waived for anyone, regardless of her prestige or position.[2]

This organization banded together the educational leaders of nursing in this country and Canada, and due to their efforts standards were established and enforced for the education of nurses. From the first meeting which aimed for better education by enriching programs, many reforms were carried out and suggested improvements were identified.

---

[2]*First and Second Annual Reports* (1894–1895) *of the American Society of Superintendents of Training Schools for Nurses*, Harrisburg, Pa., Harrisburg Publishing Company, 1897, pp. 8–9.

Nurses' Associated Alumnae of the United States and Canada

Alumnae associations felt the need to expand their efforts, to keep abreast of progress and trends, and to unite for greater control of the position of the nurse. As a result of the determination of delegates of ten alumnae associations, a meeting was convened and the outcome of this momentous conclave was the inception of the *Nurses' Associated Alumnae of the United States and Canada*. Isabel Hampton Robb was the first president and continued in this office until 1901. The chief objective of this organization was to secure legislation to differentiate the trained from the untrained nurse. Protection would thereby be provided for nurses, physicians, and the public.

In 1899 the group's name was changed to the *Nurses' Associated Alumnae of the United States*, because New York law did not permit the incorporation of representatives of two nations. State nurses' associations were organized in 1901 to work toward state legislation to control nursing practice.

International Council of Nurses

An opportunity for the union of all nurses throughout the world became a possibility through the foundation of the *International Council of Nurses* (I.C.N.). The I.C.N. is the oldest international association of professional women. It was founded in 1899 by Mrs. Bedford Fenwick, assisted by nursing leaders from many countries. Its constitution was adopted in 1900. The first meeting of the Council was held in Buffalo, New York, in 1901. Active membership was offered to self-governing national nurses' associations, and nurses in every country were encouraged to form a nurses' association in order to apply for membership, and, thereby, to contribute to elevating and maintaining the highest standards of nursing around the world as well as receiving the benefits that naturally come from such powerful joint efforts. (See Figure 12–2.) Membership in the I.C.N. consists of national associations rather than of individual members.

Since the I.C.N. was founded, quadrennial congresses have been planned at which the nurses of the world meet to discuss professional problems.

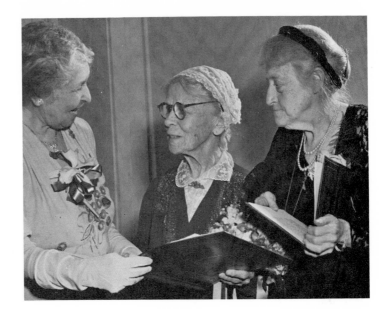

Figure 12-2. President Effie J. Taylor presenting citations from the I.C.N. to Lavinia L. Dock (center) and Annie W. Goodrich (right) on May 14, 1947.

The American Federation of Nurses was formed in 1901 by the affiliation of the American Society of Superintendents of Training Schools for Nurses and the Nurses' Associated Alumnae of the United States. The purpose of the affiliation was the opportunity it afforded for membership in the National Council of Women and participation in the proceedings of the I.C.N. In 1905 the American Federation of Nurses withdrew from the National Council of Women and joined the International Council of Nurses.

I.C.N. CONGRESSES

Year	Place	Elected President
1901	Buffalo, N.Y., U.S.A.	Mrs. Bedford Fenwick, Great Britain
1904	Berlin, Germany	Miss Susan McGahey, Australia
1909	London, England	Sister Agnes Karll, Germany
1912	Cologne, Germany	Miss Annie W. Goodrich, U.S.A.
1915	San Francisco, U.S.A.	Mrs. Henry Tcherning, Denmark
1922	Copenhagen, Denmark	Baroness Mannerheim, Finland
1925	Helsinki, Finland	Miss Nina Gage, China
1927	Geneva, Switzerland	No election
1929	Montreal, Canada	Mlle. Chaptal, France
1933	Paris, France } Brussels, Belgium }	Dame Alicia Lloyd Still, Great Britain
1937	London, England	Miss Effie Taylor, U.S.A.
1947	Atlantic City, U.S.A.	Miss Gerda Hojer, Sweden
1949	Stockholm, Sweden	No election
1953	Petropolis, Brazil	Mlle. Marie Bihet, Belgium
1957	Rome, Italy	Miss Agnes Ohlson, U.S.A.
1961	Melbourne, Australia	Mlle. Alice Clamageran, France
1965	Frankfurt, Germany	Miss Alice Girard, Canada
1969	Montreal, Canada	Miss Margarethe Kruse, Denmark

The National Association of Colored Graduate Nurses was organized in 1908 because of a need to break down discriminatory practices facing Negro nurses as well as to foster leadership in the membership. It was dissolved by legal action of the members in 1951, after contributing many sound policies for the total profession of nursing as well as many leaders whose achievements have been exemplary. At the Biennial Convention of the American Nurses' Association in Detroit in 1962, it was reported that integration has been achieved in every state in the Union so that qualified members may join their state nurses' association without discrimination due to race, creed or national background.

Canadian Nurses' Association

The *Canadian Nurses' Association* (C.N.A.), which was founded in 1908, was in reality a consolidation of the Canadian Society of Superintendents of Training Schools for Nurses, established in 1907, and the Canadian National Association for Trained Nurses, formed in 1908. The present name was adopted in 1924. The C.N.A. has been the official organization of registered nurses in Canada and is a member of the I.C.N.

American Nurses' Association

The *American Nurses' Association* (A.N.A.) was established in 1911 as a successor of the Nurses' Associated Alumnae of the United States. It is the professional organization for registered nurses in the United States and holds membership in the I.C.N. State nurses' associations of all states are constituent units of the A.N.A. As early as 1906 the Connecticut State Nurses' Association had sent protests to magazines that advertised correspondence schools of nursing; it was reported that many dropped these advertisements. This is an example of the early activity of the state associations in more than local projects.

The A.N.A. is the largest professional woman's organization in the world. Its seal has the figure of Linda Richards. The overall purposes of the association are to foster high standards of nurse practice and to promote the welfare of nurses so that all people may have better nursing care. It represents professional nurses and serves as their spokesman with allied professional and governmental groups and with the public.

The American Nurses' Foundation, Inc., was established by the American Nurses' Association in 1955 to support research and studies in nursing and to sponsor special projects. This Foundation serves as a center for the planning, guidance and coordination of nursing research and for the dissemination of research findings in the public interest.

The National League of Nursing Education (N.L.N.E.) was founded in 1912 as a successor to the American Society of Superintendents of Training Schools. In 1932 the A.N.A. and N.L.N.E. voted to make the N.L.N.E. the Department of Education of the A.N.A. Membership in the League was for educators and was to be complementary to membership in the A.N.A.

The *National Organization for Public Health Nursing* was formed in 1912. Its official journal was called *Public Health Nursing*. The membership consisted of nurses actively engaged in community nursing as well as lay members who were interested in promoting the services of public health nurses. Membership in the N.O.P.H.N. for nurses was in addition to the A.N.A. Each member received an enrollment number and a pin.

The *Association of Collegiate Schools of Nursing* was established in 1933 with the purpose of fostering nursing education on a professional and collegiate level, strengthening relationships with institutions of higher learning and encouraging research. This organization was a constituent member of the American Council on Education.

National League for Nursing

By 1952 the National League for Nursing (N.L.N.) was formed by the fusion of the following organizations: National League of Nursing Education (founded 1912), National Organization for Public Health Nursing (1912), Association of Collegiate Schools of Nursing (1933), Joint Committee on Practical Nurses and Auxiliary Workers in Nursing Services (1945), Joint Committee on Careers in Nursing (1948), National Committee for the Improvement of Nursing Services (1949) and National Nursing Accrediting Service (1949).

The *American Association of Industrial Nurses*,

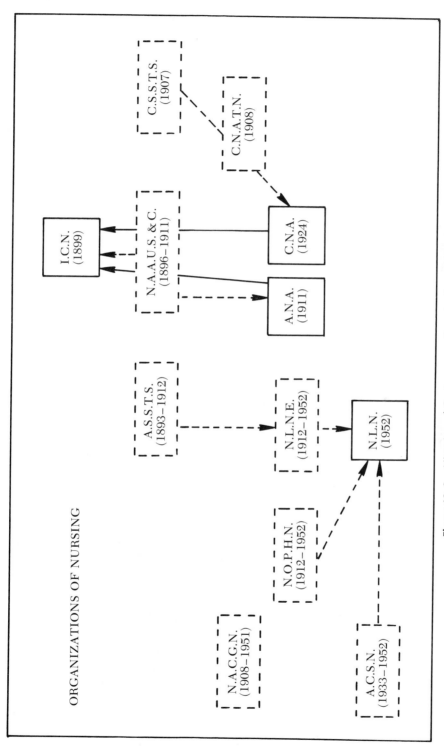

Figure 12–3. Historic and Contemporary Organizations of Nursing.

organized in 1942, has a membership of registered nurses employed in industry.

Eventually nurses felt the need to band together for the promotion of the spiritual aspects of nursing. The first of these was the *Guild of St. Barnabas for Nurses*, which was founded in England. Though now nondenominational, the American Society was organized in 1886 in Boston under the sponsorship of the Episcopal Church.

The *International Catholic Guild for Nurses* was formed in 1923 and the *National Council of Catholic Nurses* was established in 1940. The promotion of the spiritual growth of Catholic nurses was the prime purpose for these organizations. An official magazine, *The Catholic Nurse*, has been published quarterly by the latter association, which has chapters in every diocese.

The *Lutheran Nurses' Guild* was formed to foster the spiritual growth of nurses. *The Lutheran Nurse* has been published to serve as a motivating force for the members of this association.

The *National Nurses' Christian Fellowship* is another organization that aims to encourage Christian faith in daily living. A magazine, *His*, has been published by this group, as has the bimonthly N.C.F. bulletin, *The Nurse's Lamp*.

JOURNALS FOR NURSES

In America there was need for a professional magazine to establish communication between scattered groups of nurses. As early as 1896 Mrs. Robb suggested that the national association should have its own official magazine. In 1900 a stock company of nurses was organized for this purpose, and $2400 was contributed by hundreds of nurses to start the *American Journal of Nursing. Sophia Palmer*[3] (Fig. 12–4), of Rochester, N.Y., and M. E. P. Davis, of Philadelphia, both in active hospital work, made themselves personally and legally responsible for the venture. Miss

---

[3]Miss Palmer began her training in 1876 under Linda Richards at Massachusetts General Hospital. She organized schools at St. Luke's in New Bedford and at Garfield Memorial, Washington, D.C., and reorganized the school at Rochester (N.Y.) City Hospital. She helped to organize both national nursing associations, was president of the first nurses' examining board of New York, founded the *American Journal of Nursing* and was its editor for twenty years. She died in 1920.

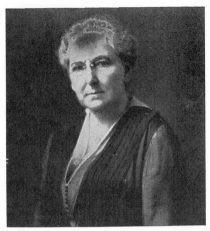

Figure 12–4. Sophia Palmer, founder of the *American Journal of Nursing*. (Portrait by Morrall, Rochester, N.Y.)

Palmer became the editor and remained in that position until 1920.

On October 1, 1900, the first issue of the *American Journal of Nursing* was published. Since 1912 the magazine has been the property of the A.N.A. and the official organ of the national nursing associations. *Mary M. Roberts* (Fig. 12–5) was editor from 1920 to 1949, when she retired after exerting remarkable influence on all fields of nursing. *Nell V. Beeby* was appointed editor of the Journal in 1949. During her administration, the duties of this office broadened in scope to include two new Journal publications, *Nursing Research* (1952) and *Nursing Outlook*

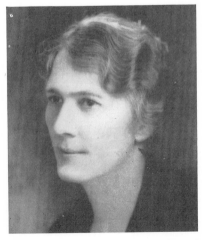

Figure 12–5. Mary M. Roberts, R.N., Editor, *American Journal of Nursing,* 1920 to 1949.

(1953). Becoming executive editor of the *American Journal of Nursing* Company as well as the editor of the *American Journal of Nursing*, Miss Beeby carried out her duties with wisdom and her death was a profound loss to the nursing profession.

Before the death of Miss Beeby in 1957, it had become apparent that the administration of the Journal Company was a heavy assignment. A new position of *executive director* was established, and *Pearl McIver* was appointed to this position in 1957. In 1959, when Miss McIver retired, she was succeeded by *Lucy D. Germain.*

The sudden death of *Jeanette White,* who replaced Miss Beeby, was another loss. *Edith Patton Lewis* (Fig. 12–6) assumed the Journal's editorial functions until December of 1959, when *Barbara G. Schutt* became editor. *Thelma M. Schorr* became editor in 1971.

The Pacific Coast Journal of Nursing was established in 1904 and continued to 1944, when it was discontinued. Its editor for many years was Genevieve Cooke.

The Trained Nurse and Hospital Review (later renamed *The Nursing World*) was established in 1888. It was the first nursing and hospital journal of national circulation in this country, and did valuable pioneer work. In 1889 it combined with the *Journal of Practical Nursing,* and later absorbed, one at a time, *The Nightingale, The Nurse, The Nursing World* and *The*

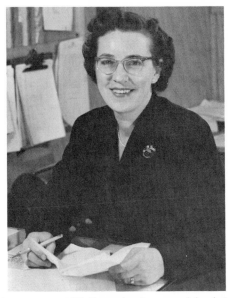

Figure 12–6. Edith Patton Lewis assumed the duties of editor of *Nursing Outlook* in 1970.

Nursing Record. This was for ten years the only nursing and hospital journal in America and was the official organ of the national societies from 1896 to 1900.

The Canadian Nurse and Hospital Review was inaugurated in 1905 through the efforts of the Toronto General Hospital Alumnae Association. It was owned by a business firm at the beginning but was purchased by the Canadian National Association of Trained Nurses in 1916. Since 1959 an edition in French has been published, *L'infirmière Canadienne.* The magazine was under the editorship of persons part-time until *Ethel Incledon Johns* became the first full-time editor. Miss Johns had held many administrative positions in Canada, served as a field director for the Rockefeller Foundation in Europe, and was director of studies of the committee for nursing organizations of the New York Hospital-Cornell Medical College Association. Miss Johns was succeeded as editor by Margaret E. Kerr. Virginia A. Lindabury has been editor of *The Canadian Nurse* since 1965, while Claire L. Bigné assumed the full-time editorship of *L'infirmière Canadienne.*

LEGISLATION FOR REGISTRATION OF NURSES

It was essential that nursing organizations protect the public from unqualified nurses. Legislation was provided that demanded the legal approval of schools of nursing, faculty preparation and the curriculum, all of which were designed to prepare the graduate to fulfill her professional responsibility. Examinations were required of graduates by a specially appointed Examining Board, which issued a certificate of licensure and identified the successful candidates as registered nurses (R.N.). Licensing examinations were constructed to test applicants who were graduates of schools of practical nursing. The letters L.P.N. refer to those candidates who have passed these examinations.

The first registration bill was passed in Cape Colony, South Africa, in 1891. By 1903 the states of North Carolina, New Jersey, New York and Virginia had passed the first laws establishing a legal system of registration. In Canada the first registration bill was enacted by the Province of Nova Scotia in 1910.

Eventually every state in the United States

and every province in Canada passed registration laws. Other countries became aware of the need for legal control of nursing practice and registration of duly qualified nurses, and took steps to fill the gap.

An editorial comment in 1902[4] presented a thought-provoking quotation from the *Philadelphia Medical Journal* of March 15, 1902.

Trained nursing is a profession, not a trade, because it involves the intelligent application of certain general principles rather than mere manual dexterity acquired by constant repetition. . . . Trained nursing is now passing through a crisis such as affects all professions at some time, whatsoever they may be. The crisis is that for purposes of profit or from motives of economy various persons and institutions are taking advantage of the desire of various women to enter by easy routes a hitherto honorable calling, and thus causing a double injury: in providing a considerable number of unqualified persons with diplomas as trained nurses, and second in so increasing the supply of nurses that the profession — just as has happened to the medical profession — is being cheapened in the eyes of the public. . . . We have found it necessary to establish a State Medical Board, which imperfect as it is, has nevertheless served a most useful purpose. We have found it necessary to prescribe a minimum term of medical instruction, because men who could perhaps in a short time acquire enough information to pass the examination of the state board would not be sufficiently familiar with disease, as such, to render them qualified to practice medicine, and this also has proved good. The question now arises whether in view of the methods by which many so-called trained nurses are educated and let loose on an unguarded public, the state should not intervene, and at least limit an abuse *which is dangerous to the sick* and an injustice to women who have conscientiously prepared themselves for their chosen calling.

In an article on the essentials of *A Good Nurse Practice Act* in 1934, Elizabeth C. Burgess suggested[5] the following:

1. That while the requirements for practice which are written into a law must be minimum, this minimum should be far above what we now accept and should be such that the person who becomes an R.N. should be a fully qualified person, safe to care for the sick.

2. That the time has passed when permissive acts meet needs. Nurse practice acts should compel all who make of nursing a profession, that is, who nurse for hire, to be licensed.

3. That in setting up provisions for much better nursing education consideration must be given to two types of qualifications: (a) personal, which relates to health, education, and character; (b) the professional preparation.

And under this heading we are concerned with the length of the course, the facilities which can be provided, the organization of the faculty and its qualifications, with resources and the curriculum.

Provision must be made for the administration of the law, for examinations, for licences and registration, for fees, for reciprocity, and provision must be made for penalties.

In answering the question of composition of the membership on the Board of Nurse Examiners she reported that "if nurses are to control the practice of their profession, physicians should certainly not be members of the board of nurse examiners."

Miss Burgess felt the need for compulsory registration and she stressed:

To me a great step forward would be taken if registration and licences were required of all professional nurses. I see no disadvantages to either the nurses or the public. . . .[6]

There were many problems inherent in interstate licensure; these have been lessened since the formation of the *Bureau of State Boards of Nurse Examiners* under the aegis of the American Nurses' Association. Since 1950 every state has used identical state board examinations, which provide one important aspect of uniformity. The tests originate from a test board pool that has been conducted by the Department of Measurement and Guidance of the National League for Nursing. By 1951 the members attending the state board conference recommended the adoption of a national minimum passing score for state board examinations.

NURSING EDUCATION

When the first three schools of nursing were started in the United States and sincerely attempted to pattern their independence in functioning after the Nightingale system, most members of the medical pro-

[4]_____ "The State Control of Trained Nurses," *American Journal of Nursing*, April 1902, p. 562.

[5]Burgess, Elizabeth C. "A Good Nurse Practice Act — What Are The Essentials," *American Journal of Nursing*, July 1934, p. 653.

[6]*Ibid.*, p. 655.

fession were vehemently opposed because of inability to *control* them. These early schools had contracted with the affiliating hospital for the provision of nursing service in exchange for educational services.

Expansion in hospital facilities occurred and forthwith a mushrooming in the development of schools of nursing resulted. It became apparent that the aims of the schools and those of the hospital were not in agreement. This conflict and confusion of trying to serve two masters—nursing education on the one hand with nursing service on the other—resulted in the union of the two areas, and schools came under the dominance of hospitals.

Due to the efforts of the stalwart, dedicated, courageous leaders from the United States and Canada, many educational reforms were initiated by the American Society of Superintendents of Training Schools.

In 1894, at the first annual convention of the American Association of Superintendents of Training Schools, the leaders stressed the importance of planning the entire educational program for the student rather than for the convenience of the hospital nursing services.

In 1895, Miss Mary Agnes Snively of Toronto presented a thought-provoking paper that emphasized the need for initiating uniformity of education for nursing through a uniform matriculation examination for admission; a requirement of specific prerequisite courses; a uniform length of the program in nursing edcuation with a shortening of the workday and week and an examination plan that indicated the possession of necessary theoretical background.

It is worthwhile to read Miss Snively's scholarly paper and note that she encouraged nurse leaders not to be frightened by "those who cry out in alarm against what they are pleased to call an attempt to educate nurses." She clearly delineated the need for a well-planned education for nurses.

At this same convention, Mrs. Isabel H. Robb, while pleading for a truly educational program, questioned the wisdom of the payment of an allowance to students. She referred to the practice of allowing eight dollars a month for the first year and 12 dollars a month for the second year. She noted: "We say in our circulars that 'this is in nowise intended as a salary but is allowed for uniforms, textbooks, and other expenses incidental to their training.'" Mrs. Robb then questioned whether this money was not intended as a remuneration for services rendered, and if so, why the amount was increased in the second year when in reality the cash expenses for the student were much greater in the first year.

Her proposal was the establishment of a three-year program of an eight-hour day on a non-payment plan. The pupils were to receive uniforms, board, room, laundry and a truly liberal education in exchange for the three years of service. She firmly believed that if schools were placed on a scholastic basis they would attract refined and intelligent students. Furthermore, if scholarships were provided, needy but highly competent women would receive an education. She commented: "I am not sure that nurses more than any others who are preparing to enter a scientific profession should expect to be self-supporting . . . and I do not believe that this arrangement would hinder any desirable additions to our numbers." Mrs. Robb believed that the money which had been given to students should be redirected to employ well-prepared head nurses.

Her constant gentle insistence that new ideas be tried is noted against illogical objections from those who were emotionally tied to the past and present.[7]

Miss Adelaide Nutting presented an electrifying report at the 1896 convention entitled, "A Statistical Report of Working Hours in Training Schools." This report revealed that work hours per day could total 15 hours with 105 hours weekly; in almost every school one lecture per week was given.

Miss Nutting asked: "Now what are training schools? Are they charitable institutions? Is it a condition of employer and employee?" She answered her questions by emphatically stating that they were really educational institutions and that it was time that this fact be better appreciated. Miss Nutting continued:

It should not be forgotten that the long hours of duty in wards may reduce pupils to a condition of servitude. It is not for the purpose of giving them more and better training that they are kept on duty so long, but rather that the amount of service rendered to the hospital may

---

[7] Dolan, Josephine A.: "Fusing the Past For Future Action." *Three Score and Ten*, New York, National League for Nursing, 1963, p. 7.

be increased and that the working force of the institution may for economy's sake be kept small. These long hours render it nearly impossible for a nurse to profit by the teaching for which her services are supposed to be given and with such long hours the teaching is merely offered as an advantage to attract applicants and is not deserving of any serious consideration.[8]

Miss Sophia Palmer inveighed against using students to maintain service and lower the costs of operation of hospitals and schools. Her resolution to this effect read:

Be it resolved. That this Society condemns the practice of utilizing pupils in training as a means of revenue to the hospital or school.[9]

The resolution was adopted unanimously. In the Address of the President in 1897, Miss Nutting made a poignant plea:

If we look into matters carefully, I think we shall find that in our profession we have still too low a standard of preliminary requirement, too short a course and too limited a curriculum, and that our examinations are somewhat superficial.

Even if a woman possesses many good qualities, without a basis of education and refinement we can never expect to obtain a training of the mind which will enable the nurse to observe, think and reason accurately.

It may be natural that all hospitals should be wise to have their nursing provided for as cheaply as possible; but the time should be over in this country when training schools are maintained with this as their main object. . . . Our training schools should lessen in number, but improve in quality. Cities that are large enough, and have material enough to support two good training schools, should not maintain a dozen inferior ones . . . this subject [is] of gravest importance to us if we are working as we say we are, for a high standard and for the best interests of the profession generally.[10]

The necessity of establishing an adequate fee for service schedule and a salary scale that would be rewarding was presented by Diana Kimber in 1897.

Miss Lucy Walker, who was Superintendent of Nurses at the Pennsylvania Hospital Training School, gave a progress report at the 1897 annual convention on the acceptance of a lengthening of the program with a shortening of the workday. She reported

"Only one school (Johns Hopkins) has adopted it in connection with the extended course. The reason for this is . . . that the three years' course is of benefit to the hospital as well as to the nurse, whereas the eight hour day system benefits the nurse only."

A quick review of comments reflects that in 1901 Dr. R. C. Cabot's article, "Suggestions for the Improvement of Training Schools for Nurses," in *The Boston Medical and Surgical Journal*, expressed dissatisfaction with the present system of training. In 1903 Dr. Francis Denny's report, "The Need of an Institution for the Education of Nurses Independent of the Hospitals," in *The Boston Medical and Surgical Journal*, stressed the benefits that might accrue if some educational institution would give instruction to the nurse before she entered the hospital. Dr. Denny encouraged nurses to be educated for a profession. He stated that "the nurse's diploma should come from this educational institution, rather than from the hospital. Its award should represent good work in the preliminary course, together with satisfactory service in a hospital in which there was a high standard of nursing."[11]

In the early period of this century the Director of Nurses taught some of the classes but the majority were given by medical practitioners and were called "doctor's lectures." The focus was centered upon hospital-based medical treatments rather than the role of the nurse in nursing intervention. Eventually textbooks for nurses were written by physicians and later on nurses were asked to collaborate with them in their authorship. However, two books were available that stressed nursing care. One was written in 1910 by Emily A. M. Stoney who had been the author of *Materia Medica for Nurses* and *Bacteriology and Surgical Technic for Nurses*. Miss Stoney, a graduate of the Training School for Nurses in Lawrence, Massachusetts, held the position of Superintendent of the Training School for Nurses at Carney Hospital in Boston and published *Practical Points in Nursing for Nurses in Private Practice*.[12] Recognizing a need for assisting all graduate nurses in

---

[8]*Ibid.*, p. 8.
[9]*Third Annual Report, AASTSN*, 1896, p. 69.
[10]Nutting, M. Adelaide: Address of the President. *Fourth Annual Report, AASTSN*, 1897, pp. 8–9.

[11]Denny, Francis P.: "The need of an institution for the education of nurses independent of the hospitals." *Boston Medical and Surgical Journal*, June 18, 1903.
[12]Stoney, Emily A. M.: *Practical Points in Nursing for Nurses in Private Practice*. 4th Ed., Philadelphia, W. B. Saunders Co., 1910.

keeping up-to-date and providing a sort of program of continuing education, her book was revised at frequent intervals. In the presentation of her data she indicated what nurses should observe and what response should be made. She indicated that a physician had a myriad of ways of attacking the problem medically but the initial nursing response should follow a certain, sound, scientific plan of action. The recall of the scientific basis of nursing was presented in a section on "Physiology and Descriptive Anatomy." The nutritive aspects of patient care were also included.

A pocket-sized reference book entitled *The Nurses' "Enquire Within,"*[13] published about the turn of the century, described *briefly* the symptoms of a condition or a disease entity and elaborated on the nurse's role. Where indicated the nursing intervention was classified further into preventive or curative nursing care.

Isabel Hampton Robb noted: "Not so long ago neither medicine nor nursing were scientific in character. But the evolution of the one created a necessity for the other."

In response to written and verbal assaults about the character of nursing, Mrs. Robb stated:

To be sure there is the side to nursing so often spoken of as menial, but nothing dominated by the mind, and dignified by the way in which it is done can be derogatory; nor need the cultured and trained woman, when the emergency arises, shrink from unpleasant tasks. The spirit in which she does her work makes all the difference. Invested as she should be with the dignity of her profession and the cloak of love for suffering humanity, she can ennoble anything her hand may be called upon to do. . . .[14]

The trained nurse, then, is no longer to be regarded as a better trained, more useful, higher class servant, but as one who has knowledge and is worthy of respect, consideration and due recompense. . . . She is also essentially an instructor; part of her duties have to do with the prevention of disease and sickness, as well as the relief of suffering humanity. In district nursing we are confronted with conditions which require the highest order of work, but the actual nursing of the patient is one of the least of the duties which the nurse is called upon to perform for the class of people with whom she meets. To this branch of our work no more appropriate name can be given than 'instructive nursing,' for educational in the best sense of the word it should be.[15]

In a period in history when nurses could not teach and answered questions with the familiar "I don't know, ask your doctor," Mrs. Robb attempted to encourage well-prepared nurses to view this expansion of their role.

She continued to widen the dimension by stating:

These are some of the essentials in nursing by which it has come to be regarded as a profession, but there still remains much to be desired, much to work for, in order to add to its dignity and usefulness. As the standard of education and requirements become of a higher character and the training more efficient, the trained nurse will draw nearer to science and its demands and take a greater share as a social factor in solving the world's needs.[16]

In the book, *A Sound Economic Basis for Schools of Nursing,* Adelaide Nutting (Fig. 12–7) reported the need for a different pattern of education:

Heavy demands of the wards made it impossible for all students to attend their weekly lecture and it was always arranged that some students would choose to take very full notes and read them later to the assembled group of less fortunate. Lectures came under the category of privileges like 'hours off duty' to be granted 'hospital duties' permitting.[17]

It appeared that an occasional class was supplementary to the work experience or clinical practice. When there was a paucity of clinical experience the philosophy of lengthening the time spent in the wards seemed a suitable solution even though it did not provide enrichment but rather "more of the same" experientially.

A scrutiny of progress in nursing education during the first 10 years reveals a change in terminology from "training" to "education," from "superintendent" to "director," from "probationer" or "probie" to "preliminary student," then to "preclinical student" and finally to "preprofessional student," and

[13]Clarke, E. M.: *The Nurses' "Enquire Within."* London. The Scientific Press, Ltd.

[14]Robb, Isabel Hampton: *Nursing Ethics.* Cleveland, J. B. Savage, 1901, p. 35.

[15]*Ibid.,* p. 37.

[16]*Ibid.,* p. 37.

[17]Nutting, M. Adelaide.: *A Sound Economic Basis for Schools of Nursing.* New York, G. P. Putnam's Sons, 1926, pp. 339–40.

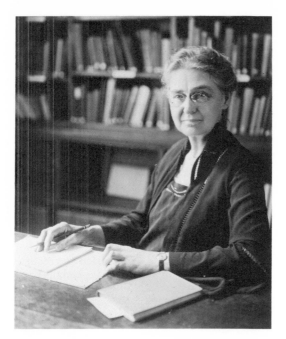

Figure 12–7. Mary Adelaide Nutting.

from "training school" to "school of nursing." The first preliminary courses varied from a few classes to a planned program lasting six months. It included biological and social sciences and practical work on the mannequin frequently called Mrs. Chase. In 1903, arrangements were made with two technical schools—Drexel Institute in Philadelphia and Pratt Institute in Brooklyn—to offer a course of instruction covering one college year for students who wanted to enter a school of nursing. A student was to live at her own expense and pay her own tuition. This came in a period when students of nursing were being paid a stipend to take the course in nursing. The stipend was for the continuous supply of service that the student provided for the hospital.

Another pioneering suggestion was presented by Isabel H. Robb; she advocated state-supported schools of nursing, but this did not materialize. The efforts of Mrs. Robb in initiating the movement for higher education for graduate nurses were brought to fruition at Teachers College, Columbia University. A one-year course in *hospital economics* was developed, and in 1907 Adelaide Nutting became the first professor of nursing in the world. Her advisory committee was a group of eminent nurses. Under her inspiration the school had a remarkable development and became a powerful influence in the nursing world.

When Miss Nutting retired in 1925, she was succeeded by *Isabel M. Stewart* (Fig. 12–8). Both these women reflected outstanding leadership in nursing education.

Miss Stewart, like Miss Nutting, was born in Canada and graduated from the Winnipeg General Hospital. She then attended Teachers College, Columbia University, after graduation becoming assistant to Miss Nutting, and in 1923 an associate professor. An authority on the history of nursing, her *Educational Status of Nursing* and *The Education of Nurses* have influenced the thinking of nursing leaders here and abroad for many years.

In 1909 *Dr. Richard O. Beard* presented a plan for a university school of nursing under the State University of Minnesota.[18]

All this is an example of the efforts of the pioneers whose vision and courage prompted a great experiment in nursing, which made the school of nursing an integral part of a university program.

An academic environment had been provided to nurture the first collegiate-type program for students of nursing. The right of the nurse to the same good education, in addition to being admitted under the same standards as all other students in college, had been achieved. The change in status was reflected in the change in title from "pupil nurse" to "student of nursing." In addition to the regular basic courses, such innovations as a course in invalid occupation was included to teach the importance of keeping convalescing patients pleasantly entertained. A manual was written at this time to assist nurses in their projects in diversional therapy.[19]

Certain learning experiences were provided, such as an observation in the dental clinics to learn the value of oral hygiene to general health. By 1917, students cared for patients in a tuberculosis sanatorium "to awaken a full understanding" of the psychological implications of illness. As Thomas Mann recounted in *The Magic Mountain*, tuberculosis imposed on its victims a special way of life.

[18] Beard, Richard O.: "The university education of the nurse." *Teachers College Record*, 11:27–40, 1910.

[19] Tracy, Susan E.: *Studies in Invalid Occupation.* Boston, Whitcomb and Barrows, 1910.

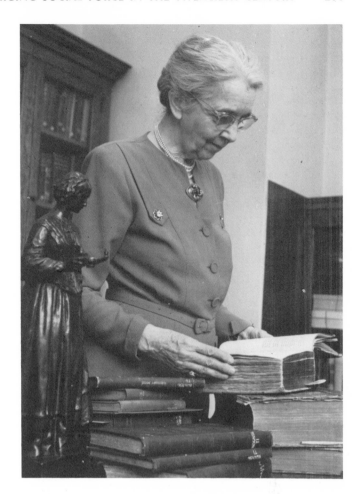

Figure 12--8. Isabel M. Stewart.

For a number of years, graduates of this program did not receive a degree.

Lip service had been paid to the need for the preparation of nurses in the cultural setting used by other professions, but when Dr. Beard urged the establishment of a university school of nursing, he rendered a monumental service to the profession of nursing.

Adelaide Nutting had been a catalytic agent in this movement because she encouraged the separation of schools of nursing from hospital control and the provision of financial support for nurse education.[20] She hoped that the importance of the profession of nursing would be recognized by universities.

Two other champions of the cause of nursing were Drs. Washburn and Burlingham,[21]

who advocated raising the whole standard of the nursing profession in the educational requirements for admission. They insisted that cultural values should be stressed.

In 1915 only 10 schools reported fulltime paid instructors; in most schools the superintendent of nurses did most of the teaching, and doctors attempted to teach anatomy and other sciences by lecture. Until about 1920 the "nursing arts" or "fundamentals of nursing" instructor did not exist; and for a long time her position and salary were lower than that of the "science" instructor who was a nurse not necessarily prepared in biological, physical or behavioral sciences.

Until state boards came into existence, each director of nursing made her own curriculum. Schools might plan and publish a program of classes and lectures, but there was often a question as to whether it was actually carried out.

One of the first publications of the *National League for Nursing Education* (N.L.N.E.), the successor of the American Society of Super-

[20]Nutting, M. A.: *Educational Status of Nursing.* United States Bureau of Education, Bulletin No. 7, 1912.

[21]Washburn, F. A., and Burlingham, L. H.: "The supply of pupil nurses and nursing standards." *The International Hospital Record,* January, 1913.

intendents of Training Schools, was the *Standard Curriculum for Schools of Nursing*. The Education Committee of the N.L.N.E. worked on this publication from 1914 until it was published in 1917. The objective of the Committee was to achieve uniformity in the programs of the schools of nursing and to assist in improvement of both content and teaching methods.

At the Proceedings of the Seventeenth Annual Convention, Miss Nutting presented a report of the Committee on Education which dealt with a particularly dismal picture of the exhaustingly long work hours of students. She commented that these

factors seem to be bound up in the relationship which the school bears to the hospital, a relationship of which the first and most far-reaching effect is that which makes it necessary for the school in order to do the work of the hospital to accept and admit in numbers candidates who do not qualify from the standpoint of age, general education, natural ability, and personal fitness for the difficult, responsible and important work of nursing.

The Committee believes that the present policy of admitting such candidates into our schools for nurses will bring about a steady deterioration in the character of nursing in hospitals, homes, and in all fields of public and private work, and that this must be the inevitable outcome of a continued policy of lowering requirements for admission in order to secure numbers to maintain an unpaid service in the hospitals. The Committee feels that the necessity for admitting such candidates is due to a system which, though sanctioned by years of custom and tradition, is one which is entirely capable of alteration and modification. They believe that in view of this a close, careful and exhaustive study is now needed on the whole question of the education of the nurse, inclusive of the fields of professional work which she occupies.

And the Committee further believes that such a study should be made by neither hospital authorities, physicians, or nurses, but by some scientific body able to bring an unprejudiced mind to the situation and to study it from the point of view of the public welfare.

The Committee therefore recommends that this Society request the Carnegie Foundation for the Advancement of Teaching to make such a study.[22]

In speaking to the recommendation of the Committee on Education, Miss Nutting so-

berly reflected on the then-current problems as being the most serious faced by the nursing leaders. It was unbelievable that they were forced to take poorly educated people to meet the quantitative demands of hospitals, and this has caused as she stated "an unrest in our field of work that is pretty general." The lack of incentive because of being unable to carry out one's goals for the expanded role of nursing care was identified when she stated

that women who enter the training school position, well qualified, full of ideals, ambition, enthusiasm, ready to give the very best that is in them, find themselves unable to go on with their work, discouraged and baffled, through nothing that they are responsible for, but through something that seems to be inherent in the situation and beyond their control.

Those who are striving to improve their training schools find themselves meeting actual conditions in the hospitals which make it extremely difficult and often impossible to carry out any reasonably satisfactory scheme of training and education. The very fact of ten hours a day duty in a school would block any good scheme of education ever suggested. A pupil who has been on duty ten hours cannot study, nor even listen intelligently.

We see hospital superintendents thinking that training schools are trying to pull away from hospitals, and we see training school superintendents struggling to be loyal to both hospital and training school and wondering how they can do well by both. In view of this unrest, and in view of the importance of the work of the nurse and the expansion of her field in the new demands that are being made upon her, we are wondering if it isn't time to make some serious study, scientifically, of this situation. Would it not be well to ask some scientific body—not hospitals, not medical people, not nurses, because we are all too deeply involved, —to make a study of the relation of the school to the hospital. Your committee therefore recommends that the Carnegie Foundation be asked to make such a study.[23]

Miss Annie W. Goodrich moved that the Carnegie Foundation be asked to study nursing and the education of nurses. The motion was approved by the membership but war was to intervene before the study could be undertaken.

In 1912 nursing leaders discussed the need for liberal arts to be available to assist students in broadening the base for the development of a professional person. An examination of the frustrations faced by able nursing

[22] *Proceedings of the Seventeenth Annual Convention of The American Society of Superintendents of Training Schools for Nurses,* Baltimore, Maryland, J. H. Furst Company, 1911, p. 75.

[23] *Ibid.,* p. 76.

leaders who tried to reform the curriculum to introduce or to enhance cultural pursuits was presented. Miss Parsons from the Massachusetts General Hospital Training School admitted that obstacles were faced when "the older schools must find themselves trying to crawl out from under the old system, where a new school starting may perhaps make its proper affiliations with a university."[24]

NEED FOR CONTINUING EDUCATION

Miss Edna L. Foley, Superintendent of the Visiting Nurses Association of Chicago, urged the leaders of nursing in 1912 to realize that expansion of knowledge and the implications for the nurse practitioner necessitated a program of continuing education as well as in-service education. She pleaded: "Is it too much to ask of nurses that they shall plan to post-graduate, or take a good university correspondence course, or at least attend a national convention once in five years?" She continued, "the training school can help in this regard very materially by offering both its pupils and graduates an annual nursing demonstration, at which old methods may be reviewed and new methods introduced and explained."[25]

In addition each of the speakers at this convention pleaded for an experience in community nursing in order to truly understand patient and family problems. Miss McKechnie regretted that "the graduate just out of the training school has the hospital point of view solely. She lacks the wider social view. I believe she will not get this point of view until she looks at her work from another side entirely; and besides a new point of view she must get a new feeling, a new attitude toward her work and toward society."[26]

Miss McKechnie probed further and prodded nurses to use their observational and intellectual skills in making a nursing diagnosis and in promoting conservation of health. Where the breadwinner was critized for unwillingness to work as "the question of a man being allowed to starve if he will not work. . . . such a case brings up the question of diagnosis and how that diagnosis shall be made. . . . because of the more intimate relation which exists between the visiting nurse and the family, the nurse is able to get at the underlying causes of a man's idleness, and often to prove that his failure to support his family is due, not so much to fault in himself as to some physical defect or weakness. I believe it is becoming more and more obvious that in relief work, the knowledge of conditions gained by the visiting nurse, and her judgment of the case, must be taken into account in the making of every diagnosis, and in planning the treatment for every dependent family."[27] She continued: ". . . the visiting nurse who believes that conservation of health and prevention of disease are the foundations upon which the wealth of the nation rests, is, while recognizing human frailties, to give friendly assistance and advice in obtaining employment, together with adequate aid,"[28] and thus the motive of helping people to help themselves was observed. In order for the nurse to be provided with the most complete plan for nursing care, it was imperative to "keep up with all the wonderful developments of her time, and be gaining knowledge every day, every month, and every year as long as she is actively at work."[29]

The nurse educators realized the need for a broad education and experiential base but reported the inability to provide these learning opportunities because of commitment to the hospitals with which they had become an integral part. They identified that when a community experience was permitted patient care improved because "it is of very great benefit to the pupils in the consideration of their patients in the hospital. They appreciated their home situation"[30] and could provide a much more meaningful plan for nursing care.

In order to provide more time and utilize it more efficiently, the question of *scientific management* was studied. The leaders of nursing were aware of the disastrous trap into which nurses were falling by assuming non-nursing tasks and leaving less time for nursing care activities. The need for nursing input into the design of buildings, equipment and

[24]*Eighteenth Annual Report of American Society of Superintendents of Training Schools for Nursing*, Baltimore, J. H. Furst, 1912, p. 37.

[25]*Ibid.*, p. 57.

[26]*Ibid.*, p. 60.

[27]*Ibid.*, pp. 60–61.

[28]*Ibid.*, p. 61.

[29]*Ibid.*, p. 62.

the new appliances and modern conveniences was discussed. Miss Giles asserted that

Scientific management can only be accomplished in a building erected on scientific lines, with the proper lighting, heating and ventilating plants, and with such arrangement of its apartments as shall best serve its purpose for the class of cases treated; the building being so constructed as to conserve the time, health, strength and nerve force of those who are engaged in this most interesting, absorbing and splendid work [of nursing].[31]

Miss Giles pleaded that the opportunity be given to nurses who know the *how* and *why* of hospital construction instead of members whose social, political or financial prominence provided this opportunity. She quoted a case of a society lady who was a member of the board of trustees of a hospital and who because of abysmal ignorance of the workings of a hospital, entered the school of nursing and completed the course. Upon graduation, she requested the opportunity of serving on the board again and was informed that "they feared her education and knowledge of hospital work would prejudice her in favor of the nursing staff. This young woman, when truly qualified . . . . was deemed unworthy by those who had been her co-workers in the days of her real ignorance of hospital management."[32]

Miss Giles concluded by requesting that nurses realize that

the structure should be an expression of its purpose; a hospital should stand for health, hygiene, strength, rest; a veritable refuge for those who seek its protection, cure, and care. . . .

As for equipment, it should be complete, and it is only complete when the institution can meet every demand made upon it. There should be everything necessary, in order that its staff of workers may use their skill and knowledge to the best advantage.[33]

In focusing on the paucity of properly prepared nurses, it was noted that it "is but false economy that the inadequate supply of nurses so often interferes with the education of the nurse, the welfare of the patient, and the reputation of the hospital."[34]

The Annual Reports are replete with those nurses who encouraged the consideration of ways of cutting costs for the hospital. The

inference of doing without things rather than wasting anything that would reflect against nursing was openly discussed. The willingness with which some nurses took on non-nursing tasks is reflected in the report of savings to the hospital by such projects as making soap and ink.[35]

The famous scientific management specialist Frank Gilbreth was invited to address the leaders of nursing and in 1912 he presented a paper on the application of scientific principles of management to the work of the nurse. He recommended that an analysis of nursing activities be conducted by an expert in time and motion study. Some nurses present felt that this would require greater speed on their part in carrying out their activities during the study. Mr. Gilbreth disabused them of this notion and emphasized the value in terms of the need for more labor-saving devices, for rest periods, for planning before performing, for assignment "to each worker of that work for which he is best suited," and said that it was waste of energy and the right incentive that prevented the production of satisfying results in one's daily work.

Some of the recurrent issues that are observed in the *Annual Reports* of these very able educators include: the need for scholarship assistance for students; importance of evaluative examinations for pre-admission as well as to measure achievement; the comparable value of theory and practice; the necessity of changing the status of the student of nursing from employee of the hospital to that of student; the disapproval of lowering nursing care by having inadequately prepared nurses encouraged by hospitals; the necessity for mandatory licensure in all states; the importance of making nursing a satisfying type of endeavor; the obligation of freeing nursing from hospital control; the desire for inclusion of programs of nursing within a university setting; and the significance of a study of nursing and nursing education by an impartial but knowledgeable group of national leaders free from paramedical or hospital manipulation.

Central schools were fairly common and successful in Europe. In them, preliminary students from several schools received class in-

[30]*Ibid.*, p. 64.
[31]*Ibid.*, p. 104.
[32]*Ibid.*, p. 105.
[33]*Ibid.*, p. 106.
[34]*Ibid.*, p. 108.

[35]Dolan, J. A.: "Fusing The Past For Future Action," *Three Score Years and Ten*, New York, National League for Nursing, 1963, p. 10.

struction at one place, often at a university, under expert teachers. In this country such schools began (1900 to 1910) as affiliations between technical schools, colleges or other nursing schools.

Early in this century New York State established certain standards for accrediting its schools of nursing. Since most of the states had no registration laws and no boards of examiners at this time, it gradually became the custom for schools in other states to apply to New York for registration, thereby enabling them to prove that they were meeting the requirements of at least one group of nursing authorities.

In 1925 a committee sponsored by the American Nurses' Association undertook a five-year study of nursing and nurse training. This was the *Committee on the Grading of Nurses*, with members who were laymen and women, and doctors and nurses; the director was an educator, May Ayres Burgess. Nurses themselves gave $115,000 to the project. The committee found it impossible to do an actual grading of schools.

The study included all schools that would cooperate in 10 states, large and small, representative of the different parts of the country. Its two reports were *Nurses, Patients and Pocketbooks* and *Nursing Schools Today and Tomorrow*. These reports exerted a remarkable influence on schools of nursing; the mere statement of unpleasant or discouraging facts stimulated action and brought marked improvement.

National accreditation was inevitable. In 1936 the *National League of Nursing Education* undertook it and in 1938 had outlined a program. Their purpose was announced: "To set up a list of good schools of nursing, judged in terms of their own stated purpose." No arbitrary standard was used and no endeavor was made to fit all schools to one pattern. Actual accrediting was begun in 1939; 50 schools were accredited in that year, which made a basis for further study of values.

In the 1930's, the financial developments of the Depression caused a great oversupply of nurses, especially for private duty. The supply exceeded the demand, causing a lowering of income throughout the nursing profession.

In 1927 a revision of the Standard Curriculum was published, entitled *Curriculum for Schools of Nursing*. Because of misinterpre-

tation the word "standard" was deleted from the title. It was apparent that the Education Committee working on this revision was striving to incorporate recommendations from the Goldmark Report. "It was definitely stipulated that the *elements* of public health nursing were to be considered as basic for *all* students regardless of the field of nursing they might plan to enter on graduation. More definite recognition was given to the care of the well child, to the health needs of the family and community and to the public health responsibilities of nurses. Psychology (including mental hygiene) was included as an essential rather than a recommended subject, and communicable disease and psychiatric nursing were both more prominently featured in the clinical program."[36]

The Depression years pointed out that where a choice for positions is possible, the better educated the person, the greater the chance of obtaining the position in question. Nurse educators realized that there were stultifying aspects to the *Curriculum for Schools of Nursing*, which was used as a bible by faculty of schools of nursing. In order to create an educationally enriched program, a guide rather than a strict rule had to be devised. In 1937 a revision of the curriculum series was published which was retitled *A Curriculum Guide for Schools of Nursing*. "It was specifically stated that the program outlined in the *Guide* was intended for students of *professional* calibre and qualifications, who were seriously preparing themselves for the practice of nursing as a *profession*. . . . A further assumption was that such schools would make every effort to adjust their programs to the resources and needs of a democratic society and to the advances of science especially in the fields of medicine and of education."[37]

The 1937 *Guide* contained a much broader and enriched presentation of scientific and nursing content. The application of social sciences to nursing received great attention. Newer approaches to teaching techniques and the role of clinical instructors were stressed. It included the use of multimedia in teaching and learning. This project was intended to stimulate creativity in the development of essential curriculum content to keep

---

[36] Stewart, Isabel M.: *The Education of Nurses*, New York, The Macmillan Company, 1953, p. 223.
[37] *Ibid.*, p. 257.

pace with societal trends and scientific progress, but for many years some schools still adhered to the suggestions in this historic document. A further revision was unwarranted.

THE ESTABLISHMENT OF MILITARY NURSING

At the close of the Spanish-American War, Dr. Anita McGee bent her efforts toward the building of the foundations for the Army Nurse Corps. It was through her efforts, with the support of the Nurses' Associated Alumnae (now the A.N.A.), that the Army Reorganization Bill was written, which, when passed by Congress in 1901, established the *Army Nurse Corps* as a branch of the Army Medical Service. Nurses received letters of appointment and agreed to serve three years, but their functions and military status were not defined.

Dita H. Kinney, who became Superintendent of the Corps from 1901 to 1909, was educated at Mills College in California and was a graduate of Massachusetts General Hospital. The second superintendent (1909–1912) was *Jane A. Delano* (Fig. 12–9), a graduate of Bellevue, where she had been superintendent of nurses. Her leadership ability was seen in many accomplishments; she organized the *American Red Cross Nursing Service*, which included the Surgeons General of the Army and Navy in its membership. She resigned from the Army Nurse Corps to become the fulltime director (without salary) of the Department of Nursing of the American Red Cross.

The major accomplishment of this Committee on Nursing Service of the American Red Cross was to develop a system by which a membership of nurses could be relied upon to form a *reserve* both for military service and emergency service with the American Red Cross. In order to join this reserve group, it was essential to be a member of the American Nurses' Association and the Army Nurse Corps, as well as the American Red Cross Nursing Service. Members had to be graduates of schools well above the minimum standards set by the state boards of nurse examiners.

By 1908 the *Navy Nurse Corps* was authorized by the Navy Appropriations Act.

In May of 1908, the *Nurse Corps* of the

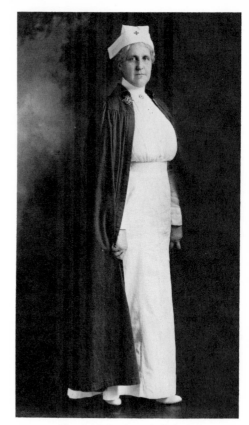

Figure 12–9. Jane A. Delano.

United States Navy was established by act of Congress. *Esther Voorhees Hasson* was appointed first superintendent in August, and by October of that year the first twenty nurses had reported to the United States Naval Hospital, Washington, D.C., for orientation and duty. The Corps grew in number and the members were assigned to naval hospitals.

By 1910, certain members of the Navy Nurse Corps were given assignments to serve outside the United States. By 1911, those nurses who were stationed at Guam established a school of nursing for young native women in conjunction with the Navy's native hospital. The educational efforts of the members of the Navy Nurse Corps have been reflected in other schools of nursing they organized, such as the one on Samoa.

WORLD WAR I

The period that followed was dominated by World War I, which was to create a huge demand for nurses, to open up new fields of specialization, to accelerate the educational processes that were already under way and to awaken in the public a consciousness of the importance of good nursing.

For the first time in history, an adequate number of carefully selected nurses was available for military service. The vision and foresight of Jane Delano of the American Red Cross Nursing Service was responsible for this reservoir of nurses.

When war broke out in August 1914, no one thought that it would last more than a few months, but the American Red Cross immediately sent units of doctors and nurses to help in six countries of Europe. When the United States came into the war in 1917, the Red Cross Nursing Service became the reserve of the Army and Navy.

Helen Scott Hay, of the Illinois Training School, Chicago, went overseas just before the World War, at the request of the Queen of Bulgaria, to establish trained nursing. She remained as chief nurse of the American Red Cross in the Balkans, and later (1921) was chief nurse of the American Red Cross in Europe.

As the war went on and country after country was drawn into it, with millions of men involved, the medical and nursing resources of the world were taxed to their utmost. Eventually, the personnel of civilian hospitals in every country were seriously depleted, and the sick civilian suffered from neglect.

The fighting was chiefly trench warfare, different from the modes used in previous wars. The wounded went in a continuous stream from first-aid station or field hospital to evacuation hospital (10 miles back), and within 24 hours to base hospitals, still farther away. There were no women nurses at the front, either in first aid stations or field hospitals. France, England and the United States maintained separate hospitals; cooperation was always good. In addition to military hospitals, there were numerous auxiliary hospitals in cities or distant villages, in the castles, chateaux or homes of the wealthy, often supported by private funds. In these the staff was composed of women, trained and untrained, and of men too old or unfit for the army, who often worked at no salary.

The *American Ambulance* at Paris, a private unit, included some famous surgeons and served throughout the war. Harvard University had a medical unit with the British in France from June, 1915, which remained even after the war. Its second unit arrived after America entered the war.

Two catastrophic episodes of World War I stand out. The epidemic of typhus in Siberia in 1915, involving half a million civilians, was a repetition of medieval days. The cause of typhus was not known, but was discovered during the epidemic by Scottish and American doctors. A unit of American nurses served through that terrible time. In 1918, an epidemic of influenza became pandemic as it reached France, the United States and other parts of the world. Army and civilian hospitals, as their doctors and nurses dropped out with the infection, struggled with a dwindling staff until the plight of both servicemen and their families at home was pitiful.

Since trench warfare was the rule, most wounds were caused by shrapnel, a few from bombs and almost none from bullets. Wounds of the head and face were common. Poison gases were used for at least three years, and the men who survived them often never recovered from the effects. Mustard gas caused the greatest agony. The Carrel-Dakin method for infected wounds was developed. Since so many supply ships were torpedoed and there was always doubt about supplies arriving, American doctors and nurses learned to economize.

The value of well-prepared nurses was demonstrated as in the days of Florence Nightingale. Graduate nurses, accustomed as they were to emergencies and to group work, stepped into war conditions and adjusted themselves unhesitatingly to a new environment. Great problems were involved in providing sanitation for armies constantly on the move, dealing with communicable diseases, caring for severely damaged tissue and coping with the unusual results of "shell shock." In previous wars there had been well-defined battles that demanded collecting and caring for the wounded and burial of the dead at the termination of the battle. In this war, the so-called battles lasted for days, the dead were buried as best they could be or not at all, and the wounded were rescued under fire. There was always a stream of wounded, sometimes swelling, sometimes thinning, but never ceasing.

The members of the Navy Nurse Corps were utilized during World War I. The first Navy nurses to be assigned for transport duty reported aboard the U.S.S. George Washington on which President Wilson sailed to France in 1918. The first Navy nurses to serve on board a hospital ship did so in 1920 aboard the U.S.S. Relief.

In order to recruit many women who were motivated to study nursing, the *Army School of Nursing* was organized in 1918 with *Annie W. Goodrich* as dean. For those interested in meeting the nursing needs at home, classes in "Home Hygiene and Care of the Sick" were formed.

Annie W. Goodrich was the originator of the plan for an Army school of nursing. Anna Jammé was her assistant in 1918. Begun in 1918 as a war measure, the school was also designed to be a permanent organization. The course lasted for three years, and nine months' credit was given to college graduates. The work was centered in the Army hospitals, with affiliations in civilian hospitals. At the height of war enthusiasm, the applicants numbered in the thousands.

The first graduating class, in 1921, numbered 500, with 400 graduating at the Walter Reed Hospital, Washington, D.C., and 100 at Letterman Hospital, San Francisco. It was unquestionably the largest class of nurses ever graduated at one time in the world's history. The school continued, but with smaller classes. It was discontinued in 1932 for economic reasons, and the last class graduated in 1933. This school was organized in an excellent fashion and set a superb example for all other schools to emulate.

Since Canadian nurses had had officers' rank since 1906 and other countries gave their nurses a semi-official status, American nurses felt the need of rank. In 1920, after the war was over, enough pressure was made so that "relative rank" as officers was granted to nurses.

Julia Stimson (1881–1948) graduated from Vassar before entering the New York Hospital School of Nursing. She succeeded Miss Goodrich as dean of the Army School of Nursing. Miss Stimson then held the position of superintendent of the Army Nurse Corps. She agreed with the concern felt by the members of the nursing profession at the lack of rank for military nurses. When relative rank was awarded to nurses through the Army Reorganization Act of 1920, she became *Major Stimson*. She served later as president of the American Nurses' Association.

On November 11, 1918, the armistice was signed. Troops and medical units began to return home.

Although the nurses of World War I seemed to receive less recognition in the United States than elsewhere, they had in their hearts the consciousness of work well done, of the gratitude of the men and of what they felt was great fortune—to have been able to serve in this historic war. "Never before had such a thing occurred, the sending across three thousand miles of danger-strewn seas of ten thousand soldier-women, to be part of a great expeditionary force."

World War I made both military authorities and the public conscious of their dependence on nurses. The epidemic of pneumonia in 1917–1918 and the pandemic outbreak of influenza in 1918 emphasized the need for well-prepared nurses.

EVALUATION OF NURSING

The war had terminated, the ghastly influenza pandemic had subsided, and a hopeful, peaceful country could now assess strengths as well as areas needing strengthening.

Many leaders in nursing had pleaded for improvement of the educational programs for nurses in a milieu that provided a sound, broad preparation for living as well as earning a living. Many leaders, utilizing data-collecting skills, eloquently presented facts that reflected a need for change. Miss Nutting's recommendation for a careful and exhaustive study of the education of the nurse— "... by some scientific body able to bring an unprejudiced mind to the situation and to study from the point of view of public welfare ..." was reconsidered.

The *Rockefeller Foundation* financed a survey of nursing education headed by *Dr. C. E. A. Winslow.*

The findings and conclusions of this survey were published in February 1923 in a book called *Nursing and Nursing Education in the United States.* This remarkable report, frequently referred to as the *Goldmark Report,* should be read in its entirety for many of its suggestions have not yet been comprehended.

The members of this committee were aware of many of the weaknesses in the educational preparation of nurse practitioners. It was evident that nursing in 1922 was still on an apprenticeship basis of an earn-while-you-learn-system. This type of preparation had been abandoned by other professions that demanded specialized professional or technical education. It was apparent that nursing was still struggling with the problem of serving two masters: the care of the sick in the hospital and the education of the nurse. In stressful situations the first assumed the more important role while the latter was neglected.

Many of the instructors were poorly prepared as was illustrated thus: In one hospital, the course in anatomy and physiology, which was of nine months' duration, was interrupted seven times by the entrance of a new class that studied the subject at whatever point it was being presented. The instructor explained that "it makes no difference in anatomy, as one part is not dependent on another."[38]

The lack of well-prepared teachers was a problem, as was the quaint custom of admitting a student to replace every student who withdrew from the school.

The following conclusions are noteworthy:

Conclusion 1. That, since constructive health work and health teaching in families is best done by persons:

(a) capable of giving general health instruction, as distinguished from instruction in any one specialty; and

(b) capable of rendering bedside care at need; the agent responsible for such constructive health work and health teaching in families should have completed the nurses' training. There will, of course, be need for the employment, in addition to the public health nurse, of other types of experts such as nutrition workers, social workers, occupational therapists, and the like.

That as soon as may be practicable all agencies, public or private, employing public health nurses, should require as a prerequisite for employment the basic hospital training, followed by a post-graduate course, including both class work and field work, in public health nursing.

Conclusion 2. That the career open to young women of high capacity, in public health nursing or in hospital supervision and nursing education, is one of the most attractive fields now open, in its promise of professional success and of rewarding public service; and that every effort should be made to attract such women into this field.

Conclusion 3. That for the care of persons suffering from serious and acute disease the safety of the patient, and the responsibility of the medical and nursing professions, demand the maintenance of the standards of educational attainment

now generally accepted by the best sentiment of both professions and embodied in the legislation of the more progressive states; and that any attempt to lower these standards would be fraught with real danger to the public.

Conclusion 4. That steps should be taken through state legislation for the definition and licensure of a subsidiary grade of nursing service, the subsidiary type of worker to serve under practising physicians in the care of mild and chronic illness, and convalescence, and possibly to assist under the direction of the trained nurse in certain phases of hospital and visiting nursing.

Conclusion 5. That, while training schools for nurses have made remarkable progress, and while the best schools of today in many respects reach a high level of educational attainment, the average hospital training school is not organized on such a basis as to conform to the standards accepted in other educational fields; that the instruction in such schools is frequently casual and uncorrelated; that the educational needs and the health and strength of students are frequently sacrificed to practical hospital exigencies; that such shortcomings are primarily due to the lack of independent endowments for nursing education; that existing educational facilities are on the whole, in the majority of schools, inadequate for the preparation of the high grade of nurses required for the care of serious illness and for service in the fields of public health nursing and nursing education; and that one of the chief reasons for the lack of sufficient recruits, of a high type, to meet such needs lies precisely in the fact that the average hospital training school does not offer a sufficiently attractive avenue of entrance to this field.

Conclusion 6. That, with the necessary financial support and under a separate board or training school committee, organized primarily for educational purposes, it is possible, with completion of a high school course or its equivalent as a prerequisite, to reduce the fundamental period of hospital training to 28 months, and at the same time, by eliminating unessential, non-educational routine, and adopting the principles laid down in Miss Goldmark's report, to organize the course along intensive and coordinated lines with such modifications as may be necessary for practical application; and that courses of this standard would be reasonably certain to attract students of high quality in increasing numbers.

Conclusion 7. Superintendents, supervisors, instructors, and public health nurses should in all cases receive special additional training beyond the basic nursing course.

Conclusion 8. That the development and strengthening of University schools of Nursing of a high grade for the training of leaders is of fundamental importance in the furtherance of nursing education.

Conclusion 9. That when the licensure of a sub-

---

[38] Winslow, C. E. A., et al.: *Nursing and Nursing Education in the United States.* New York, The Macmillan Co., 1923, p. 224.

sidiary grade of nursing service is provided for, the establishment of training courses in preparation for such service is highly desirable; that such courses should be conducted in special hospitals, in small unaffiliated general hospitals, or in separate sections of hospitals where nurses are also trained; and that the course should be of 8 or 9 months' duration; provided the standards of such schools be approved by the same educational board which governs nursing training schools.

Conclusion 10. That the development of nursing service adequate for the care of the sick and for the conduct of the modern public health campaign demands as an absolute prerequisite the securing of funds for the endowment of nursing education of all types; and that it is of primary importance, in this connection, to provide reasonably generous endowment for university schools of nursing.

DEVELOPMENT OF ENDOWED UNIVERSITY SCHOOLS OF NURSING

Two of the history-making results of the Rockefeller study were the establishment of two famous collegiate schools of nursing and a re-emphasis on the need for commitment to education and service in public health nursing. In 1897, Miss Nutting had asked the members to reflect upon the relationship of nursing to the community. She felt that the nurse touched the social fabric at every point in her endeavors. As early as 1905 nursing leaders recommended that community nursing (district nursing) be incorporated into the curriculum. *Yale University School of Nursing,* financed by the Rockefeller Foundation, with *Annie W. Goodrich* as dean, and *Western Reserve University School of Nursing,* endowed by Frances Payne Bolton, with Miss *Carolyn E. Gray* as dean, were consequently opened.

Yale University School of Nursing was established in 1923 on the fiftieth anniversary of the founding of the Connecticut Training School for Nurses, which it succeeded. Provision for *educational leadership* as well as a background in *public health nursing* was incorporated into the curriculum. The degree of Bachelor of Nursing was given to graduates from 1926 to 1936; then, the degree of Master of Nursing was awarded until this famous school was closed in 1958.

Annie W. Goodrich felt collegiate nursing education was the preferred type of education for all nurses: "It is desirable that nursing education should find its place in the university, which is another way of saying

that it belongs where all educational expressions have been increasingly placed, and for the reason that universal knowledge is here assembled and distributed in accordance with the needs of the students as future builders of the community."[39]

Miss Goodrich was succeeded by *Effie J. Taylor,* a Canadian by birth, who graduated from Johns Hopkins School of Nursing. She had received her degree from Columbia, had been on the staff of the Phipps Psychiatric Institute at Johns Hopkins, had served in the First World War and went to Yale in 1923. She was president of the I.C.N. during World War II. Elizabeth Bixler, a graduate of Yale University School of Nursing, succeeded Miss Taylor as dean until the closing of the basic program.

At the end of the 1920's, there was marked expansion in the development of the field of nursing.

In 1900 there were 160 medical schools and 432 schools of nursing. By 1926, there were 79 medical schools and 2155 schools of nursing.

The medical profession had responded to the suggestions of the Flexner Report. There were fewer schools, but the schools had been enriched and improved.

The recommendations of the Goldmark Report were being initiated by the nurse leaders. Many substandard schools had closed; high school graduation as a requirement for admission was becoming uniform; the 48-hour week was beginning to be maximum with 44 hours and 40 hours accepted in many areas.

HOSPITAL NURSING SERVICE

Another major breakthrough in nursing care of patients and education for students of nursing came as a direct result of the Goldmark Report. It emphasized the obvious need for the employment of a general staff of graduate nurses to care for patients and thus release the student from the roles of supervisor, head nurse and general duty nurse.

A position of significance was that of the head nurse. She had the opportunity to become an influence in the management of the

---

[39] Goodrich, Annie W.: *Social and Ethical Significance of Nursing.* New York, The Macmillan Co., 1932.

unit and the care of each patient, a model for students of nursing and a dependable associate of the physicians. The constant development of scientific procedures in the treatment and care of patients has demanded a highly specialized preparation for such a nurse. Scientific progress has expanded, bringing with it the need for special patient care, including well-planned patient teaching; head nurses have released the business detail to unit managers and the secretarial aspects to unit secretaries.

With the inception of a stable staff of nursing personnel, many patients with diseases such as pneumonia and typhoid fever were referred to as nursing care problems because their recovery was partly a result of excellent nursing care. Patients were bedridden for long periods of time and it was a reflection of poor nursing care if patients developed decubitus ulcers.

HOSPITAL SOCIAL SERVICE

"Social service" is a term that covers the whole field of philanthropy. Including all activities whereby men serve their fellow men, it is defined as "those activities which deal directly with personality, family and community, and are not strictly medical nor educational. . . . It helps adjust the lives of human beings who are unable to take advantage of what is offered, to lead the life they must lead with the resources at hand." *Hospital social service* limits the work to whatever may be done toward establishing the patient's bodily health, and involves questions not only physical, but moral and spiritual as well.

In 1902 some of the students of Johns Hopkins Medical School organized friendly visiting in connection with the Charity Organization of Baltimore, thus recognizing early the social side of illness. In 1904 the National Conference of Charities invited the visiting nurses of the country to join with the "other social workers" at their annual meeting. Nurses expressed concern about the instructive aspects of patient care taking priority over skilled nursing.

In 1905 Dr. Richard Cabot, an eminent medical man, seeking to improve outpatient practice in Boston, founded at the Massachusetts General Hospital a hospital social service department. This established the principles and set the standards for the whole country and has influenced the entire world.

Dr. Cabot was assisted capably by *Ida M. Cannon,* a nurse who became an authority on hospital social service.

In 1906 the work was established at Bellevue Hospital, New York, by Mary A. Wadleigh, a nurse, with the help of Lillian Wald of the Henry Street Settlement. In 1925 it was reported that 600 hospitals had social service departments. This department is now considered to be an essential part of every hospital in every community, and has been adopted abroad.

PRIVATE DUTY NURSING

For many years far more nurses went into private duty than into any other field. This was partly because the demand was great and there were few opportunities in other fields, and partly because private duty did not demand and was not supposed to need any preparation beyond the nurse's basic training.

Even before the depression of the 1930's, it was recognized that the situation of the private duty nurse presented a problem. The difficulties were largely economic, both for patient and nurse. Surveys were made in the 1920's that showed that about 10 per cent of all the sick were cared for in hospitals and about 10 per cent had paid nurses at home or received some care from public health nurses. *Eighty per cent* were cared for as they were centuries ago, by members of their families or untrained neighbors.

Private duty nursing came to be recognized as a highly irregular job, one in which both work and salary were unpredictable. It became a job without supervision, without opportunity for advanced study and one in which experience was uncompensated.

In the work of the Committee on the Grading of Nurses, private duty was found to be one of the major problems that affected both nurses and the public and in which there was deep dissatisfaction on both sides. This committee ably analyzed the problem but did not attempt to suggest remedies.

Private duty was usually for 24 hours in homes, and might be the same in hospital "specialling." Often the nurse slept on a cot in the patient's room. Doctors and nursing superintendents could offer no help since the matter was entirely economic. Hospital trustees and the public had no understanding of the situation.

BALANCING NURSING SERVICE AND EDUCATION

More than 90 years ago Miss Nightingale's foresight made her found the school at St. Thomas' as an *educational institution.* Its features were: Nurses were primarily students. Heads of departments were chosen for their teaching and organizing ability. The school was liberally endowed and thus in control of its own activities.

Though Miss Nightingale stated her principles clearly, they have been largely misunderstood. In consequence, many schools of nursing, from her time until now, have been organized with the purpose "to provide better nursing for the hospital." Even now these two different ends, nursing service and nursing education, are misunderstood. It is a well recognized fact that there is *no other educational project in which students carry responsibility for the work* of an organization.

Economic pressure had been the chief cause of this confusion, though that idea was discussed for at least two decades before any analysis of it was made.

Administrative Cost Analysis for Nursing Service and Nursing Education, 1940, was a study made under the American Hospital Association and the National League of Nursing Education. It greatly clarified the chaos of ideas existing on the monetary value of student nurses' work. It worked out the number of hours' care given in each 24 hours to different types of patients, the cost of housing, feeding and educating student nurses, and arrived at definite conclusions.

For more than half a century, directors of schools of nursing have been perplexed by the problem of trying to educate their nurses and at the same time with the same personnel getting the patients in hospitals cared for. As a rule, the two aims came into sharp conflict, and since the care of patients was of paramount importance, it was nursing education that assumed second place. For many years hospitals absorbed the nurse's whole time, always her social life; often her health was affected; her personal life was given little consideration.

In the past, the educational foundation for all professions was not well defined.

NURSING AND WORLD WAR II

World War II had a profound influence on nursing. In the United States almost revolutionary changes came about as a direct result of it. In other countries the same was true.

Early in 1941 the United States had begun to draft men by the thousands. Many nurses were needed for the great army camps established throughout the country, and many responded to the Government's appeal.

As early as 1940 two American medical units went to help the Allies, one sent by Harvard University to England, and an American-Scandinavian unit to Poland.

Even earlier, in the spring of 1940, our nursing leaders had comprehended the potential need and had formed the *Nursing Council of National Defense,* composed of representatives from all the national nursing bodies (the A.N.A., the N.L.N.E. and the N.O.P.H.N.), the Red Cross Nursing Service, the Federal nursing services, the Association of Collegiate Schools of Nursing and the National Association of Colored Graduate Nurses. Major Julia Stimson was chairman of this Council. Plans were made to cooperate with Canada and Central and South America.

In 1942 this body became the *National Nursing Council for War Service.* In order to increase the number of nurses for military service and at the same time to see that civilians were cared for, it planned refresher courses for graduate nurses, pooled teaching staffs, and was available for consultant service.

From 1940 there was a National Nurses' Committee on Procurement and Assignment, with branches in each state, which *classified* nurses as essential or nonessential, about 300,000 in all being considered individually.

Wartime Nursing Education

In the summer of 1941, the U. S. Congress was induced to appropriate $1,250,000 for nursing education, and in 1942, $3,500,000 —an epoch-making action. This was accomplished by a laywoman, Frances Payne Bolton (Fig. 12–10), Congresswoman from Ohio, under what is known as the Bolton Bill. This provided for: refresher courses for graduate nurses, assistance to schools of nursing so that they might increase their student body (nurses' homes, classrooms, laboratories), postgraduate courses, preparation for in-

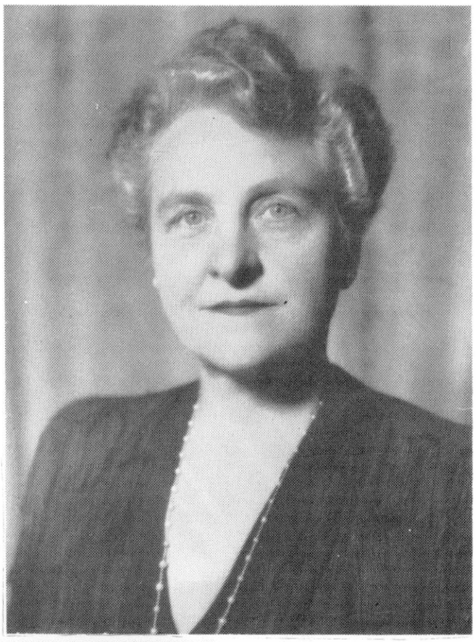

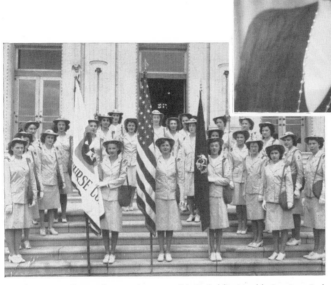

Figure 12–10. Hon. Frances Payne Bolton, sponsor in U. S. Congress of the bill that created the U. S. Cadet Nurse Corps.

Figure 12–11. U. S. Cadet Nurse Corps, first anniversary. (U. S. Public Health Service, Federal Security Agency.)

structors and other personnel and training in midwifery and other specialties.

Never before had the Government recognized nurses as a group; still less had it concerned itself with their advancement. This was an important milestone in the history of American nursing.

In 1942 Mrs. Bolton sponsored in Congress a second bill, creating the *U.S. Cadet Nurse Corps* (Fig. 12–11). This had been carefully planned by the *National Nursing Council for War Service*, and it aimed to increase as rapidly as possible the number of nurses in the country.

In June, 1943, the Bolton Act was passed by Congress, and the Corps became a fact. It was placed under the Division of Nurse Education of the U. S. Public Health Service. The Bolton Act created a great system of scholarships given by the Government to qualified young women—those who met the requirements of their respective state boards and of the schools to which they might apply. It was the largest project for nursing education ever planned.

From that time, about 95 per cent of all nursing students were enrolled in the Cadet Corps. Much publicity was given the Corps, and during its first year 65,000 students enrolled in it. The total number who joined the Corps was 179,000. The first two schools to enroll in the Corps were Freedman's (Negro) and Providence (Catholic) of the District of Columbia.

"Relative" military rank had been granted to both Army and Navy nurses by which they had the authority of officers, though they were not commissioned. On June 22, 1944, President Roosevelt signed an executive order making the Corps an integral part of the army, its personnel to receive the same pay and prerogatives as other officers. This order became effective on July 12, when the Corps numbered approximately 40,000 nurses. On April 16, 1947, the *Army-Navy Nurse Act* (Public Law 36) was enacted, which authorized permanent commissioned status for Army nurses. Florence A. Blanchfield became the first woman to be given a permanent commission in the regular Army as "Colonel."

The Army nurses were assigned to nine stations and 52 areas throughout the world; the Navy nurses, to a dozen hospital ships and more than 300 naval stations.

Some nurses did not go overseas, but worked in the 80 Army hospitals of the home country. (There were about 600 Army hospitals abroad with 18,000 beds, and 43 Navy hospitals and 10,000 berths on hospital ships.)

Hospitals requested, and got, thousands of untrained *volunteers*, both men and women, for all sorts of tasks. Many business and professional men spent their evenings as orderlies. The American Red Cross, under the U. S. Director of Civilian Defense, did an outstanding piece of work in training aides.

On July 1, 1949, a separate *Air Force Nurse Corps* was established with a transfer of Army nurses desiring this assignment.

All through the war the work of nurses had special attention from both the government and the public. Hundreds of significant decorations and citations were bestowed on them; 1619 nurses (approximately one out of every 40) were decorated with such medals as the Army Commendation ribbon, the Bronze Star, the Air Medal, the Distinguished Service Medal, the Silver Star and the Distinguished Flying Cross.

Regret was expressed by the Government that no way was found, other than public commendation, to reward the no-less-heroic services of instructors and thousands of personnel who remained on duty in civilian hospitals. Dr. Parran of the U. S. Public Health Service gave certificates "for meritorious service" to the instructors of more than a thousand schools who "prepared the largest classes of student nurses in history."

Generals and medical officers gave high praise. "Those who know the record of the Army nurses since the days of the Crimea are not surprised that they proved themselves the equal of men under combat conditions."[40]

"Their untiring service, their professional skill, and their ability to sustain the unparalleled morale of the wounded in their care will always reflect the highest credit to the Nurse Corps, U. S. Navy."[41]

PRACTICAL NURSING

The designation of *practical nursing* has long been under discussion. Nurses who practice without full training had been called attendants, subsidiary nurses, auxiliary nurses or assistant nurses. The formal definition of a practical nurse is: A person trained to care for subacute, convalescent and chronic patients in their own homes or in institutions, who works under the direction of a licensed physician or a registered professional nurse and who is prepared to give household assistance when necessary.

Both the American Nurses' Association and the American Hospital Association had been advocating short courses of training in nursing for women not eligible for the full course. It is known that from about 1880 there were attempts at training practical nurses or attendants. In this century there have been a few excellent schools giving short courses in nursing. Two of the pioneers were the Ballard School, New York, and the Household Nursing Association, Boston; they taught cooking, care of the house, diet theory, simple science classes and hospital experience in the simpler nursing procedures.

For over 40 years there have been *correspondence* schools of nursing, and their "graduates" have numbered in the thousands. Attempts to close them have not been completely successful.

In 1941 an organization was formed of those engaged in training practical nurses, the *National Association for Practical Nurse Education.*

In 1949 the *National Federation of Licensed Practical Nurses* was formed to foster high standards of practical nursing and to promote the welfare of the practical nurse to the end that the public will be served with the highest possible care. The State Board Test Pool provided examinations for practical nurses.

---

[40] Editorial, *New York Tribune*, 1943.

[41] Adm. William F. Halsey.

NURSING PROGRAMS FOR MEN

For many years certain hospitals accepted men in programs, though most of them gave the men a short course. The men were frequently not called "nurses," but "attendants."

In 1888, at Bellevue Hospital in New York, the Mills School was established with a two-year course; its graduates were called attendants, following the custom of the time. Bellevue has for a long time given a full course so that its graduates are registered nurses. Frederick Jones, director of the school from 1921 to 1929, not only developed this school, but did much to promote the preparation of male nurses.

Other early schools were at Grace Hospital, Detroit, and Battle Creek Sanitarium, Mich.; Boston City Hospital, Carney and St. Margaret's Hospital, Boston; St. Joseph's Hospital and the Pennsylvania Hospital in Philadelphia; and the Alexian Brothers in Chicago and St. Louis (Figs. 12–12 and 12–13).

In 1943 there were four schools of nursing for men only: the Mills School, New York, the Pennsylvania Hospital School of Nursing for Men and the two Alexian Brothers' hospitals in Chicago and St. Louis. Now many more men are interested in nursing. Since 1948 the number of male student nurses has increased.

AEROSPACE NURSING

Aerospace nursing is one of the newer specialties in nursing practice. Nurses are receiving educational experiences to assist man in adapting to a space environment. Nurses are assigned to the Air Force's *Bioastronautic Operational Support Unit* (B.O.S.U.). Bioastronautics is the study of the effects of space travel on life to assure that man will be able to function effectively in extraterrestrial environments. *Major Pearl E. Tucker* directed the B.O.S.U. nursing staff.

LATER DEVELOPMENTS

In 1946, the *Hospital Survey and Construction Act*, also called the Hill-Burton Bill, was signed by the President. This provided a five-year federal grant-in-aid program to the states for the purpose of surveying needs,

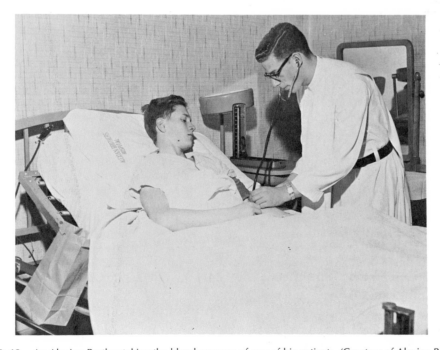

Figure 12–12. An Alexian Brother taking the blood pressure of one of his patients. (Courtesy of Alexian Brothers.)

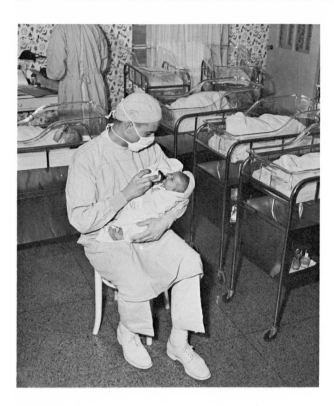

Figure 12–13. The nursery in Pennsylvania Hospital, Philadelphia. (Courtesy of Public Health Service, U. S. Department of Health, Education and Welfare.)

planning and constructing necessary hospitals and health centers. The Federal government paid one third of the cost for the survey and construction; the other two-thirds were assumed by the individual states.

This was a challenging opportunity for nurses to be consulted and to make suggestions for the planning of work areas in which they would carry out their duties. This was stressed by Louise Waagen,[42] Chief of the Hospital Nursing Section, Division of Hospital Facilities of the United States Public Health Service.

The search for better methods of doing things, for labor-saving and step-saving devices, for the application of the principles of work simplification, had long since been utilized in agriculture, industry and the home. Yet, while nursing assumed new functions, it still clung to old methods, and nurses worked frequently in antiquated work areas, walking miles and carrying heavy things.

In 1947, a book was published entitled *Nursing in Modern Society,*[43] which made the

members of the nursing profession aware of their present role and which set the stage for a period of critical analysis of nursing and of nursing education. The foreword to this erudite work states that the book "constitutes a natural introduction . . . for it presents an enveloping concept of the true place of nursing today in the social background of which it is a part."

Miss Chayer stressed that: "A revolution is needed in nursing today. One is being experienced whether it is being recognized or not. Our time-honored methods of serving the public are no longer adequate." She continued: "Any institution that has permanence centers its activities around fundamental human needs."

Miss Chayer further indicated that as times changed and new knowledge was assembled, new techniques and skills should be developed to satisfy these needs. "What was good enough, or at least tolerated at one stage of development, is not good enough for another. The 'horse and buggy age' gives place to the 'atomic age,' with its new responsibilities and dangers."

The present problem is then crystallized:

Never before in our history have so many persons been the recipients of so many hours of

[42]Waggen, Louise: The Hospital Survey and Construction Act. *American Journal of Nursing,* 48:361–363, 1948.

[43]Chayer, Mary Ella: *Nursing in Modern Society.* New York, G. P. Putnam's Sons, 1947.

nursing care; yet even now only a small fraction of the people most in need of nursing care are receiving its benefits. What are the social forces that have increased the demand for nursing services at a time when death rates are lower, fewer people are acutely ill, the duration of illness has been lessened, and the duration of bed care shortened? . . . Whatever the causes . . . the problem is ours as a professional group to solve, with the inestimable help . . . of the consumers of nursing service.

The *National Nursing Council for War Service* was organized in 1942 as a coordinating council for the fourteen national organizations concerned with nursing. This council's achievements were remarkable, and at the end of the war it continued as the *National Nursing Council*, for the purpose of sponsoring three studies: a history of its own accomplishments, presented in *The History of the National Nursing Council* by Hope Newell; an economic survey of the nursing profession, compiled and distributed by the Bureau of Labor Statistics of the United States Department of Labor; and a *study of nursing education.* The National Nursing Council felt that the deficiencies in nursing service in quantity and quality resulted from the prevailing system of nurse education.

NURSING EDUCATION

A financial grant was obtained from the Carnegie Foundation, and *Esther Lucile Brown* (Fig. 12–14), Director of the Department of Studies in the Professions at The Russell Sage Foundation, was appointed to carry out the study of nurse education. Miss Brown was well prepared to conduct the survey, since she had conducted studies and published findings on the role of education in the essential professions of social work, engineering, medicine and law and how this education could be molded to meet the needs of society.

The problem for the study of nurse education revolved around the question: *How should a basic professional school of nursing be organized, administered, controlled and financed to prepare its graduates to meet community need?*

It was essential to consider the function of the nurse and her place in society before recommendations could be made for her preparation. Three subproblems were set up.

1. What will be the probable nature of health services during the second half of the twentieth century and what nursing services

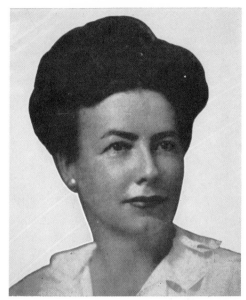

Figure 12–14. Esther Lucile Brown. (Courtesy of *American Journal of Nursing.*)

will meet the needs of society most adequately?

2. What kind of education and training will prepare nurses most effectively to render these services?

3. How should this education be organized, controlled and financed?

Miss Brown visited about fifty schools and held three regional conferences of nursing leaders in San Francisco, Chicago and Washington, D.C.[44] Her findings were interpreted and discussed, and in 1948 recommendations were published in *Nursing for the Future.* These 28 recommendations could be briefly summarized as follows:

Need for nurses to study and analyze nursing functions.

Need for nursing functions to be carried out by nursing service teams.

Need for clarification of the use of the term "professional," which should be used as the term is understood by educators.[45]

---

[44]An account of these conferences may be found in *A Thousand Think Together.* New York, National Nursing Council, 1948.

[45]"Careful consideration should be given to the fact that professional schools in most other fields have already come within degree-conferring institutions to such an extent that possession of a degree is fast becoming a criterion of a person's having received professional as contrasted with vocational training." Brown, Ester L.: *Nursing for the Future.* New York, The Russell Sage Foundation, 1948, p. 77.

Need for university schools of nursing to be autonomous, improve their programs, obtain a better prepared faculty, seek the best available clinical facilities, and have contracts between the degree-granting institution and the clinical agency stating the privileges and obligations of both the institution and the agency and including a statement concerning the use of the students' time exclusively for purposes of education.

Need for positive steps to be taken by the nursing profession to create an atmosphere that attracts a carefully selected segment of the population.

Need for provisions to be made within the university for distinguished hospital schools of nursing.

Need for experimentation in shortening the course in other hospital schools and at the same time making provisions for enriching their course of study. (A vast number of schools conducted by hospitals offer, in spite of improvements, apprenticeship training.)

Need to consider the use of psychiatric hospitals as agencies for affiliation in psychiatric nursing, rather than have these institutions conduct their own schools.

Need to conduct a periodic examination of schools, to publish and distribute lists of accredited schools and to plan for periodic reexamination of schools.

Need for the public to assume greater financial responsibility for nursing education.

Need to provide a more substantial academic preparation for leadership in nursing education and in clinical nursing specialties.

Need for improved programs in the educational preparation of the graduate nurse.

Need for a study to plan for the distribution of schools on local and regional bases to serve the needs of the entire country.

Need to improve in-service education and to achieve better interpersonal relationships within the hospital.

Need for better interprofessional team relationships in more congenial hospital atmospheres.

Need to increase the use of trained practical nurses, to improve their educational preparation and enact sound legislation to safeguard their practice.

Need for the greater use of men as nurses and for the employment of married nurses.

Need for hospitals to assume a positive health function in the community and to have an increased awareness of the importance of the social and emotional factors involved in illness.

This study, the *Brown Report* as it has been called, presented findings that challenged action in securing these long-range goals. The necessity of being aware of the needs of society in the second half of the twentieth century and the preparation of nurses to meet these needs were emphasized. The Brown Report quotes from the proceedings of a workshop organized by the National Nursing Council, which defines the place of the future professional nurse in her field of nursing and in our larger society:

It is the opinion of this group that in the latter half of the twentieth century, the professional nurse will be one who recognizes and understands the fundamental (health) needs of a person, sick or well, and who knows how these needs can best be met. She will possess a body of scientific nursing knowledge which is based upon and keeps pace with general scientific advancement, and she will be able to apply this knowledge in meeting the nursing needs of a person and a community. She must possess that kind of discriminative judgment which will enable her to recognize those activities which fall within the area of professional nursing and those activities which have been identified with the fields of other professional or nonprofessional groups.

She must able to exert leadership in at least four different ways: (1) in making her unique contribution to the preventive and remedial aspects of illness; (2) in improving those nursing skills already in existence and developing new nursing skills; (3) in teaching and supervising other nurses and auxiliary workers; and (4) in cooperating with other professions in planning for positive health on community, state, national, and international levels.

In defining nursing itself, the Brown Report quoted Sister M. Olivia (Gowan) of the Catholic University of America:

Nursing in its broadest sense may be defined as an art and a science which involves the whole patient—body, mind, and spirit; promotes his spiritual, mental and physical health by teaching and by example; stresses health education and health preservation, as well as ministration to the sick; involves the care of the patient's environment—social and spiritual as well as physical; and gives health service to the family and community as well as to the individual.

The function of the professional nurse, and that of professional nursing, has been more than just the carrying out of treatments and the assistance of members of other professions. This function should be that of *assisting patients*. Miss Brown was impressed by the universal desire of nurses to nurse: "Nurses both want and like" to care for patients. She also noted that a challenging opportunity was not satisfied because nurses were involved with non-nursing activities in archaic, energy-depleting hospital units.

With the publication of the Brown Report in 1948, the National Nursing Council, having achieved its last objective, dissolved.

While the Brown Report was being made another study was being analyzed by the *Committee on the Function of Nursing* appointed by the Division of Nursing Education of the Teachers College, Columbia University. The aim of this committee was to review "a selected group of problems centering around the current and prospective shortages of nursing personnel."[46] The results of the discussion of this group were published in a thought-provoking and worthwhile book entitled *A Program for the Nursing Profession*.

The proposals of this committee, which were summarized briefly at the end of the book, were that:

a. The nursing function be subdivided among two groups of personnel—professional and practical nurses.

b. Relations be clarified and improved between the nurse and the other members of the medical and health team.

c. Suitable relations be developed among the various groups of nursing personnel who together comprise the nursing team.

d. The professional nurse complete a four-year course in a college- or university-affiliated school of nursing.

e. The practical nurse be graduated from a 9- to 12-month program in an approved school for practical nursing.

f. A goal of approximately 200,000 professional nurses for 1960 be established.

g. A goal of approximately 400,000 practical nurses for 1960 be established.

h. Conditions of pay and work in nursing be substantially improved and differentials in reward be instituted.

i. Research receive a heightened emphasis.

It was interesting that these recommendations in the main parallel those of the Brown Report.

The national nursing organizations formed a *Committee on Implementing the Brown Report*, with representatives from allied professional groups. The committee was eventually called the *National Committee for the Improvement of Nursing Services*. One of the important projects sponsored by this group was the *School Data Analysis*: by means of a questionnaire, a report of the practices in schools of nursing in 1949 was procured.

The schools cooperated wholeheartedly and 97 per cent responded. The data were analyzed and the schools were classified against other participating schools, rather than against other criteria.[47] In November of 1949, the classification of schools appeared in the *American Journal of Nursing* under the heading "Interim Classification of Schools of Nursing Offering Basic Programs."

The Interim Classification was published again in *Nursing Schools at the Mid-Century*,[48] together with a complete analysis of the data presented in an informative, graphic manner.

The nursing education programs of Canada have also faced scrutiny. For many years nursing leaders have voiced criticism of service-oriented programs for the preparation of nurses.

The first definitive survey of such programs was co-sponsored by the Canadian Nurses' Association and the Canadian Medical Association and was completed in 1931 by Dr. G. M. Weir, professor of education at the University of British Columbia. His report, published the following year, revealed many weaknesses in the system of nurse preparation and suggested remedial courses of action.

In the mid-1940's, Nettie D. Fidler, a member of the nursing faculty at the University of Toronto, was representative of those who continued to voice concerns of the nursing profession. In her 1944 report to the CNA general meeting, she identified three problem areas: the need for factual knowlege of the nursing requirements of the country; the probability that these would reveal the need for varied types of nursing services and of preparation for them; and the need for educational, i.e., financial, independence of nursing schools.[49]

In 1956, the Canadian Nurses' Association inaugurated and financed a project to identify the strengths and weaknesses of the existing schools of nursing. The need for studying the value and feasibility of a national, voluntary accreditation program for schools of nursing was carried out. This study became the Pilot Project for the Evaluation of Schools of Nursing in Canada, which was completed in 1960. Projects were undertaken to develop school improvement programs and to evaluate the quality of nursing service

[46]The Committee on the Function of Nursing: *A Program for the Nursing Profession*. New York, The Macmillan Co., 1948, p. ix.

[47]Diploma and degree programs were graded separately.

[48]National Committee for the Improvement of Nursing Services: *Nursing Schools at the Mid-Century*. New York, Osmond-Johnson, 1950.

[49]Canadian Nurses' Association. *The Leaf and the Lamp*, Ottawa, 1968, p. 5.

as well as continue the thrust toward an accreditation program.

These large and expensive programs occupied the energies of the national association during the years 1960–1966, and the conclusions drawn from them form the philosophical and practical base from which the CNA now functions. Essentially, the CNA is committed to provide all reasonable help for effecting curriculum improvements in all schools of nursing. A consulting service is provided by national headquarters to work on request with provincial groups seeking to examine and improve educational processes.

Meanwhile, through provincial and national associations, nursing educators seek general acceptance, within and beyond the profession, of the principle that nurses should be prepared in educational institutions. Inseparable from this objective is the necessity of having educational programs developed and conducted primarily by educators and separated entirely from the requirement of providing service in exchange for training—an outmoded practice in conflict with modern concepts of education. Measurable evidence of progress towards this end was observed in 1966 when the Saskatchewan legislature made nursing education a responsibility of the province's educational system.[50]

The members of the nursing profession, realizing that in unity there was strength, began studying the possibility of substituting one or two organizations for the six already existing ones. The possibility of reorganizing for the greater unified action of a more effective professional association was realized in 1950 when the proposal for the *American Nurses' Association* (A.N.A.) and the *National League for Nursing* (N.L.N.) was endorsed. The change was completed in 1952.

At the biennial convention of 1952, another milestone was reached when the students of nursing voted to form a *National Student Nurse Association* under the sponsorship of the Coordinating Council of the American Nurses' Association and the National League for Nursing. This association is composed of students enrolled in state-approved schools of professional nursing.

It was amazing that, in less than ten years after the completion of our so-called professional stock-taking, so many suggestions and solutions for our problems had crystallized.

A step forward was taken by the nursing profession when its members requested a study of all phases of nursing care. This request was approved by the House of Delegates at the 1950 Convention, and it endorsed the *A.N.A. Program of Studies of Nursing Functions*. Thus was launched the five-year plan for research in nursing, which was financially supported from voluntary membership contributions. The earnest wish of all nurses seemed to be that nursing continue to be an important link in the chain of total health care.

In assuming its professional responsibility of undertaking research in nursing functions, the A.N.A. had a threefold purpose:

1. To determine the functions and relationships of institutional nursing personnel of all types—professional nurses, practical nurses and auxiliary workers—in order to improve nursing care and to utilize nursing personnel most economically and effectively.

2. To determine what proportion of nursing time should be provided by each group in various situations.

3. To develop techniques for achieving the first two statements of purpose, which can be applied to all types of hospitals, and thus obtain a national picture.

Studies have been made during a six-year period. Clara A. Hardin, Associate Executive Secretary of the American Nurses' Association, was appointed Director of the Research and Statistics Unit, and at the 1956 American Nurses' Association convention the preliminary report, *Nurses Invest in Patient Care*, was released.

The American Nurses' Association also stimulated the study of functions, standards and qualifications (F. S. & Q.)[51] for the practice of nursing. Such statements are invaluable guides[52] for those who are planning curricula for future practitioners, those who are constructing job specifications and qualifications, those who are struggling to construct an acceptable definition for nursing, those who are trying to explain our profession to the general public and even those who are striving to defend an acceptable standard of conduct in nursing to lawyers and to courts.

---

[50]*Ibid.*, p. 6.

[51]American Nurses' Association statements of functions, standards and qualifications. *American Journal of Nursing*, 56:898, 1027, 1165, 1305, 1586, 1956.
[52]McIver, Pearl, and Anderson, Bernice: Functions, standards and qualifications. *American Journal of Nursing*, 57:748–750, 1957.

In contemplating the study of the functions and standards of nursing care, the area of nursing service was scrutinized. Many studies have been made and are still being carried out in this area. Notable among these has been the investigation on interpersonal relations and their effect on patient recovery done by Leo Simmons[53] at the New York Hospital. Another point of interest was in determining how many non-nursing tasks were being carried out by nurses. The Division of Nursing Resources of the U.S. Public Health Service conducted a study in this at the Massachusetts General Hospital.[54]

Another study in this category was an investigation into the misuse of professional nursing personnel, with suggestions for using this personnel more effectively to achieve greater satisfaction. This project was carried out at Harper Hospital in Detroit,[55] and the emphasis seemed to be that nursing be given back to nurses.

Also studied were the formations and uses of *nursing teams*, including the development of the philosophy of team work, the methods of planning for and the acceptance of this philosophy and, finally, implementing these principles in practice.[56]

The educational preparation of the practitioner also received attention and two books presented the studies in two areas: university preparation,[57] and the preparation of *nursing technicians*.[58] The latter was a description of an experimental program established to educate and prepare a group to function at a level beyond that of the practical nurse and be certified as semiprofessional. This program was placed under the aegis of a junior college. The graduate of this program could assume the intermediate range of functions between the simple ones carried out by the aide and the complex ones assumed by the professional nurse only.

Experimental programs on a two-year basis had been appearing for some time. These programs stressed the value of educational control in an education-centered agency rather than a service-centered agency. Not just time, but *better educational use of time* was needed; thus, a shortened program might result. In 1946, the Canadian Red Cross Society made a financial grant to the Canadian Nurses' Association to establish the Metropolitan School of Nursing.[59] This program was financially and administratively independent of any hospital, and lasted two years. Enrichment of the learning experiences for the student was paramount.

The need for a single professional nursing accrediting agency was finally realized in January, 1949 when the joint boards of directors of the six national nursing organizations merged to form the *N.N.A.S.*, the *National Nursing Accrediting Service*. Since its inception this group has carried on the important function of visiting, evaluating and accrediting schools of nursing. The accrediting service has also carried out a program of guidance to the faculties of schools of nursing by conducting workshops and conferences. It publishes lists of accredited schools for the public, for prospective students of nursing and for guidance counselors in high schools.

Accreditation has not been an end in itself, but has been a means of stimulating schools to improve their programs.

Legislation on local and federal planes was enacted to encourage students to enter schools of nursing, and to prepare all nursing personnel—faculty members and nursing service staff members—to become better prepared in their particular area of specialization. On the local level, many states[60] have passed bills for scholarship aid for nurses.

The most gratifying legislative accomplishment was the passage of the *Health Amendments Act* in 1956, which provided for nurses to obtain advanced preparation for positions in administration, supervision and teaching and in traineeships for public health personnel. It also provided for financial support

[53]Simmons, Leo W.: *Studies in the Application of Social Science in Medicine and Nursing at New York Hospital—Cornell Medical Center.* New York, The Russell Sage Foundation, 1950.

[54]Olson, Appollinia F., and Tibbitts, Helen G.: *A Study of Head Nurse Functions in a General Hospital.* Public Health Monograph, No. 3 (P.H.S. publication, No. 107), Washington, D. C., United States Government Printing Office, 1951.

[55]Wright, Marion J.: *The Improvement of Patient Care.* New York, G. P. Putnam's Sons, 1954.

[56]Newcomb, Dorothy P.: *The Team Plan.* New York, G. P. Putnam's Sons, 1954.

[57]Bridgman, Margaret: *Collegiate Education for Nursing.* New York, Russell Sage Foundation, 1953.

[58]Montag, Mildred: *The Education of Nursing Technicians.* New York, G. P. Putnam's Sons, 1951.

[59]Fidler, Nettie: The Metropolitan School of Nursing. *American Journal of Nursing, 51*:51, 1951.

[60]Connecticut's scholarship aid program. *American Journal of Nursing, 54*:200–202, 1954.

in the expansion and improvement of practical nurse programs in the states, under the direction of vocational education. The success of this program in encouraging more academic preparation for leadership has been apparent.[61]

On August 9, 1955, President Eisenhower signed the Bolton Amendment to the Army-Navy Nurses Act of 1947. This made it possible for qualified male nurses to become commissioned officers in the Army Nurse Corps Reserve.[62]

In 1953, the first patients were admitted to the Clinical Center for Medical Research at Bethesda, Maryland. In this center, scientific research projects are conducted in many areas of medicine and nursing. This research center operates under the administration of the Department of Health, Education and Welfare and is one of the sections of the National Institutes of Health of the U. S. Public Health Service. This provided a challenging opportunity for the well-prepared professional nurse who was research-minded.[63]

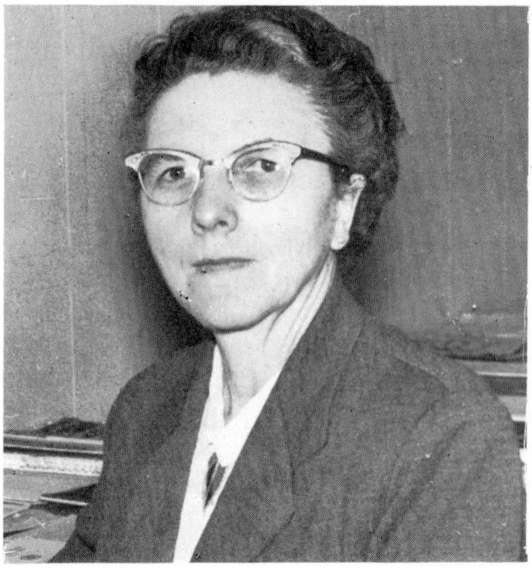

Figure 12–15. Lyle Creelman, who succeeded Olive Baggallay as Chief of the Nursing Section of the World Health Organization.

INTERNATIONAL RELATIONS

With the inception of the Nursing Section of the World Health Organization in 1949, *Olive Baggallay* was appointed chief and continued in this office until 1954. Miss Baggallay graduated from St. Thomas' in London and had been secretary of the Florence Nightingale International Foundation from 1934 to 1949. She had served also as chief nurse consultant for UNRRA in Greece. Her contributions to the welfare of mankind have been manifold.

In July, 1954, *Lyle Creelman* (Fig. 12–15), a graduate of Vancouver General Hospital School of Nursing, who received a B.S. degree from the University of British Columbia and a M.A. degree from Teachers College, Columbia University, became chief of the Nursing Section of the World Health Organization. She had been public health nursing administrator in the Nursing Section of W.H.O. since 1949. Her guidance and counsel had been extended in the area of public health nursing to all throughout the world. Miss Creelman had just completed a study on public health practice in Canada previous to her new assignment.

Mention has been made of heroes and heroines in the care of sick whose valor and devotion under difficult circumstances have merited world-wide acclaim. Such opportunities present themselves daily for the nurse, even though she does not receive international tribute. The world is ready to cheer, however, when the spotlight does fix itself on such a heroine.

PROJECT HOPE

In 1960, a floating medical center sailed on a one-year journey to Indonesia and Southeast Asia, including South Vietnam, to attempt a personal approach to bring about a healthier, happier and probably a more peaceful world. The medical center is situ-

---

[61] Jenney, Mary O., and Wehrwein, Annabel: Federal traineeships—the first year. *American Journal of Nursing,* 57:726–728, 1957.

[62] Male nurses were not eligible, under the present law, for a commission in the regular Army Nurse Corps.

[63] Johnson, Ruth L., Dilworth, Ava S., and Fagin, Claire M.: Nursing in a clinical center for medical research. *American Journal of Nursing, 53*:1329–1332, 1953.

ated on a renovated, rechristened former naval hospital ship now called the *S.S. Hope*. The *Hope* signified *Health Opportunity for People Everywhere* and reflects the desire of professional people to share their knowledge in a person-to-person relationship. The director who brought this project to fruition was Dr. William B. Walsh, a Washington, D.C. physician.

The staff of this 800-bed medical center has consisted of 15 fulltime physicians, 2 dentists, 22 registered professional nurses and about 20 other medical personnel. Additional physicians and surgeons were flown to the ship on a short-time basis. The latest medical equipment and teaching facilities were installed on the ship, including closed circuit color television for enrichment of teaching. The American doctors and nurses shared their latest information, new techniques and methods of treatment, and their Indonesian counterparts explained diseases unfamiliar to Americans and displayed cases, mainly tropical diseases, to support this information. By working together as well as playing together much was accomplished in gaining the trust and friendship of the people of these newly developing countries.

Project Hope is a shining example of service to humanity through the sharing of modern health care techniques with disadvantaged societies.

THE PEACE CORPS

In his Inaugural Address on January 20, 1961, President John F. Kennedy urged: "Ask not what your country can do for you — ask what you can do for your country." The Peace Corps has presented an opportunity for citizens to represent their country while working directly with peoples of other countries to provide economic, social and educational assistance and to stress the cause of peace through personal sharing and the encouragement of mutual understanding.

The Peace Corps was launched on March 1, 1961, when President Kennedy issued an executive order establishing the Corps on a temporary basis. The Peace Corps is an independent agency within the State Department. Through the Corps a pool of trained manpower is made available to help other countries meet pressing problems. Volunteers function as teachers, nurses, doctors, librar-

ians, social workers, laboratory technicians, community development workers, agricultural extension workers, sanitary engineers and in various other occupations.

The volunteer is desirous of elevating the standards of living, and of improving educational and social levels in the newly developing areas of the world. Peace Corps members go to these areas to teach, to build, to work, and to live in the communities to which they are sent. In the Corps nurses really have an opportunity to participate actively in what President Kennedy called "a long twilight struggle . . . a struggle against the common enemies of man: tyranny, poverty, disease and war itself."

MEDICARE—A CHALLENGE FOR NURSING

Former Secretary of Health, Education and Welfare John W. Gardner urged Governors to take maximum advantage of expanded Federal aid authorized for state health and welfare programs under the Social Security Amendments of 1965. In his letter, Secretary Gardner stated, "The new law lays the foundation for a medical care program for public assistance recipients and other low income persons that, within the next ten years, could go far to reduce one of the major causes of poverty and other social problems — the disabilities resulting from preventable or remediable health problems among persons in all age groups who cannot afford the medical care they need." Noting A.N.A.'s long-term backing of the extension of Social Security, President Johnson asked A.N.A.'s president and the director of the Washington office to join the official party of 200 to be present for the signing of Medicare on July 30, 1965 at the Truman Library in Independence, Missouri.

The starting date for Medicare was July 1, 1966; services in extended care facilities were not covered until January 1, 1967. Additional provisions specifically designed to benefit future generations include: increased authorization for maternal and child health, crippled children and child welfare services; increased funds for grants to help colleges and universities train more professional personnel to work with crippled children, particularly the mentally retarded and the multiple handicapped; and a five-year program of special project grants to provide comprehensive health care and services for preschool and school-age children, particularly in areas with concentrations of low-income families.

To date, two A.N.A. statements have spelled out nursing's concerns in the implementation of Medicare. The first statement noted that: "Nurses must now help to assure the health services provided through this legislation are of high quality. Nursing is an essential component of modern patient care. It must be available to all patients in the amount, character and place consistent with their nursing needs. The responsibility for standards of nursing care is vested in the profession itself. This basic responsibility can neither be delegated to others nor can it be assumed by outside interests. Therefore, if acceptable levels of health care are to be achieved, nurses must be involved in the planning, implementing and evaluation of health care service provided through Medicare."

A second statement, "Nursing Concerns in the Home Health Services in Health Insurance for the Aged," discussed the relationships of public health nurses and home health aides.

SELF-EVALUATION IN THE SIXTIES

On May 4, 1960, at the forty-second convention of the American Nurses' Association held in Miami Beach, the delegates voted to accept from the Committee on Current and Long Term Goals a report that was to become the basis for continued discussion in the states. Included in this report was a section referred to as Goal Three that stated:

To insure that, within the next twenty to thirty years, the education basic to the professional practice of nursing for those who then enter the profession shall be secured in a program that provides the intellectual, technical and cultural components of both a professional and liberal education. Toward this end, the ANA shall promote the baccalaureate program so that in due course it becomes the basic educational foundation for professional nursing.

Many states appointed committees to study the progress of nursing and nursing education in each state.

In the clinical setting at the turn of this century, the patient, the students of nursing, the director of nursing and, of course, the patient's physician were the members of the team. Many members of other professions have joined the health team. They, too, have gone through the evolutionary process toward professional status. The problems have been comparable, and they are still comparable. It is through the united efforts of all that problems are identified, analyzed and solved. Thus is history written.

FUNCTIONS AND PURPOSES OF NURSING ORGANIZATIONS

The American Nurses' Association

The purposes of the American Nurses' Association are to foster high standards of nursing practice, and to promote the professional and educational advancement of nurses and the welfare of nurses to the end that all people may have better nursing care. These purposes are unrestricted by considerations of nationality, race, creed or color. A.N.A. represents nurses and serves as their spokesman with allied national and international organizations, governmental bodies and the public.

The A.N.A. *Committee on Nursing Education* has the following as its functions: to study and develop standards for nursing education and methods for their implementation, to evaluate scientific and educational developments as well as changes in health needs and practices, to determine implications for nursing education and to encourage and stimulate research in all areas of nursing education.

A.N.A. Position Paper of 1965

Acting in the role of implementing these purposes, the Committee on Nursing Education prepared *A Position Paper* in 1965, which had as its major thesis that "education for those who work in nursing should take place in institutions of learning within the general system of education."

This paper was of tremendous historic significance because it was proposed by the American Nurses' Association and was approved by the membership of this association, meeting in biennial assembly in San Francisco in 1966.

Nursing practice has become exceedingly complex. The conditions of nursing are determined by the structure of society and its prevailing values. Nurses are required to master a complex, constantly enlarging body of knowledge and to make critical, independent judgments about patients and their care.

The essential components of professional nursing are care, cure and coordination. From the early Judeo-Christian base in nursing we know that the care aspect is more than "to take care of," it is "caring for" and "caring about" people in the broadest dimension. It is dealing with human beings under stress and, on occasion, this occurs over long periods of time. Other dimensions include comfort and support in times of anxiety, loneliness and helplessness. It involves listening, evaluating and intervening when necessary.

The cure aspect involves the promotion of health and healing. It requires assisting patients to understand their health problems, and, through teaching, to cope with them. It includes carrying out a prescribed plan for care of the patient, but it shares the burden, with the community, of the responsibility for the health and welfare of all by participating in programs to prevent illness and maintain health. It also encompasses the supervising and teaching of those who give any aspect of nursing care, as well as providing the ability to participate in research or to collaborate with those in other disciplines in research that results in more satisfying, scientific and better nursing care.

This rationale prompted the A.N.A. Committee on Nursing Education to recommend that:

1. Minimum preparation for beginning professional nursing practice should be baccalaureate degree education in nursing.
2. Minimum preparation for beginning technical nursing practice should be associate degree education in nursing.
3. Education for assistants in the health service occupations should be short, intensive preservice programs in vocational education institutions rather than on-the-job training programs.

The technological advances in medicine that have stimulated incredible innovations in mechanical devices compel the profession to demand a scientific but humanistic nurse who can function in this environment and, in addition, provide compassionate personal care.

Colleges have been charged with designing programs to provide master clinical practitioners to assume faculty positions, with developing programs for continuing education, and with encouraging research in nursing to expand the boundaries of nursing as an art and a science.

The ultimate aim of nursing education and nursing service is the improvement of nursing care.

The primary aim of nursing education is to provide an environment in which the nursing student can develop self-discipline, intellectual curiosity, the ability to think clearly and acquire knowledge necessary for practice. Nursing education reaches its ultimate aim when recent advances in knowledge and findings from nursing research are incorporated into the program of nursing study.

The primary aim of nursing service is to provide nursing care of the type needed, and in the amount required, to those in need of nursing care. Nursing service reaches its ultimate aim when it provides a climate in which questions about practice can be raised and answers sought, in which nursing staffs continue to develop and learn, and in which nurses work in collaboration with persons in other disciplines to provide improved services to patients.

These aims—educating nurses and providing patients with care—can only be carried out when nurses in education and in service recognize their interdependence and actively collaborate to achieve the ultimate aim of both—improved nursing care.

The American Nurses' Association adopted structural changes due to the action of the House of Delegates in 1966. The *Nursing Practice Department* devises plans to advance the clinical competence of practitioners of nursing. Provision for recognition of professional achievement and research relative to the practice of nursing has been fostered. With the approval of the statements of standards of practice, *certification* will be earned.

In March of 1967 the newly established *Commission on Nursing Education* of the A.N.A. identified four areas of need:

1. The need to delineate the "sphere of influence," responsibility and authority of nurses.
2. The need to identify inadequacies in

the current system of education and health care.

3. The need to define the purpose and essential characteristics of education for nurse practitioners.

4. The need to identify functions for baccalaureate and associate degree graduates.

A prime A.N.A. task is the implementation of the education position. To accomplish the orderly transition of nursing education into educational institutions, the Association has issued several major statements calling for community planning for nursing education throughout the United States.

A.N.A. works to set standards and policies for nursing education. Activities of the A.N.A. Commission on Nursing Education include the evaluation of relevant scientific and educational developments, changes in health needs and practice as they apply to nursing education; the encouraging and stimulating of research in all areas of nursing education and formulating policy and recommending action concerning federal and state legislation in the field of education.

Through the A.N.A.–N.L.N. Nursing Careers Program qualified people are recruited into nursing education programs. Particular emphasis is given to the career development of the registered nurse.

The Council of State Boards of Nursing, which includes one representative from each State Board of Nursing, establishes policies for the development and use of the State Board Test Pool Examination for nurse candidates in all states. State Boards are authorized by state law to license nurse practitioners.

The Council also recommends methods and procedures to encourage reasonable uniformity in state board standards and practice to facilitate interstate licensure. Another Council activity includes developing materials for use by boards in the approving of basic nursing education programs.

Through national annual meetings and education conferences A.N.A. provides Council members with information on national trends and changes in nursing education, nursing practice and nursing services.[64]

Nursing Practice

There are five divisions on nursing practice, each responsibile for advancing the

standards, knowledge and skills in one of these areas: community health nursing, geriatric nursing, maternal and child health nursing, medical-surgical nursing, psychiatric nursing and mental health nursing.

An executive committee of expert practitioners in each division gives assistance to nurses interested in that area of practice through dissemination of current information relevant to practice, and by conducting various educational conferences. Each executive committee has appointed a standards committee to develop and implement written standards for practice in its area of concern and a certification board to develop and implement recognition of excellence in practice through the process of certification.

A Congress for Nursing Practice establishes the scope of nursing practice, evaluates relevant scientific and educational developments, encourages research, recommends action concerning federal and state legislation related to nursing practice, provides guidance to state committees or councils on practice regarding ethical, legal and professional aspects of practice, coordinates the work of the A.N.A. divisions on practice. The Congress is composed of the chairman of each A.N.A. division on nursing practice and four members who are appointed by the A.N.A. board. An Academy of Nursing is to be established for the advancement of knowledge, education and nursing practice. Fellows will be selected for an outstanding contribution to nursing.[65]

Nursing Services

The A.N.A. Commission on Nursing Services works to develop standards and guides, and to assist in other ways to bring about improvements in the organization and management of nursing services. The Commissioners are responsible for evaluating scientific and educational developments, changes in health needs and practices and their implications for nursing services, changes in health needs and care and estimating requirements for nursing manpower and resources. It formulates and recommends policy related to federal and state legislation where it affects the organized nursing services.

A.N.A. maintains liaison with allied health groups such as the American Hospital Association, the American Society of Hospital Pharmacists, and the National Federation of Licensed Practical Nurses.

Plans for essential nursing services in the event of natural or man-made disaster have been developed by the A.N.A. Committee on Emergency

---

[64]American Nurses' Association, *This Is A.N.A.*, Seventy-fifth Anniversary—1896–1971. New York, A.N.A., 1972. p. 2.

[65]*Ibid.*, pp. 1–2.

Health Preparedness and National Defense. This committee has developed criteria and guidelines for utilization of registered nurses in the event of disaster and has enumerated nursing functions that should be expanded during national emergency.

[The program of Economic and General Welfare is] based on the principle that nurses have the right as well as the the the duty to participate in determining their salaries and conditions of employment. The program is carried out on local, district, state and national levels. The aim is to assure that (1) nurses receive fair compensation and benefits for their professional services, (2) employment conditions are conducive to providing high quality nursing care and (3) the number of qualified nurses necessary to meet the nation's health care needs is recruited and retained. To this end A.N.A. advises and assists the constituent state nurses associations (S.N.A.'s) which in turn act as the representatives of nurses in all employment settings.

The A.N.A. Commission on Economic and General Welfare formulates policies of the economic security program and has a program which provides direct assistance to S.N.A.'s on projects related to organizing and representing nurses. Commission responsibilities include developing and implementing general economic standards and an economic education program; formulating policy and recommending action related to federal and state economic security legislation interests; and studying and evaluating the economics of health care as well as the economics of nursing.[66]

Research and Statistics

A.N.A. studies are made relating to the program interests and needs of the Association. Current and comprehensive manpower and economic data are compiled and analyzed. Information about A.N.A. and its membership, informational support to all A.N.A. departments and programs, and information to nurses and the public is disseminated through *Facts About Nursing* and other reports.

The A.N.A. Commission on Nursing Research encourages and stimulates research in all areas of nursing. Its responsibilities include participating in the establishment of standards of nursing research; recommending priorities for the profession's research concerns; assisting organizational units in identifying research needs to expand nursing knowledge; assisting constituents in developing nursing research programs; developing and disseminating research-related documents; assisting in the dissemination of nursing research findings; conducting nursing research workshops; developing and maintaining liaison with appropriate groups, such as the American Nurses' Foundation.

A.N.A. sponsors the American Nurses' Foundation which was established in 1955 and which has as its objectives conducting and promoting scientific nursing research in patient care, providing financial support for research, providing interdisciplinary research experience, disseminating and promoting dissemination of research findings, and conducting experimental investigation in methods of implementing research results.[67]

In 1969 the American Nurses' Association issued a *Statement on Graduate Education in Nursing*: "The major purpose of graduate study in nursing should be the preparation of nurse clinicians capable of improving nursing care through the advancement of nursing theory and science."

The assumptions which moved the membership of the A.N.A. Commission on Nursing Education to prepare the preceding statement were:

Graduate education is a more intensive and analytic extension of undergraduate education, enabling students to perceive and develop new relationships among the various factors and forces that affect nursing.

There is now available an increasingly large body of nursing knowledge which appropriately and logically belongs in graduate education.

Nursing must further develop and structure its body of knowledge, and add new knowledge that is relevant to both general and specialty practice.

Corporate responsibility for the education of nurse clinicians capable of advancing nursing theory and science rests with institutions of higher learning.

Nurses prepared at graduate levels can assume leadership in assessing the role of nursing in relation to changing concepts of health care, delineating action to bring about change, selecting that action most feasible at any given time, implementing decisions, and evaluating results in order to achieve quality nursing care.[68]

National League for Nursing

The National League for Nursing is a membership organization to improve nurs-

---

[66]*Ibid.*, p. 3.

[67]*Ibid.*, p. 4.
[68]American Nurses' Association. *Statement on Graduate Education in Nursing*, New York, A.N.A., 1969, p. 2.

ing, and thereby health services, through a coalition of community leaders, nurses, allied professionals, nursing service agencies, and schools of nursing. N.L.N. fosters community planning for nursing as a primary component of comprehensive health care, the development of nursing manpower, and high standards of nursing service and education.

At the biennial convention of this community organization for nursing, in May of 1967, a new structure was adopted. The new bylaws of the National League for Nursing, amended in 1967, were designed to provide a greater degree of flexibility in the structure of the organization. It was hoped that through this new form both the national board of directors and the constituent leagues could achieve a closer working relationship to reinforce each other's goals and objectives.

Greater freedom was afforded the constituent leagues to determine boundaries. State boundaries could define the limits of a constituent league, or a section of a state or a union of several states might be chosen in order to provide the best milieu for the consideration of "area" needs.

The principal framework of the National League for Nursing now consists of individual members and agency members; the *Assembly of Constituent Leagues for Nursing* together with six regional assemblies which provide coordination of planning and action among the constituent leagues; the councils of: Associate Degree Programs, Baccalaureate and Higher Degree Programs, Diploma Programs, Practical Nursing Programs, Hospital and Related Institutional Nursing Services and Home Health Agencies and Community Health Services.

The League's Council of Hospital and Related Institutional Nursing Services has been active in providing continuing education workshops for agency as well as individual members. A leadership workshop series focuses on the development of continuity of service—from hospital to continuing care facility to community health facility.

The Council of Home Health Agencies and Community Health Services assists agency members to meet problems faced by

them and individual nurses in the delivery of health services on the local level.

Open Curriculum in Nursing Education

In February 1970, the Board of Directors approved the following statement:

An open curriculum in nursing education is a system which takes into account the different purposes of the various types of programs but recognizes common areas of achievement. Such a system permits student mobility in the light of ability, changing career goals, and changing aspirations. It also requires clear delineation of the achievement expectations of nursing programs, from practical nursing through graduate education. It recognizes the possibility of mobility from other health related fields. It is an interrelated system of achievement in nursing education with open doors rather than quantitative serial steps.[69]

The Board of Directors approved the following *Statement of Concern About Degree Programs for Nursing Students That Have No Major in Nursing* in October 1971.

The National League for Nursing notes with concern the growth in the number of collegiate programs that have no major in nursing but are designed to appeal specifically to potential and enrolled nursing students and registered nurses. Publicity about these programs leads students to believe that they offer preparation for advanced positions in nursing or provide the base needed for further education in nursing when this is not the case.

The programs in question lead to associate or baccalaureate degrees in such fields as applied science, biology, education, health science, occupational therapy, psychology, and sociology. Large blocks of credit are promised the student for nursing education obtained outside the college. The collegiate programs may provide the student with increased knowledge in the specified area of the major, but they do not offer additional preparation in nursing.[70]

At the meeting of the Board of Directors in February 1972, a statement pertaining to *Nursing Education in the Seventies* was approved.

---

[69]National League for Nursing. *The Open Curriculum in Nursing Education*, New York, N.L.N., 1970.

[70]————. *A Statement of Concern About Degree Programs For Nursing Students That Have No Major in Nursing*, New York, N.L.N., 1971.

REFERENCE READINGS

Addams, Jane: *Forty Years at Hull House.* New York, The Macmillan Co., 1935.

American Journal of Nursing: *The Story of the Journal.* New York, American Journal of Nursing, 1950.

Anderson, Bernice E.: *Facilitation of the Interstate Movement of Nurses.* Philadelphia, J. B. Lippincott Co., 1950.

Boyd, Louie Croft: *State Registration for Nurses.* 2nd ed., Philadelphia, W. B. Saunders Co., 1915.

Breay, Margaret and Fenwick, Ethel Gordon: *The History of the International Council of Nurses, 1899–1925.* Geneva, The International Council of Nurses, 1931.

Bridges, Daisy C.: *A History of the International Council of Nurses 1899–1964.* Philadelphia, J. B. Lippincott Co., 1967.

Burgess, May Ayres: *Nurses, Patients and Pocketbooks.* New York, National League of Nursing Education, 1928.

Burgess, May Ayres: *Nursing Schools Today and Tomorrow.* New York, National League of Nursing Education, 1934.

Cannon, Ida M.: *Social Work in Hospitals: A contribution to progressive medicine.* New York, Russell Sage Foundation, 1923.

Committee on Nursing and Nursing Education in the United States: *Nursing and Nursing Education in the United States.* New York, The Macmillan Co., 1928.

Committee on Structure of National Nursing Organizations: *New Horizons in Nursing.* New York, The Macmillan Co., 1950.

Gardner, Mary S.: *Public Health Nursing.* 3rd ed. New York, The Macmillan Co., 1936.

Gelinas, Agnes: *Nursing and Nursing Education.* New York, Commonwealth Fund, 1946.

Gibbon, John Murray and Matthewson, Mary S.: *Three Centuries of Canadian Nursing.* New York, The Macmillan Company, 1947.

Giles, Dorothy: *A Candle in Her Hand, A Story of the Nursing Schools of Bellevue Hospital.* New York, G. P. Putnam's Sons, 1949.

Goodrich, Annie W.: *The Social and Ethical Significance of Nursing.* New York, The Macmillan Co., 1932.

Gray, James: *The University of Minnesota, 1851–1951,* Minneapolis, University of Minnesota Press, 1951.

Johns, Ethel and Pfefferkorn, Blanche: *An Activity Analysis of Nursing,* Committee on the Grading of Nursing Schools, New York, 1934.

Lee, Eleanor: *History of the School of Nursing of the Presbyterian Hospital, New York, 1892–1942.* New York, G. P. Putnam's Sons, 1942.

Lesnik, Milton J. and Anderson, Bernice L.: *Legal Aspects of Nursing.* Philadelphia, J. B. Lippincott, 1947. 292

_____. *Manual of Public Health Nursing.* Prepared by the NOPHN. New York, The Macmillan Company, 1926.

Marvin, Mary M.: "Research in Nursing—The Place of Research and Experimentation in Improving the Nursing Care of the Patient." *American Journal of Nursing,* 27:331, 1927.

Munson, H.: *The Story of the National League of Nursing Education.* Philadelphia, W. B. Saunders Co., 1934.

NACGN—*Four Decades of Service.* New York, The National Association of Colored Graduate Nurses, Inc., 1945.

_____. *Nursing Schools Today and Tomorrow.* Final Report of the Committee on the Grading of Nursing Schools, New York, 1934.

National League of Nursing Education. *A Curriculum Guide for Schools of Nursing.* New York, National League of Nursing Education, 1937.

_____. *Curriculum for Schools of Nursing.* New York, National League of Nursing Education, 1927.

_____. *Essentials of a Good School of Nursing.* New York, National League of Nursing Education, 1936.

_____. *Essentials of a Good School of Nursing.* Rev. ed. New York, National League of Nursing Education, 1942.

_____. *Standard Curriculum for Schools of Nursing.* New York, National League of Nursing Education, 1917.

National Organization for Public Health Nursing: *The Public Health Nursing Curriculum Guide.* New York, National Organization for Public Health Nursing, 1942.

Nutting, M. Adelaide: *A Sound Economic Basis for Schools of Nursing.* New York, G. P. Putnam's Sons, 1926.

Rathbone, William: *The History and Progress of District Nursing.* New York, The Macmillan Co., 1890.

Roberts, Mary M.: *American Nursing.* New York, The Macmillan Company, 1954.

Stewart, Isabel M.: *The Education of Nurses.* New York, The Macmillan Company, 1943.

Thoms, Adah B.: *Pathfinders—A History of the Progress of Colored Graduate Nurses.* New York, Kay Printing House, 1929.

Wayland, Mary M.: *The Hospital Head Nurse.* New York, The Macmillan Company, 1938.

Winslow, C. E. A.: "The Role of the Visiting Nurse in the Campaign for Public Health." *American Journal of Nursing,* Vol. 11, 1911.

CHAPTER 13

Nursing as a Continuing Social Force in Health Care in the Twentieth Century

NURSING—A DEFINITION

Virginia Henderson has defined nursing practice in the following way:

The unique function of the nurse is to assist the individual (sick or well), in the performance of those activities contributing to health or its recovery (or to peaceful death) that he would perform unaided if he had the necessary strength, will, or knowledge. And to do this in such a way as to help him gain independence as rapidly as possible.[1]

In reviewing the accomplishments of nursing it has been noted that nursing has not been restricted to a patient-centered approach but has included family-centered and community-oriented care. The location of the practice of the nurse has been found within the fabric of life itself. The significant difference has not been *where* the nurse practiced but the *quality* of *what* she did as a nurse practitioner. Cooperation and coordination between nurses in different settings as well as with all health workers has increased the value of the care received by the individual family and community.

In retrospect some of the highlights of nursing in this century will be reviewed against the background of Virginia Henderson's definition of nursing.

---

[1] Henderson, Virginia: *The Nature of Nursing.* New York, Macmillan, 1966.

NURSING—WHERE THE ACTION HAS BEEN

Nursing in the Community

The emphasis of the Goldmark Report on public health nursing focused attention on the need for inclusion of community nursing as a learning experience for well-prepared nurses.

The first nurses' settlement was the well known Henry Street Settlement in New York City, founded in 1893 by Lillian D. Wald.

At the close of the nineteenth century, sanitary inspectors visited schools and carried out a program of anticontagion service. Thousands of children were excluded from school because of pediculosis, ringworm, scabies, impetigo and trachoma.

Lillian Wald recognized the need for the well prepared nurse to play a dynamic role in the detection of illness, and the provision of care for these persons and their families, as well as prevention of disease and promotion of health.

Lillian Wald's first assignment as a graduate nurse was at the Juvenile Asylum in New York City where she discovered the treatment of the children to be abysmally cruel. She enrolled at the Women's Medical College and in her free time conducted classes in home nursing for immigrants. The critical need for help on the part of the poor and her strong interest in the role of the nurse caused her to terminate her medical educa-

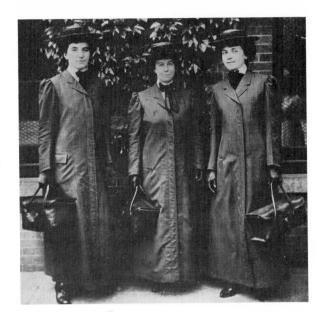

Figure 13–1. The official uniform adopted by the Henry Street Visiting Nurse Service in 1908.

tion and concentrate on the now world-famous project of developing the "House" on Henry Street that became the Henry Street Visiting Nurse Service (Figs. 13–1, 13–2 and 13–3).

Due to her motivation, lectures on public health nursing were inaugurated at Teachers' College, Columbia University in 1899. The Instructive District Nursing Association of Boston offered a postgraduate course in public health nursing in 1906. The first university course in public health nursing was given by Columbia University in 1910.

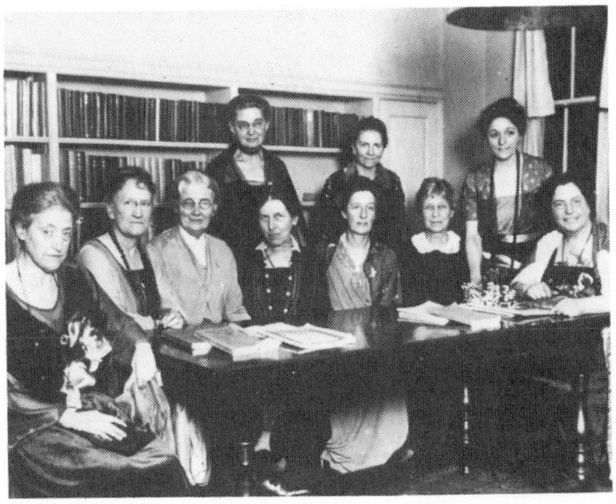

The Board of Education of the City of New York established the first class of ungraded pupils for the retarded children in 1900, which resulted in the creation of a separate department for special education for the mentally retarded in 1908.

Public health nursing began under voluntary philanthropic organizations that employed one or two nurses. Their service demon-

Figure 13–2. A group of nurse leaders at the opening of the Henry Street Visiting Nurse Service. Left to right: Annie W. Goodrich, Jane E. Hitchcock, Georgiana B. Judson, M. Adelaide Nutting, Henrietta Van Cleft, Rebecca Shatz, Mary Magonn Brown, Lavinia L. Dock, Elizabeth A. Frank, and Lillian D. Wald.

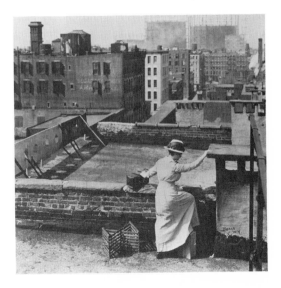

Figure 13–3. A nurse from the Henry Street Visiting Nurse Service takes a shortcut over the roofs of the tenements in New York's Lower East Side (ca. 1908). (Courtesy of Visiting Nurse Service of New York.)

strated their value and attracted public attention and support, including that of local and state Boards of Health who began to employ nurses.

In 1891 at the International Congress of Hygiene and Demography, Dr. Malcolm Morris proposed that a staff of specially educated nurses should visit the elementary schools regularly to examine the children. In 1892 *school nursing* was introduced into the school system in London. *Amy Hughes* accepted the invitation to become the first school nurse. She had been superintendent of the Queen's Nurses. It was not until 1907 that an act was passed which provided for medical inspection of school children in England.

In her book, *Practical Hints on District Nursing*, she discusses the power of the movement of nurses in the community. "The power of keeping a home together, when the alternative is the workhouse, is a social question with far-reaching consequences. To shorten the bread-winner's illness. . . . to save mothers of families from life-long effects of ignorance and neglect, to teach the proper management of infants and children, are gains to the community at large."[2] She states further: "The true way to help the poor is to teach them to help themselves."

By 1902, Lillian Wald encouraged the use of nurses to supplement the work of doctors in the schools of New York. *Lina Rogers* was sent from the Henry Street Settlement to a school on a one-month trial basis. She visited four schools a day, spending about one hour in each school with follow-up visits in the homes. This experiment was a successful one and dispensaries were improvised with supplies being furnished by the Board of Education. The nurses who were sent to assume this assignment felt the need for better education.

As early as 1903, New York City established the first municipally sponsored nursing service for children in schools. *Miss Lina L. Rogers* was employed by the Board of Health to direct this program. The area selected encompassed four schools with 4500 pupils in the worst slum areas of the city. In this setting Miss Rogers carried out a program of communicable disease control. It has been recorded that she visited the poor in crowded,

unhealthy tenements, and instructed both parents and children in personal cleanliness, demonstrated simple treatments that improved patients and prevented the spread of contagious diseases. Statistics reveal that as a result of this nurse leadership there was a marked reduction in the number of children absent from school. The identification of health needs and follow-through on the provision of necessary health facilities as well as the utilization of the nurse as a health teacher, contributed to the success of the project and the better health of the community. With the addition of many more nurses to this department, treatment clinics were established in the schools; this permitted students to receive care while attending school. School nurses visited newborn babies and mothers during the summer months, which had been such a hazardous period of the year for developing "cholera infantum" which caused a high infant mortality rate. It has been estimated that 1200 more babies survived that first summer. These creative nurses recognized the importance of the application of their knowledge to health teaching. Pamphlets were written as another tool for dissemination of important health information.

By 1907, inspection for communicable diseases among school children was delegated to the school nurse and school health programs were expanded.

"Little Mother's Leagues" (Fig. 13–4) were formed in the schools. Girls eight years old and over assumed the roles of little mothers and were taught how to care for their younger brothers and sisters. This opportunity was received with enthusiasm and was a valuable asset to the health of this community.

In 1905 school lunch programs were initiated by Miss Wald and the Board of Education of New York City served the lunches, which were available to all children in the public school system. The same year she realized the need for a Federal Children's Bureau; this became a reality in 1912 with a federal agency established to care specifically for children. Miss Wald was also instrumental in encouraging the organization of study halls because she and her staff realized the inadequacy of most homes for study.

The nurse in a school setting has been employed by one of three agencies: a board of education, a local health department or a community nursing service. Certification

---

[2]Hughes, Amy: *Practical Hints on District Nursing.* London, The Scientific Press, Ltd., pp. 2–3.

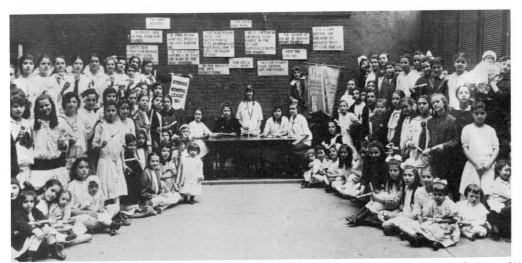

Figure 13–4. A positive and enthusiastic response to a call to participate in a Little Mother's League. (Courtesy of New York City Department of Health.)

requirements for nurses in a school system were enunciated without consultation with representatives of the nursing profession so that a foundation in education rather than a good preparation in nursing has been required. It cannot be denied that the educational requirements of certification broadened the background of school nurses.

In 1961, the American Nurses' Association and, in 1962, the National League for Nursing, recommended that school nurses have a baccalaureate degree and field experience in school nursing at the undergraduate or graduate level. Elizabeth Stobo's efforts as director of a study by the National League for Nursing resulted in guidelines for the preparation of school nurses.[3]

The California State Legislature passed the Fisher Bill in 1960 which lengthened the time required to prepare teachers from four years to five. This had a profound influence in the need for reevaluation of methods of preparation for the nurse in a school setting as well as that of the classroom teacher.

This was followed by two significant documents, one by Anne Marks[4] on the delineation of guidelines for content of graduate programs in school nursing, and the other by Helen Florentine[5] which discussed the preparation and role of the nurse in a program of school health.

San Francisco State College developed a supplementary program of 30 credits for graduate nurses who had earned a baccalaureate degree. Gudrun Burtz described this program as well as the role for which the students are being prepared.

The comprehensive role of the school nurse is one of an educator, which includes health counseling and guidance. She is the liaison between the school and the home. She works as a member of the health team in the school and . . . has special knowledge of . . . health problems. She interprets school problems to parents, and brings back to the teachers and principals the concerns of parents which affect the child's health.[6]

This highlighted a need for knowledge and understanding of the educational process.

The University of Colorado offers a program for school nurses who have baccalaureate degrees to become school nurse practitioners. The nurse practitioner is expected to assess psychological, neurological and

[3] Stobo, Elizabeth: *Findings of a Study Designed to Assist in the Development of Guidelines for the Preparation of Nurses for School Health Work.* New York, National League for Nursing, 1961.

[4] Marks, Anne P.: *School Nursing; Guidelines for Content of Graduate Programs of Study in the Specialty of School Nursing.* San Francisco, University of California School of Nursing, 1962.

[5] Florentine, Helen G.: *Preparation and the Role of Nurses in School Health Programs.* New York, National League for Nursing, 1962.

[6] Burtz, Gudrun S.: "A Fifth Year for School Nurse Preparation." *Nursing Outlook,* October 1969, pp. 38–40.

other problems that can affect the normal behavior of the child and his ability to learn. In addition to taking histories, doing physical examinations and giving immunizations and treatments for minor illnesses, the School Nurse Practitioner will supervise tests to detect and evaluate evidence of problems of speech, sight, hearing, posture or drug abuse.

Nursing's War Against Tuberculosis

Communicable diseases still continued to plague persons, families and communities at the turn of the century. Community nurses visited patients to assess their needs, and patients suffering from "consumption" or tuberculosis, which was the white plague in the early part of this century, received special attention. They distributed free milk and eggs to needy patients with tuberculosis. Because of the efforts of these nurses, a tuberculosis pavilion was opened in Riverside Hospital and a tuberculosis dispensary was organized with nurses in charge. The need for instruction by the visiting nurse was essential for preventive as well as curative measures. It was declared necessary to detect cases of tuberculosis in order to prevent the spread of the disease, and Dr. William Osler was the motivating force behind a project to carry out plans to do this.

In 1899, one of the women medical students at Johns Hopkins was selected to do follow-up work with dispensary patients in their homes. Through Dr. Osler's prompting, in 1900 the *Laënnec Society of Baltimore* was founded. It disseminated information of the disease to the public. By 1903, a nurse replaced the medical student and gave complete home care, which included instruction for the patient and his family. In 1910, work with tuberculosis patients was absorbed by the City Boards of Health. By 1904, the National Association for the Study and Prevention of Tuberculosis had been organized; by 1907, the Boston Consumptives' Hospital had developed a tuberculosis visiting nursing group within its Out-Patient Department; and, by 1908, an affiliation had become effective between the nursing staff and the Boston School for Social Workers.

Another specialized service within the overall coverage of nursing in the community was that of orthopedic nursing. In the late thirties,

Marguerite Wales in her well-known book *The Public Health Nurse in Action*, estimates that there were "between 400,000 and 500,000 children under twenty-one years of age who were crippled by disease or conditions such as poliomyelitis, tuberculosis of bones and joints, birth injuries, injuries due to accidents, and congenital deformities. . . ."[7] *Jessie L. Stevenson*, consultant in orthopedic nursing for the National Organization for Public Health Nursing stressed that nursing care of patients with orthopedic problems should be part of all nursing whether in the home or the hospital.

The dilemma of generalized nursing services in contrast to specialized nursing services was studied in the twenties by the American Red Cross. It was decided that specialized services isolate and concentrate on specific health entities while deleting the broader approach to the total physical, social, emotional and economic family problems embraced by the generalized type of service.

Even insurance companies became involved in the new aspects of community-based nursing. In 1909 the *Metropolitan Life Insurance Company* offered home nursing to its countless numbers of industrial policy-holders in the United States and Canada. The visiting nurse associations were enlisted to furnish the nursing with payment based upon the exact cost of the visits. In 1925 the *John Hancock Mutual Life Insurance Company* contracted for similar service. The value of health teaching and care in the conservation of life had been recognized.

In 1912, Miss Wald prevailed upon Mr. Jacob Schiff to donate money to the Red Cross for the purpose of inaugurating a system of *rural nursing*. This department was called Rural Nursing Service but the name was changed to *Town and Country Nursing*. Its service reached vast neglected areas of the country.

Miss Wald recognized that nursing leadership could penetrate any area where health needs of people were in jeopardy. She became a member of the New York State Immigration Commission in 1909 and upon making an inspection trip to two engineering projects revealed the exploitation of immigrant workers and deplorable living and

---

[7] Wales, Marguerite. *The Public Health Nurse in Action.* New York, The Macmillan Company, 1941, p. 252.

working conditions. She pleaded their cause which resulted in better enforcement of labor laws and health and sanitary facilities.

This kind of experience led Miss Wald to work for labor codes which were enacted in 1910. That same year she was appointed to membership on the New York Joint Board of Sanitary Control. The first inspection revealed that two-thirds of the 1243 shops visited were defective in fire protection, sanitation or both. As a result standards were delineated which eliminated sweat-shops in tenements. Due to her efforts as a member of the Factory Investigating Committee fire drills became mandatory.

When illness invaded the home, a family of moderate means needed nursing service to make the ill person comfortable and permit the family to continue their work program. A solution to this problem appeared in 1909 in Brattleboro, Vermont under the name of *Household Nursing*. There were three types of workers in this program: graduate nurses, supervised non-graduate nurses who performed household duties in addition to caring for the sick, and women who did housework in the homes of people with illness. This was an early professional nurse, practical nurse and homemaker aid team plan.

In 1912, when the *National Organization for Public Health Nursing* (NOPHN) was instituted, Lillian Wald was elected the first president. Membership in this organization was conferred only upon nurses possessing specified professional qualifications. Agencies could possess corporate membership only if organizations employed nurses of whom a given percentage were eligible for membership. One of the chief aims was to raise the educational standards for the practice of community nursing.

The U.S. Public Health Service openly proclaimed its dependence on the public health nurse. General Thomas Parran, when head of this service, said, "In this country more than any other, with the possible exception of Canada, there is almost complete recognition among public health officers and citizens alike of nursing as the spearhead of the whole public health movement. Dependence is placed upon it to advance new causes and to serve new needs."

The great foundations have aided materially in setting patterns and aiding public health work; they did not replace government projects, but supplemented them by providing services not undertaken by state and federal agencies.

The *Rockefeller Foundation*, established in 1913, has as its stated goal "To promote the well-being of mankind throughout the world."

Many leaders in the nursing field were staunch pacifists. Lavinia Dock worked ardently for world peace as did Annie W. Goodrich. In 1914 Lillian Wald was elected chairman of the American Union Against Militarism. Yet when the United States declared war, they all made every effort to bind up the wounds of suffering humanity.

When an epidemic of poliomyelitis struck New York City in 1916, the Henry Street Nursing Service gave meritorious service. At the termination of the war when the Spanish influenza epidemic occurred nurses were needed and responded.

The plight of all communities and their response to human need is reflected in reports about the afflictions of the Flu Epidemic of 1918. In one city, Lawrence, Massachusetts, the first case was reported on September 8 and lasted to the latter part of October. The devastation was unbelievable. Pneumonia became a serious complication.

At the outbreak of the epidemic in that city, the Armory was used as a temporary hospital and then an emergency open-air settlement was erected on the summit of Tower Hill overlooking the Merrimac River (Fig. 13–5). This settlement consisted of 100 tents furnished by military authorities and housed two patients in each tent. Many public health nurses were joined by volunteers, both lay people and members of religious orders. The method of protection for the nurses, in addition to washing their hands, frequently appears to have been wearing of masks (Fig. 13–6).

It is reported that the Surgeon General ordered wooden buildings to be erected on a hill for the treatment of the patients with pneumonia. The chairman of the Health Department in Lawrence, Massachusetts received orders at noon on a Sunday and by six o'clock, forty carpenters had started work erecting the building, which was 180 feet long and 15 feet wide and was ready for occupancy the following afternoon.

During this period in the city of Lawrence, 3155 cases were reported with 215 deaths from influenza and 247 deaths from pneumonia.

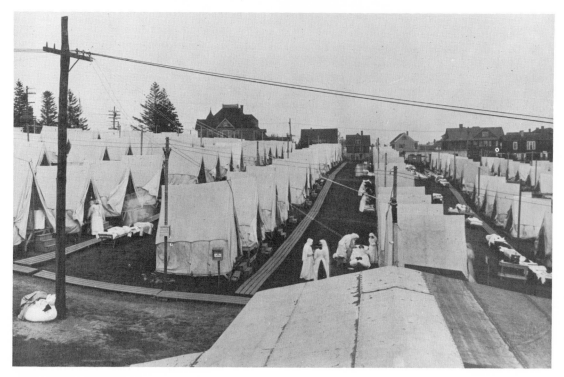

Figure 13–5. Tent City at Tower Hill (Emery Hill) in Lawrence, Massachusetts on May 29, 1919. This reveals the special hospital for victims of epidemic influenza. (Courtesy of American Red Cross.)

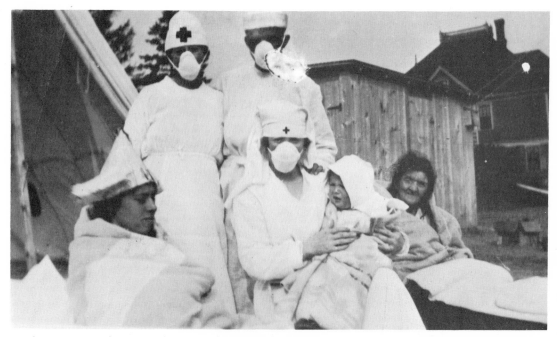

Figure 13–6. A closer view of Tent City shows the nurses and doctors wearing masks as a means of prevention. (Courtesy of Yvonne Charpentier, R. N.)

The disease was called Spanish Influenza because members of the royal family of Spain were purported to be the first victims of this outbreak. The last recorded appearance of the disease was in 1889.

Mary S. Gardner (Fig. 13–7) (1871–1961) of Providence, R. I., founded an outstanding visiting nurse organization there. Her book on the subject was the first and for long the only text available. She was for many years recognized as a national authority in public health nursing, and is internationally known.

Miss Gardner, R.N., M.A., graduated from Newport (R. I.) Hospital, and was director of the Providence District Nursing Association until 1931. During part of this time she assisted the Red Cross in Washington and Italy (with Edna Foley) and inspected Red Cross child welfare work in Europe. She was the second president of the N.O.P.H.N. and chairman of the public health nursing section of the I.C.N. She has written *Public Health Nursing, So Build We* and *Katherine Kent*, the last two being novels of public health nursing.

Lavinia Lloyd Dock was another pioneer in public health nursing. She came from a cultured philanthropic family. She and her brother shared an interest in the medical fields of endeavor. This brother became a professor of medicine in the schools of medicine at the University of Michigan and Washington University.

Miss Dock entered Bellevue Training School for Nurses from which she graduated in 1886. Her first assignment was with a pioneering effort called the United Workers of Norwich, Connecticut. This group wanted to try a three months' experiment whereby a trained nurse would take care of the sickness in the community. Through her efforts it was a successful experiment. She volunteered for service during a yellow fever epidemic, was one of the group of visiting nurses with the New York City Mission and finally became assistant to Miss Hampton (Mrs. Robb) at Johns Hopkins Hospital. After a brief experience as principal of the Illinois Training School for Nurses in Chicago, she joined the Henry Street Settlement in New York City to work with Lillian Wald. Interest in her patients prompted Miss Dock to spend her free time studying languages.

It was the belief of Lavinia Dock that a public health movement on a world basis would emphasize prevention, thereby creating a need for a better educated nurse than the bedside nurse of the time.

Miss Dock was the first secretary of the American Society of Superintendents of Training Schools for Nurses. In addition, she was the first secretary of the I.C.N. The nurses of the United States and the world profited by her wisdom and guidance as an officer of both organizations and a contributor of many articles to the early issues of the *American Journal of Nursing*. Her gift for writing has been preserved in her early textbooks: *A Materia Medica for Nurses* and *Hygiene and Morality*, as well as the magnificent contribution of the four-volume *History of Nursing*, which she authored in collaboration with M. Adelaide Nutting. This remains a lasting memorial to two brilliant, scholarly and gifted leaders of nursing.

Mary Beard was a member of the international health committee of the Rockefeller Foundation and was head of the American Red Cross Nursing Service. Ella Phillips Crandall, Edna Foley, Elizabeth G. Fox, Marguerite Wales, and Harriet Fulmer were also prominent in public health nursing early in this century.

Community health needs continued, on occasion manifesting unusual aspects. The 1930's brought stress and distress in many

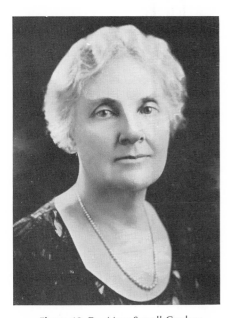

Figure 13–7. Mary Sewall Gardner.

forms with poverty and unemployment as a consequence. Low-cost housing was built on the Lower East Side due to the vision and prodding of Miss Wald.

In addition to housing, the ancient system of almsgiving was reintroduced and agencies gave food to the "bread lines" of people. The *Works Progress Administration* (WPA) utilized the human resources of our country to assist in many welfare services.

A highly respected author, *Faith Baldwin*, wrote a popular book[8] which she dedicated to "The V.N.A. and Welfare Nurses Everywhere." This was widely read and served in its way to assist in appreciating the nurse in the community.

The Department of Philanthropic Information of the Central Hanover Bank and Trust Company issued a brochure on *The Public Health Nurse.* The purpose was to pay tribute to the unprecedented accomplishments of public health nurses and to broaden their contributions by encouraging anyone interested in "wise public giving" by presenting a "bird's-eye view of current activities and needs in that field." In urging financial support the bank officials quoted Dr. Howard W. Haggard:

You who have done the work, and I who have watched as an interested spectator, do not need to have our emotions aroused. We have seen and we have heard. We know the stories of the tragedies averted and lives saved behind the bare records of those 29,000,000 visits last year. We have heard the sound of hoofbeats and creak of leather as a nurse on horseback rides alone at night over a rough mountain trail to a cabin, and there in the uncertain light of an oil lamp helps to bring a new life into the world. . . . The future of an American family has hung on her help and on her gift of the priceless knowledge of feeding, care, cleanliness, disease prevention.

And again, in surroundings perhaps less picturesque, but none the less vital, we have heard the footsteps—often weary ones—of the nurse and the creak of the tenement stairs she mounts, and from above we have heard the cry of a fretting, feverish child to whom the nurse brings the soothing hand of comfort; and the sigh of a desperate mother to whom the nurse brings the clear, cold knowledge to solve those problems from which the tragedies of a home may come.

You have heard those sounds for the millions of visits you have made; but there are a hundred million of our people who have not heard them.

They have not seen, or felt, or known. Is it not then your duty to amplify these sounds so familiar to you until they reach the ears of every citizen, and reaching them, stir sentiment until a hundred million strong they join with their support to the work you carry out.[9]

A well-respected nurse, Mary S. Gardner, wrote of the high place nursing took in the life of our country:

We see that she has had her effect on city and state legislation, and has influenced public opinion to effect non-legislative reform. We find her valued as a preventive agent and health instructor by municipalities and state bodies, and the usefulness of her statistics acknowledged by research workers. . . . She is found in the juvenile courts and public playgrounds, in the department stores and big hotels, in the schools and factories, in the houses of small wage-earners and in the swarming tenements of the very poor. We find her in the big cities, the small towns, and to a limited extent in the rural districts and the lonely mountain regions. We find her dealing with tuberculosis, babies, mental cases, industrial workers, expectant mothers, and housing conditions.[10]

MATERNAL AND CHILD HEALTH NURSING

In the area of maternal and child health nursing, many changes have taken place since the inception of the twentieth century. At the turn of the century the nurses needed to know: the hygiene of pregnancy; how to recognize approaching labor; how to help the doctor and comfort the mother during that labor; what supplies were necessary and how to prepare them; how to prepare the patient; how to examine and when and why; how to prevent septic infection; how to guard against hemorrhage; what symptoms precede eclampsia; what to do at a normal birth (with or without a doctor); what to do at an instrumental delivery; how to prevent attacks of puerperal fever; the aftercare (with or without complications); and the care of the new baby.[11]

In the 1920's a maternity center was run by nurses. The nurse examined, taught, visited and helped the mother. She referred

---

[8] Baldwin, Faith: *District Nurse.* Philadelphia, The Blakiston Company, 1932.

[9] Dr. Howard W. Haggard in *Public Health Nursing,* April, 1936.
[10] *Ibid.,* pp. 39–40.
[11] Keith, Mary L.: "Preliminaries of Obstetric Nursing," *American Journal of Nursing,* January 1901, Vol. 1, p. 257.

women to the obstetrician and coordinated all other facilities.[12]

In the 1930's three phases of maternal care were recognized—pre-natal, labor and delivery, and postnatal. The nurse now had an expansion in her role. In addition she was the one who gave the pre-parent education. The literature indicates that German and Russian obstetricians were reported to be using hypnosis to ease the pains of childbirth. In 1933, *Dr. Grantly Dick Read* introduced a form of *natural childbirth.* Read believed that if fear and tension could be eliminated, the pain would be eliminated or minimized. The women were taught the physical facts of childbirth and how to relax, exercise, concentrate and breathe properly. The nurse took an active role in the classes for prepared childbirth.

Many women were anesthetized very heavily for the delivery process during this period and many hospital policies excluded fathers from the labor and delivery rooms.

By 1950, in many schools of nursing, a practice was instituted whereby a student was assigned to a mother for whom she cared during labor and delivery (Fig. 13–8). She helped with breathing exercises, back rubs and supported her patient emotionally. Many nurses and doctors realized that individual care was more important than a strict routine.[13]

In this fifth decade, Grace-New Haven Hospital launched a pioneer experiment in which many mothers attended antepartal clinics during their entire pregnancy. The Clinic provided classes given by obstetricians and obstetrical nurses which included exercise classes and a tour of the obstetrical department. Everything was done to eliminate her fears. Husbands were permitted to be with their wives in the labor and delivery room to provide emotional support and to assist in elimination of fear. After the delivery, the infant was placed in a plastic crib by the mother's bed. During the rooming-in period the mother and father became acquainted with and learned to care for their child. Individualized care was given to mother

---

[12]Stevens, Ann: "Maternity Center Work." *American Journal of Nursing*, Vol. XX, March 1920, pp. 456–457.

[13]Corbin, Hazel: "Maternity Care Today and Tomorrow." *American Journal of Nursing*. Vol. 53, February 1953, pp. 201–204.

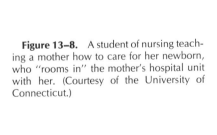

Figure 13–8. A student of nursing teaching a mother how to care for her newborn, who "rooms in" the mother's hospital unit with her. (Courtesy of the University of Connecticut.)

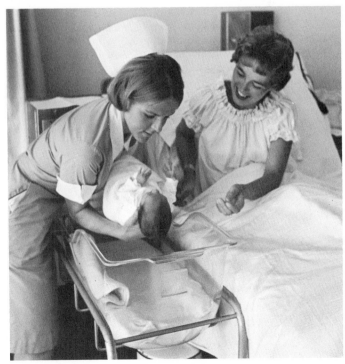

and baby and the family as a unit was emphasized.[14]

In Europe *midwifery* has been considered an important specialty, with a two-year course commonly required. Formerly in England nearly all state-registered nurses were registered midwives as well.

In the United States the subject had been neglected despite the fact that the maternal death rate had been high and that a considerable number of untrained, ignorant midwives were practicing. The training of nurses in midwifery had been prevented by the attitude of the medical profession, which held the ideal that every woman should be aided in delivery by a physician. In actual fact, thousands of women live where no doctor is available; other thousands employ incompetent midwives. In rural districts the need for the midwife nurse is especially apparent. One million women annually in the United States have deliveries without the aid of a physician and a quarter of a million are attended by untrained women.

In 1911, Bellevue Hospital founded a *school of midwifery* to help care for the 40,000 mothers per year in New York who were assisted in delivery by untrained women. For many years there were nine centers offering courses and granting certificates in nurse-midwifery such as Maternity Center Association in New York City, which opened the first school for nurse-midwives in the United States, in cooperation with the Lobenstine Clinic; Tuskegee Institute, Alabama; Mary Breckinridge's Frontier Nursing Service, Kentucky and the Catholic Maternity Institute, Santa Fe, New Mexico.

The Catholic Maternity Institute is under the Medical Mission Sisters, a Catholic organization founded in 1925, which has centers in England, Holland and India. The sisters are fully trained doctors, pharmacists, nurses and technicians who do missionary work at home and abroad.

There are six schools which offer the certificates in conjunction with a master's degree —Yale, Johns Hopkins, New York Medical College, Catholic University, Columbia University, and the University of Utah.

The first organized *midwifery service* in this country was conducted by *Mary Breckinridge*

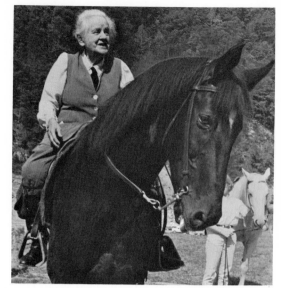

Figure 13–9. Mary Breckinridge at age 82 on her horse "Doc." (Courtesy of *Courier-Journal* and *Louisville Times*.)

(Fig. 13–9), a graduate of St. Luke's, New York, who had organized public health nursing in France. Until recently Miss Breckinridge used English-trained nurse midwives since there were so few in this country. Her nurses travelled on horseback to assist women in childbirth who live in remote places, but jeeps have now replaced the more traditional vehicle of travel. Miss Breckinridge's goal to provide a program of good health care for all persons in an area of severe social and economic deprivation has been realized. Her original plan of family-centered care prompted the need for her nurses to be well prepared and this included certification as a nurse midwife for each of her nursing staff.

She implemented her philosophy of helping people to help themselves by including the people in the community in planning the programs given by the Frontier Nursing Service.

Dr. Gertrude Isaacs, who was the first nurse to earn a *Doctor of Nursing Science* degree, is now in charge of the Family Nurse educational program.[15]

Vanderbilt University School of Nursing

---

[14]Jensen, Faith E.: "Having a Baby is a Family Matter." *American Journal of Nursing*, Vol. 50, October 1950, pp. 674–675.

[15]Schutt, Barbara G.: "Frontier's Family Nurses." *American Journal of Nursing*. Vol. 72, No. 5, May 1972, pp. 903–909.

has inaugurated an eight-week field experience at the Frontier Nursing Service in their master's program in Family Nursing.

Maternity care is again being provided with nurse-midwifery services. Dorothea Lang, who directs the Nurse-Midwifery Program in the New York City Department of Health, describes the current role and function[16] of the nurse-midwife as a specialist who combines two disciplines—nursing and midwifery. The maternity program in New York City provided services in the community health centers of the Department of Health which then affiliated with a nearby hospital. The nurse-midwife becomes incorporated in the clinic-hospital affiliation program and "acts as a liaison between the clinic and hospital teams and may serve as a 'ombudsman' for patients."[17] The care of the newborn is an essential aspect of the service.

The interdisciplinary and interdependency function is described as:

The Certified Nurse-Midwife assumes many of the functions of the physician as they relate to the medically uncomplicated patient. However, she does not assume the ultimate responsibility, which continues to rest with the medical staff. Neither does she assume the responsibility of the nursing care of the patient, which falls within the realm of nursing but rather she extends and supplements some of the nursing services so that patients may benefit more fully from the existing maternity, new-born, and interconceptional care programs.[18]

Referrals play an important role in the functions of the nurse midwife, who refers her patients for continuity of care from the public health nurse, nutritionist, social worker or dentist, if needed, and even specialized services of the affiliating hospital are utilized.

In a *Symposium on Maternity Nursing*[19] the changing role of the maternity nurse and maternity nursing to patient-focused and "family-centered" nursing care is described. That change has been needed is reflected in one fact alone: that many countries have a lower infant mortality rate. Hilliard reports[20] that in 1951 there were five countries while in 1966, sixteen countries reported lower infant mortality rates than in the United States.

CARE OF CHILDREN

In 1865 an unusual charity known as *St. John's Guild* was founded by Rev. Alvak Wiswall. It carried out an extensive program among the poor in the crowded areas of New York City. The plans included a volunteer visitor for every block of tenement houses so that in times of great destitution or sickness every family could be visited and cared for. In 1874 the Guild established a floating hospital (Fig. 13–10) so mothers could take sick children from their "dens" to the cool breezes of the river to breathe fresh air. The members of the Guild could not refuse certain elderly people who pleaded for this healthful opportunity.

Another interesting and important nursing contribution to child care took place when the *Boston Floating Hospital* (Fig. 13–11) had its origin in 1894. It began its tour of duty as a rented excursion boat towed around Boston Harbor to give indigent mothers and their sick babies relief from the summer heat. From its inception it has provided substantial knowledge of infant feeding and problems of disease in children, especially of infectious summer diarrhea and dysentery.

The story of the Boston Floating Hospital is an interesting one. In the 1890's when humanitarianism was reflected in organized philanthropic enterprises, certain writers had served as catalysts. *Edward Everett Hale* (1822–1909) exemplified this type of person and two of his books, *Ten Times One Is Ten* and *In His Name*, stimulated the formation of several groups dedicated to helping the destitute, the sick, the aged, and the malnourished. It is reported[21] that on a hot summer night in 1893, the Rev. Rufus Toby, a close friend of Mr. Hale, was returning home from an exhausting day in Boston. He noted the large numbers of mothers who were carrying infants across the South Boston Bridge trying to escape the heat and con-

[16]Lang, Dorothea: "Providing Maternity Care Through a Nurse Midwifery Service Program." *The Nursing Clinics of North America*. Philadelphia, W. B. Saunders Co., Vol. 4, No. 3, September 1969, pp. 509–520.

[17]*Ibid.*, p. 516.

[18]*Ibid.*, p. 512.

[19]Rains, Anna P., et al.: "Symposium on Maternity Nursing." *The Nursing Clinics of North America*. Philadelphia, W. B. Saunders Co., Vol. 3, No. 2, June 1968, pp. 275–365.

[20]*Ibid.*, p. 277.

[21]Beaven, Paul: "A History of the Boston Floating Hospital." *Pediatrics*. Vol. 19, No. 4, April, 1957.

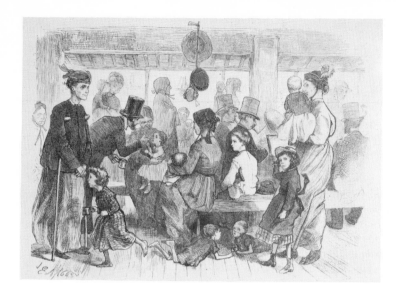

Figure 13–10. The Floating Hospital of St. John's Guild. (Author's collection.)

gestion of their tenement dwellings. It occurred to him that an excursion boat might be a suitable solution. Money was obtained through the efforts of many influential persons such as Edward Everett Hale for five trips.

The first trip took place on July 25, 1894 when the rented barge, *Clifford,* was towed away from Pickett's Wharf in East Boston. In order to obtain passage aboard this boat, an admission ticket had to be obtained from a physician by a mother for herself and her sick child. The *Clifford,* which was used ordinarily for Sunday excursions and moonlight cruises, underwent a transformation when the cruise furniture was removed and cots, bassinets, and equipment for sterilizing milk

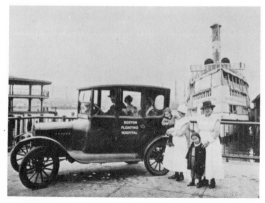

Figure 13–11. Returning children to their homes from a day's health care on the Boston Floating Hospital facilities. (Author's collection.)

were installed. The project was a success and money was obtained for continued service.

This project was tremendously important in coping with the care and treatment of infants with infectious summer diarrhea, frequently referred to as cholera infantum. The infant mortality rate was exceedingly high. Parents felt that if they could keep children alive through their second summer then chances of survival increased remarkably.

The need for a staff of physicians and nurses to diagnose and treat the various pediatric disorders became of paramount importance. In 1897 the hospital became incorporated and very sick infants began to be kept on board as in-patients. The Boston Floating Hospital now provided care for sick infants, a learning experience for students of nursing and medicine, and an opportunity for research in the problems of the sick child.

Among the assigned duties of the nurse in 1900 were to provide instruction for mothers on care of well children, preparation of formulas, in addition to the care and treatment of sick ones (Fig. 13–12). The nurse participated in many research projects. The first recorded research involved the observation and treatment of diarrhea. It attracted the notice of Dr. Simon Flexner of the University of Pennsylvania who came on board to observe this research.

With the purchase and commission of a new 170 foot boat in 1905, the larger hospital and laboratory facility increased the research activities and assisted many more sick infants.

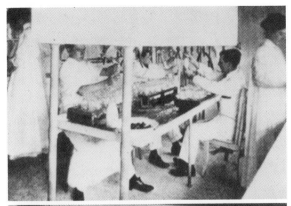

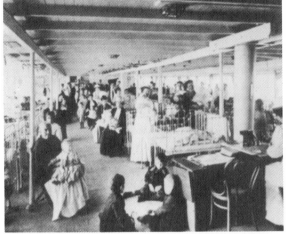

Figure 13–12. Scenes aboard the Boston Floating Hospital. (*Above*) Using a "mechanical cow" in the formula room, the staff prepared dozens of formulas prescribed for individual infants each day. (*Below*) The effects of various formulas were examined clinically on the hundreds of children on the decks of the hospital.

The study focused on the causation, recognition and treatment of diarrheal diseases of infancy. The research findings were most rewarding.

In 1921 a law was passed in Boston that required pasteurization of milk, and a downward trend was noted in the incidence of summer diarrhea. This development focused attention on infant nutrition. Human milk banks were instituted and research commenced on the chemistry of milk and suitability of formulas.

One morning in June, 1927 when the boat had been refurbished for another season, a fire destroyed the entire structure, including records. This institution had served a vital need at a time of urgency, so it was decided to build a permanent hospital and to join with Tufts Medical School and the Boston Dispensary to become the New England Medical Center.

Only in the last 100 years have we had children's hospitals and separate departments for the care of children in general hospitals. (See Figure 13–13.) Many a child with a childhood affliction was cared for at home. Emphasis was on the disease rather than the child.

In 1908, *Sister Amy* (Fig. 13–14) of the Sisters of St. Margaret presented a program of specialization in nursing care for sick children at the Fourteenth Annual Meeting of the Superintendents of Training Schools. In carrying out the program, a study of the normal growth and development of the child was proffered.

In reviewing the development of nursing in child care Blake states that:

Recognition of the need for special instruction of nurses in the care of children roughly parallels the development of separate units for the care of children which appeared first in foundling homes, then in the children's hospitals and finally in the pediatric units within general hospitals. Associated with some of the earliest children's hospitals—

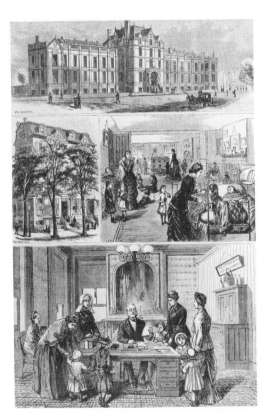

Figure 13–13. Early beginnings of the Children's Hospital in Boston as seen in 1881. The Huntington Avenue Hospital; the Rutland Street Hospital; a ward in the Rutland Street Hospital; the out-patient department on Washington Street. (Courtesy of The Children's Hospital, Boston.)

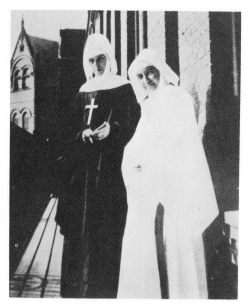

Figure 13–14. Sister Amy and Sister Lucilla of the Episcopal Sisters of St. Margaret, who first directed and staffed the Children's Hospital in Boston.

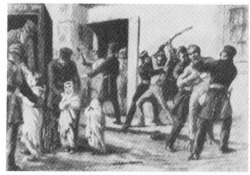

Figure 13–15. During the outbreak of smallpox in Montreal in 1885, fathers fought police officers while children were herded into a van which took them to a pest house.

those in Philadelphia, Denver, Boston and New York—schools were established which were devoted to the training of nurses in the care of sick children. But it was not until departments of pediatrics were firmly established in medical schools that pediatrics became a compulsory part of the undergraduate nursing school curriculum. University graduate study of pediatric nursing did not appear until the fourth decade of this century. Supplementary courses for registered nurses were given in many children's hospitals, but the development of university programs of study leading to specialization in the field are of comparatively recent origin.[22]

The well-prepared nurse in a child care setting joins with many other specialists such as child psychologists, psychiatrists and nutritionists in providing health care delivery and in the identification of new knowledge. The nurse not only gives nursing care but acts as a "liaison between children, doctors, parents and other professional and ancillary workers who are involved in the provision of care."[23]

At the beginning of the twentieth century, the causes of many diseases, most of them communicable, were unknown. Illnesses were prolonged and serious, were a medical chal-

lenge, and necessitated skilled nursing care during the lengthy illness which was given in the home. Parents fought against members of their families being sent to general hospitals or isolation hospitals for care. The frightening aspects of the isolation procedures with techniques coupled with limited visiting hours and a general discouragement of members of the family coming in contact with the ill member produced serious emotional stress (Figs. 13–15 and 13–16). In a period when antibiotics were nonexistent, the time-consuming aspects of isolation techniques minimized the consideration of the child's need for emotional support from his family and the need of companionship and toys.

The discovery of antibiotics, the advances in medical knowledge, including that of nutrition and psychology, plus a marked change in all aspects of health care delivery and hospitalization have produced demands for a new role for nursing practice.

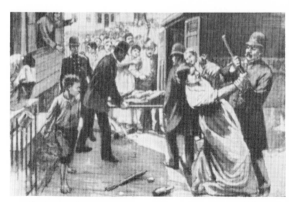

Figure 13–16. Families resisting police in Milwaukee in 1886 during a typhoid epidemic. Patients were brought to the isolation hospital.

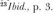

[22] Blake, Florence G., and Wright, F. Howell: *Essentials of Pediatric Nursing.* 7th ed. Philadelphia, J. B. Lippincott, 1963, p. 2.
[23] *Ibid.,* p. 3.

Clinical Nurse Specialist in Child Care

In discussing this pediatric nurse specialist role, Wingert indicates:

Increased use of immunizations and better control of communicable diseases have shifted emphasis in child health to prevention of illness, interpreting growth and development, and management of behavior problems . . . child health is no longer a luxury but rather a necessity, calling not for episodic care but for preventative, continuous, and comprehensive attention. Each child must be allowed to grow and develop physically, socially, and emotionally to his full capacity, and parents must have access to continuing guidance to help him reach this goal by using appropriate community resources. This means that child health must be family-centered, not child-centered, and it covers a more inclusive time span from conception through adolescence, rather than birth to twelve years.[24]

Wingert states further:

The nurse specialist's actions are based on a depth of knowledge in her particular field. In child health this knowledge includes advanced preparation in child, family, and community patterns of adaptation, health care, and growth and development. Emphasis is placed on the interactions between individuals, within families, and in the community; communicating with children at their level; and increasing observation, interviewing, and counseling skills. This knowledge is used to ascertain physical, developmental, social, and emotional health, and to promote or change existing patterns of adaptation. The nurse specialist has a higher level of skill in decision making . . .[25]

The nurse specialist incorporates a greater depth of knowledge of the behavioral, biological and physical sciences into the family-centered child care.

Another view of a nurse clinical specialist is presented by Miss Barnes. In describing a psychiatric cardiac team which was formed to explore the needs of cardiac children, Miss Barnes[26] described that team as consisting of a child psychiatrist, a nurse clinical specialist and a psychiatric social worker. In describing the role of the *nurse clinical specialist,* three areas are encompassed: service, education and research, but the key role is

care of the child, which includes support of the anxious parents.

Miss Barnes related that from the initial cases this professional team studied, they learned the following:

1. Each of the children underwent a critical experience or was the victim of severe anxiety preceding his admission.
2. All of the parents were unable to communicate with their children and to allay their fears before admission and before surgery.
3. These anxious children could be helped to express their fears by a nurse clinical specialist and these children had the strength to endure stress if they were given support and could be helped to focus attention on the cause of the fear.
4. The parents needed as much help from the nurse clinical specialist as the children in overcoming their own fears.

Child Care Philosophy

At the beginning of the century the philosophy of child care involved strict discipline. In the school setting if one spared the rod it was felt that the child would be spoiled. Even when parents loved their children they were careful not to indulge them. The care of infants and children was marked by strict adherence to a time schedule, and individual growth patterns and needs were not considered.

In childhood, obedience to parents and teachers was mandatory and "self expression" was not encouraged. Slow learners were subjected to cruel treatment by adults and to ridicule by their peers.

Friedrich Froebel, born in Thuringia in 1782, believed children belonged to society as well as their parents. It was he who introduced the kindergarten (children's garden) system which emphasized that education could be enjoyable as well as informative. It was he who stressed: the baby has not become a child, nor has the child become a youth, by reaching a certain age but only by having lived through childhood, and on through youth, true to the requirements of his mind, his feelings, and his body. Froebel's educational goal was designed to strengthen their bodies, educate their senses, awaken their minds and acquaint them with nature and their fellow men.

School was not a pleasant experience for many children. Mothers of impoverished

[24]Wingert, Patricia: "The Pediatric Nurse Specialist in the Community," *Nursing Outlook,* 17 (Dec., 1969), p. 28.
[25]*Ibid.,* p. 30.
[26]Barnes, Corinne M.: "Working with Parents of Children Undergoing Heart Surgery." *Nursing Clinics of North America,* Vol. 4, No. 1, March, 1969.

families kept children at home because of ragged clothing which brought shame and scorn on the children. Many children were placed in factories at an early age with very little schooling.

In 1896, Maria Montessori was the first woman to earn the degree of doctor of medicine in Italy, having graduated from the Medical College of the University of Rome. She was a woman of intelligence, compassion and strong spirituality and was a staunch humanitarian. She was chosen to represent the women of Italy at a feminist congress in Berlin.

Dr. Montessori studied the health needs of individuals and recognized that if society was to be healthy, children should be taught how to live as well as how to learn. She was appalled at the treatment of the mentally retarded while she was participating in a residence program in a psychiatric institution. She championed the need for education and rehabilitation of the retarded. A state school was founded called the *Orthophenic School,* where under her guidance retarded children from schools and psychiatric institutions received a carefully planned program of education. She was successful and these students, many of whom had been referred to as idiots, surpassed so-called normal children on regular examinations.

Maria Montessori then pressed the need for all children to have a different educational program. Her method of education, the Montessori Method, has had wide acceptance and has been most successful. Not all programs identified as "Montessori" follow the educational pattern she developed.

Dr. Montessori had a great influence on child care in the home, school and hospital and played an important role in eliminating the rigidity of child health practices. She assumed the roles of both nurse and physician when rendering health care.

Modern Child Health Care

In focusing on child health needs in the latter part of the twentieth century, many programs and resources are available to assist in the provision of child care. Even the hospital setting has returned to a family-centered form of care but with the enriched dimension of the application of behavioral, biological and health science principles. Provision for permitting mothers or a member of the family on a rooming-in basis has been available for some time. In addition there has been a trend toward relaxation in the schedule of visiting hours.

In a *Symposium on Family-Centered Care in a Pediatric Setting*[27] the benefits of the delivery of care in a milieu which is geared to a more healthful life for the child and his family are presented as are the role of the nurse and the components of nursing in such a family-centered setting. Coping with the problem of death and dying for a child and the family; assisting the adolescent's quest for self-identity in family-centered care; finding ways of introducing programs for staff development to encourage implementation of family-centered nursing care between the hospital and home complete the presentation of ways of planning for the most satisfying and therapeutically sound child care.

Yet, not all children receive this kind of satisfaction in living because of inability to receive the benefits of a program in good health care. Another tragic plight which afflicts many children during these last years of the twentieth century is that of the "battered child" syndrome. Joan Hopkins urges the nursing profession to "assume its role in the tremendous responsibility of case-finding, prevention and treatment of the abused and neglected child. No other profession has the opportunity to spend as much meaningful time with these patients and their families as does the nurse."[28] The members of the health professions are protected by law in many states and nurses are being called upon to testify in cases of child neglect and child abuse.

Many infants and children need and receive very special and complicated health care. Many of these clinical settings, technical procedures and nursing skills are presented in a "Symposium on Care of the Infant and Young Child."[29]

In an article entitled "The Pediatric Nurse

---

[27] Beatty, Audry, et al.: "Symposium on Family-Centered Care in a Pediatric Setting." *The Nursing Clinics of North America,* Philadelphia, W. B. Saunders Co., Vol. 7, No. 1, March 1972, pp. 1–93.

[28] Hopkins, Joan: "The Nurse and the Abused Child." *Nursing Clinics of North America.* Philadelphia, W. B. Saunders Co., Vol. 5, No. 4, December 1970, pp. 589–598.

[29] Rothrock, E. Cleves, et al.: "Symposium on Care of the Infant and Young Child." *Nursing Clinics of North America.* Philadelphia, W. B. Saunders Co., Vol. 5, No. 3, September 1970, pp. 373–448.

Practitioner," appearing in the March, 1971 issue of the *American Journal of Nursing*, the developmental sequence of the concept of the role of the pediatric nurse practitioner, guidelines on short-term programs for continuing education for pediatric nurse associates and description of such a practitioner in a neighborhood center were presented. In perusing the literature from 1963 to 1970, the authors reviewed "only the studies of pediatric primary care (ambulatory) settings in which registered nurses . . . assumed broad responsibilities in collaboration with practicing pediatricians." The gradual expansion of the role of the nurse from her traditional early twentieth century one is apparent. Proponents and opponents have reacted to the concept of the nurse practitioner, but the authors, Andrews and Yankauer, feel that the major obstacles are: concept confusion, disagreements about content and method of training, and problems in the adaptation of both nurse and physician to the role changes and collaborative working relationships demanded of them.

In examining the current role of the pediatric nurse practitioner the opposition from nurse leaders is reflected as follows:

Some nursing leaders charge that such a nurse practitioner has abandoned her identity as a professional nurse to become a physician's assistant. Other nursing leaders are concerned that a variety of continuing education and in-service programs conducted outside graduate schools of nursing claim to prepare such a nurse practitioner. Differences of opinion center on the length of training and the legitimacy of including medical as well as nursing faculty in teaching and in supervision of clinical practice. Some nursing educators believe the baccalaureate program already prepares a nurse to assume the pediatric nurse practitioner role: others believe that only a master's degree program can do so.

Despite the objections which have been presented, Andrews and Yankauer held that: "The effects of current shortages in pediatric manpower can be expressed in terms of human need and suffering. The pediatric nurse practitioner appears to offer an acceptable, practical, and workable contribution toward alleviating the manpower shortage."

A joint statement was issued by the American Nurses' Association and the American Academy of Pediatrics:

The American Nurses' Association and American Academy of Pediatrics recognize collaborative

efforts are essential to increase the quality, availability and accessibility of child health care in the U.S.A. In order to meet the health care needs of children, it is essential that the skills inherent in the nursing and medical professions be utilized more efficiently in the delivery of child health care.

Innovative methods are needed to utilize these professional skills more fully. One such innovative approach is the development of the Pediatric Nurse Associate program. (The titles "Pediatric Nurse Associate" and "Pediatric Nurse Practitioner" are used interchangeably.) This program will enable nurses, both in practice and reentering practice, to update and expand their knowledge and skills. It is essential that physicians become more aware of the skills and abilities of the nursing profession and that such skills be expanded in the area of ambulatory child health to enable both the nurse and the physician to devote their efforts in the delivery of child health care to the areas of their respective professional expertise.

ROLE OF THE PSYCHIATRIC-MENTAL HEALTH NURSE

In tracing the historical development of psychiatric and mental health nursing, the changes that took place in the role of the nurse, in the inception of hospitals devoted exclusively to the care of the mentally ill, and the beginning foundation of psychiatry and psychology as fields of endeavor all played a significant role.

An illuminating view of the care received by a person who was mentally ill is available through the indefatigable efforts of *Clifford W. Beers* (1876–1945).

Mr. Beers, when a young graduate of Yale, attempted to commit suicide by jumping from the fourth story window of his home. He was rescued; though seriously injured, he was alive. He was incarcerated for three years in various institutions for the mentally ill. His treatment vacillated between indifference and cruelty. At one period, he was kept in a strait jacket for 21 consecutive days and nights. It was his firm determination to devote his energies to the improvement of the care of the mentally ill. His chance came after he was discharged in 1903, cured only by the processes of nature.

In 1908, Clifford Beers published his epoch-making book, *A Mind that Found Itself*. This book was a frank, disarming picture of his illness, the way he was treated and the unbelievable sufferings to which he was subjected. In 1908 in his native state of Connecticut, he founded a *Society of Mental Hy-*

giene, whose purposes were "to work for the conservation of mental health, to help prevent nervous and mental disorders, and mental defects and to help raise the standards of care for those suffering from any of these disorders."

In 1909, a *National Committee of Mental Hygiene* was established through his efforts and with essentially the same purposes. In 1930, in Washington, D.C., the representatives of 53 nations joined in establishing the *International Committee for Mental Hygiene.*

The prevention, early detection and acceptance of prompt psychiatric care has been advocated. The public has developed a greater acceptance of this illness as one of the illnesses of the body rather than as an isolated punitive illness of which one is ashamed.

When Nicholas Brown died in 1841, he left a bequest of $30,000 for a retreat for the insane; thus, in 1844, the Rhode Island legislature issued a charter for the building of a "Rhode Island Asylum for the Insane." Butler Hospital was constructed and became one of the foremost institutions of its kind in the United States; it continued to treat the mentally ill until 1955 when it was closed. Because of public pressure, a new board of directors and a successful financial campaign, the institution was reopened in 1957 as the Butler Health Center for various health and welfare agencies. In its modern approach to the problems of the mentally ill, Butler Hospital is carrying on the great tradition it established almost a century and a half ago.

This modern service seems far broader in scope and seems to have followed the pattern of psychiatric hospitals that have been replaced in many areas by community mental health centers. A better understanding of emotional problems, psychiatric disorders, medications and treatments by better prepared psychiatrists, clinical psychologists and professional nurses have contributed to the progress made in this area of health care.

The position of the nurse was not on a very high level because many nurses had a very meager background in basic principles of psychology and psychiatry and their tasks became custodial. This condition reflected the philosophy and policies of the institutions for the mentally ill. Physical restraints produced an intolerable condition for both patients and attendants. Increased agitation, injury to skin surfaces, inability to eat, all

produced pathetically unhappy patients. Methods of forced feedings increased the discomfort and the resultant "cerebral congestion" was supposedly relieved by cold wet therapy followed by the administration of sedatives.

The first school to educate nurses with a psychiatric preparation was established at McLean Hospital in Waverly, Massachusetts in 1882. Gradually there was a growing appreciation of the therapeutic role of the psychiatric nurse. Santos relates that:

Paralleling the growth of psychiatric thought, psychiatric nursing by 1900 had become an organized discipline with its own body of knowledge and techniques, and with its emphasis on the nursing of the whole person. Nevertheless, it was suffused with the static custodial concepts of the psychiatric treatment of the time that it served.[30]

A growing concern developed of the influence of forces affecting a person within and from outside his body which could produce a pathological process within the person. *Psychoanalysis* gradually evolved. In addition, an increasing awareness of the extent of mental illness as a national health problem focused on the magnitude of the emotional needs of all people and the obligation of all health workers to understand human behavior.

The National Mental Health Act of 1946 provided funds for the improvement of mental health through research, education of professional personnel and to upgrade the treatment of the mentally ill. Schmahl has written:

After years of struggling to retain the integrity of nursing . . . nursing leaders suddenly found support for their efforts from a new development in the medical field—the recognition of the contributions that psychiatry could make to the care of all patients.[31]

The integration of psychiatry with medial treatment enhanced the role of the psychiatric nurse. Nursing contributions were also recognized due to the increased use of somatic treatments such as insulin shock,

---

[30] Santos, Elvin and Stainbrook, Edward: "A History of Psychiatric Nursing in the Nineteenth Century." *Journal of the History of Medicine and Allied Sciences,* Winter 1949, p. 59.

[31] Schmahl, Janet: *Experiment in Change.* New York, The Macmillan Co., 1966, p. 12.

electroshock, sleep therapy and psychosurgery.

Now the psychiatric nurse had become a member of a professional team in a therapeutic community. Her therapeutic role has been reputed to be to "support and encourage the patient in his participation in the total treatment by acting as a clarifier and interpreter when the patient encounters difficulty, collaborate with the doctor in therapy, and most importantly, to serve as the transmitter of the therapeutic culture to the patient."[32]

Nurse educators began to encourage all students of nursing to receive preparation in this field because patients of all ages, in homes, in general hospitals, as well as in psychiatric institutions needed psychiatrically oriented nursing care. Attempts were made to integrate psychiatric principles into the curriculum of professional schools of nursing with financial support from the government. Many collegiate schools responded to this challenge but a five-year study at the Skidmore College Department of Nursing "to investigate and demonstrate the ways in which the various resources at the department's command could be utilized to foster the student's awareness of psychiatric concepts and techniques and to help her apply them in the nursing care of all patients," was reported by Jane Schmahl. The title of this report was *Experiment in Change; An Interdisciplinary Approach to the Integration of Psychiatric Content in Baccalaureate Nursing Education.*

The psychiatric nurse aims to create an environment in which the patient can develop new behavior patterns and work out his own problems. Mental illness is overcome by a growth process, so experiences promoting the growth process are encouraged and interpersonal relationships provide the learning experiences necessary for growth.[33]

Federal legislation in 1963 authorized funding for community mental health centers. Provision for *preventive* services was an essential part of this legislation.

The nurse with psychiatric-mental health preparation functions in more than psychi-

atric and general hospitals. This specialist participates in community involvement in half-way houses, community health clinics and community mental health centers. The skills of such a person are used to help combat particular mental health problems such as drug addiction, suicide, child abuse, juvenile delinquency, alcoholism and many other emotional disturbances.

A presentation of the extending role of the psychiatric-mental health nurse is presented in a *Symposium on the Nurse in Community Mental Health.*[34]

Many modalities have been used in patient care, among them recreational therapy, art therapy, music therapy, occupational and recreational therapy, and dance therapy. Marion Chace at St. Elizabeth's Hospital in Washington was one of the first dance therapists to report her use of the dance as therapy including its use in nonverbal communication.

The task of demonstrating competence as a psychotherapist "on the same level and with the same type of patient" as her co-workers — psychiatric social case workers, clinical psychologists and psychiatrists — still confronts psychiatric nurses.[35]

The role of the nurse who is responsive to community needs and striving for mental health for members of the community must become involved in social change.

NURSING IN OCCUPATIONAL HEALTH

It is difficult to trace the actual beginnings of the field of *"industrial nursing"* because many isolated firms had for years employed a single nurse. A few employers established *hospitals* for injured employees. The Manufacturing Company of Lowell, Massachusetts had such a hospital in 1859. The next one was probably a log cabin in Lead, South Dakota, which from 1877 cared for persons with mining injuries. In 1881 the Colorado Fuel and Iron Company of Pueblo estab-

[32] Kalkman, Marion: *Psychiatric Nursing*, New York, McGraw-Hill, Inc., 1967, p. 10.

[33] Gregg, Dorothy: "The Psychiatric Nurse's Role." *Psychiatric Nursing.* Dubuque, Iowa, William C. Brown Co., 1966, p. 178.

[34] Fischer, Lorene R., et al.: "Symposium on the Nurse in Community Health." *The Nursing Clinics of North America*, Philadelphia, W. B. Saunders Co., Vol. 5, No. 4, December 1970, pp. 631–712.

[35] Stokes, Gertrude: "Extending the Role of the Psychiatric-Mental Health Nurse in Community Mental Health." *The Nursing Clinics of North America*, Philadelphia, W. B. Saunders Co., Vol. 5, No. 4, December 1970, p. 639.

lished an industrial hospital which was staffed by male nurses. Even the Union Pacific Railroad established a hospital in 1893.

In 1895 the Proctor Marble Company in Vermont was purported to be the first industrial plant to employ a nurse to visit and give nursing care to sick employees. Her name was *Ada Stewart* (Mrs. Markoff).

Another early project was the Employees Benefit Association of John Wanamaker's department store in New York City which was established in 1897.

The term industrial nursing has been supplanted by a broader concept—that of the nurse in the field of occupational health. The nurse in the field of *occupational health* has been employed in factories, department stores, telephone companies and in many industrial enterprises.

Health care has been largely a twentieth-century development, and until about 1920 there was little general interest in it. Even now some employers do not realize that half-sick men do not produce as much as expected, that absence from illness cuts into profits and that it pays to care for the health of workers. Insurance companies first called attention to this, and when workmen's compensation laws came into force, employers realized the value of health care. The National Safety Council has done much in the prevention of accidents and occupational hazards and illnesses.

Boston University, in 1917, was probably the first college in the United States to give a *course in industrial nursing.* Simmons College established such a course in 1919 (for college graduates), discontinued it, and began it again in 1942. The University of Minnesota, Wayne University, Detroit and Columbia Universities also gave courses.

The nurse in occupational health needs to know not merely her basic work and prevention of disease but must also have a knowledge of industrial hazards, safety rules, labor laws (including her own legal limitations), plant hygiene, community hygiene and whatever health programs are being undertaken. She may be consultant to state hygiene departments in the U.S. Public Health Service.

The American Association of Industrial Nurses was formed in 1942. In 1944 the American Nurses' Association created a section for industrial nurses. The U. S. Public Health Service has nurse consultants in occupational health.

The nurse leadership in occupational health nursing has been recognized. *Mary Louise Brown*, as a faculty member in the Graduate School of Public Health at Yale and later as chief of the Occupational Health Nursing Section of the United States Public Health Service, has contributed much through guidance and her literary efforts in the development of occupational health nursing and improvement of the role of the nurse in such a program.

Many others have given direction and leadership in this field. A contribution of significance was Marjorie Keller's four-year study which resulted in the identification of occupational health content for the professional nursing curriculum.[36] The suggested approach for this curriculum integrates Leavell and Clark's concepts of levels of prevention with Maslow's theory of a hierarchy of needs while superimposing the nursing process.

In a "Symposium on Occupational Health Nursing"[37] key issues were identified and proposals for their solution were presented.

An important milestone occurred when the *Occupational Safety and Health Act* was signed by President Nixon on December 29, 1970. This act, which became effective in July of 1971, had implications for nurses as employees as well as health professionals. The purpose of this act was:

To assure safe and healthful working conditions for working men and women; by authorizing enforcement of the standards developed under the Act; by assisting and encouraging the States in their efforts to assure safe and healthful working conditions; by providing for research, information, education and training in the field of occupational safety and health; and for other purposes.

NURSING CARE OF THE ELDERLY

Dr. Howard Rusk has said: "We have added years to life, now add life to the years." Life has been lengthened in the twentieth century and we have greater numbers of older citizens due to many factors, among

---

[36] Keller, Marjorie J. in association with May, W. T.: *Occupational Health Content in Baccalaureate Nursing Education.* Cincinnati, U.S. Department of Health, Education, and Welfare, Environmental Control Administration, 1970.

[37] Keller, Marjorie J., et al.: "Symposium on Occupational Health Nursing." *The Nursing Clinics of North America.* Philadelphia, W. B. Saunders Co., Vol. 7, No. 1, March 1972, pp. 95–182.

them the control of communicable diseases, lowered infant mortality, improved child care, increased nutritional information and better balanced diets.

The addition of the spark which can enrich and enliven the extension of life has been the role of the nurse. Geriatric nursing has been a relatively new field in our contemporary society, in fact geriatrics was not established as a medical specialty until almost 1940. Yet historically and culturally, the elderly have received reverential treatment; nursing care of the elderly was developed as a special field of endeavor by St. Helena, the Dowager-Empress of the Roman Empire.

In the early part of this century the elderly who were also poor were sent to a "poorhouse" or "almshouse" where what nursing was available was limited to the infirmary. Caroline Barlett Crane vividly describes the pathetic conditions in 1907.[38] She states: "And of all that motley assemblage of human beings who were once carelessly consigned to oblivion in the county poorhouse, presently none will be left except—the aged and infirm. . . . Homeless, friendless poor old men and women: these are—and will become more and more—the great body of our almshouse population." Miss Crane explained that the insane were removed to asylums and the children to special hospitals based on their needs but the aged were left to deteriorate in these bleak, cheerless surroundings.

The feelings of despair and rejection of the elderly when they had to leave family, friends and possessions was depicted in the poignant ballad by Will Carleton, "Over the Hill to the Poorhouse." A striking comparison can be noted between the feelings of an elderly woman of the late nineteenth century with those of many older people who face admission to convalescent homes at this point in time.

It was gradually recognized that nursing of the elderly requires special skills, a sense of humor, modification of the patient's diet, and provision for regular exercise in fresh air. Recreational therapy received emphasis.[39]

The word "geriatrics" was first used in 1909 in a New York medical journal in an ar-

ticle written by Dr. Nascher who wrote the first textbook in this country on geriatrics in 1914. The first university course in the problems of the aged was offered in 1933 by the University of Minnesota in the program of Human Development. A group of physicians formed the American Geriatric Society in 1942 to promote the organized study of medical problems of older people and in 1945 physicians, biologists and psychologists organized the American Gerontological Society to sponsor research on the problems of aging.

The first textbook devoted to an understanding of the nursing contribution to the care of the aged was written by Kathleen Newton.[40]

In 1970[41] a definition of geriatric nursing was enunciated as follows: "Geriatric nursing is concerned with the assessment of nursing needs of older people, planning and implementing nursing care to meet these needs, and evaluating the effectiveness of such care to achieve and maintain a level of wellness consistent with the limitations imposed by the aging process." The geriatric nurse must be sensitive to the special problems of the elderly, appreciating their basic desire to be accepted as useful, contributing members of society. (See Figure 13–17.) In carrying out this definition, the nurse is challenged to use her skills and ability to preserve the proper functioning of the mind and body as long as possible.

The A.N.A. developed nine standards for the practice of geriatric nursing in 1968.

Standard I: The nurse observes and interprets all signs and symptoms associated with normal and abnormal aging and institutes appropriate nursing measures.

Standard II: The nurse differentiates between pathologic social behavior and the normal life style of each individual.

Standard III: The nurse demonstrates an appreciation for the heritage, values and wisdom of older persons.

Standard IV: The nurse supports and promotes normal physiologic functioning of the older person.

Standard V: The nurse protects aged persons from injury and excessive stress, and supports them through stressful experiences.

[38] Crane, Caroline Barlett: "Almshouse Nursing: The Human Need; The Professional Opportunity." *American Journal of Nursing.* July 1907, pp. 874–877.

[39] Breeze, Jessie: "The Care of the Aged." *American Journal of Nursing.* Vol. 9, No. 7, July 1909, pp. 826–828.

[40] Newton, Kathleen: *Geriatric Nursing.* St. Louis, C. V. Mosby Co., 1950.

[41] "Standards for Geriatric Nursing Practice." *American Journal of Nursing,* September 1970, p. 1894.

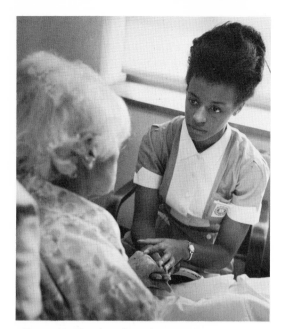

Figure 13–17. A student of nursing listens with compassion to her patient, who squeezes her hand appreciatively. (Courtesy of University of Connecticut.)

Standard VI: The nurse employs methods to promote the communication and social interaction of the aged with other individuals and with his family.

Standard VII: The nurse together with the older person designs and adapts the physical and psychosocial environment to meet his needs within the limitations of the situation.

Standard VIII: The nurse assists older persons to obtain and use devices which help them function on a higher level and sees to it that these devices are kept in good repair.

Standard IX: The nurse seeks to resolve her conflicting attitudes regarding aging and death so that she can assist the elderly patient and his relatives to maintain life with dignity and comfort.

The Nursing Clinics of North America presented a symposium on implementing these geriatric nursing standards in nursing practice.[42] In this symposium the contributors of each article elaborated on each standard and gave examples of ways in which each one could be carried out by the nurse practitioner.

———

[42] Knowles, Lois, et al.: "Symposium on Putting Geriatric Nursing Standards into Practice." *Nursing Clinics of North America*, Philadelphia, W. B. Saunders Co., Vol. 7, No. 2, June 1972, pp. 201–309.

There are institutions whose philosophy of patient care coincide with the aforesaid standards and have achieved the comfort, satisfaction and praise of patients and families. "The nurse, in caring for the geriatric patient can be the enabler who, on the strength of her beliefs, provides the impetus for drive in the patient, the motivation for self-realization."[43]

Remotivation therapy is being tried which encourages group interaction designed to help patients toward reality. After several sessions it was evaluated that "...a positive change in the mood tone of older patients occurred when new, younger, and concerned people took them out of their rooms and involved them in group interaction.... If nursing is to be more than meeting patients' physical needs, it is necessary to increase our understanding of older peoples' need for psycho-social stimulation."[44]

Many elderly people stay in their homes and nursing care may be provided by community nurses from Visiting Nurses Associations (Fig. 13–18). Her special skills beyond meeting the actual nursing care needs can involve her abilities as a resource person as needed. She can assist in obtaining additional funds; in finding suitable housing; in join-

———

[43] Dupuis, P. H.: "Old is Beautiful." *Nursing Outlook,* August 1970, p. 26.

[44] Moody, L., et al.: "Moving the Past into the Present." *American Journal of Nursing,* November 1970, p. 2356.

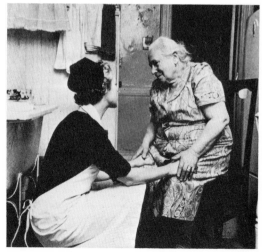

Figure 13–18. A community health nurse listens attentively to her patient's tale of distress.

ing Senior Citizen or Golden Age groups; in encouraging the spiritual advisor who is needed; in contracting with the Meals-on-Wheels project and in many other ways.

The challenge of the well-prepared nurse in meeting the needs of the elderly remains one of infinite and compassionate concern.

NURSING CARE OF THE DYING

Throughout the ages, persons have needed a special kind of assistance when they faced the dying process and the cessation of life. Henry Fielding in his *Amelia* suggested: "It hath often been said . . . that it is not death, but dying that is terrible."

Florence Nightingale pleaded for a nurse to use special skills in meeting the needs of a dying person when she wrote:

But the long chronic case, who knows too well himself, and who has been told by his physician that he will never enter active life again, who feels that every month he has to give up something he could do the month before . . . oh, spare such sufferers your chattering hopes. You do not know how you worry and weary them.

Almost a century later a student of nursing who was dying wrote a poignant plea to nurses when she said:

I am a student nurse. I am dying. I write this to you who are, and will become, nurses in the hope that by my sharing my feelings with you, you may someday be better able to help those who share my experience.

I'm out of the hospital now—perhaps for a month, for six months, perhaps for a year . . . but no one likes to talk about such things. In fact, no one likes to talk about much at all. Nursing must be advancing, but I wish it would hurry. We're taught not to be overly cheery now, to omit the "Everything's fine" routine, and we have done pretty well. But now one is left in a lonely silent void. With the protective "fine, fine" gone, the staff is left with only their own vulnerability and fear. The dying patient is not yet seen as a person and thus cannot be communicated with as such. He is a symbol of what every human fears and what we each know, at least academically, that we too must someday face. What did they say in psychiatric nursing about meeting pathology with pathology to the detriment of both patient and nurse? And there was a lot about knowing one's own feelings before you could help another with his. How true.

But for me, fear is today and dying is now. You slip in and out of my room, give me medications and check my blood pressure. Is it because I am a student nurse, myself, or just a human being, that I sense your fright? And your fear enhances mine. Why are you afraid? I am the one who is dying!

I know, you feel insecure, don't know what to say, don't know what to do. But please believe me, if you care, you can't go wrong. Just admit that you care. That is really for what we search. We may ask for why's and wherefores, but we don't really expect answers. Don't run away . . . wait . . . all I want to know is that there will be someone to hold my hand when I need it. I am afraid. Death may get to be a routine to you, but it is new to me. You may not see me as unique, but I've never died before. To me, once is pretty unique!

You whisper about my youth, but when one is dying, is he really so young anymore? I have lots I wish we could talk about. It really would not take much more of your time because you are in here quite a bit anyway.

If only we could be honest, both admit of our fears, touch one another. If you really care, would you lose so much of your valuable professionalism if you even cried with me? Just person to person? Then, it might not be so hard to die . . . in a hospital . . . with friends close by.[45]

Rose Hawthorne Lathrop (1851–1926), the brilliant and beautiful daughter of Nathaniel Hawthorne, has been credited with carrying on the most successful campaign in the interests of patients suffering with cancer. In the early 1890's, she visited her seamstress, who was dying of cancer on New York's Welfare Island. She was appalled at the poor care these victims received, at their anguish, which was not relieved by any kind of emotional support, and at the absence of human love throughout their days of illness, and especially at the time of death.

It became apparent that patients afflicted with cancer that was incurable were not wanted in hospitals and in many instances were not permitted to remain in their own homes.

Rose Hawthorne Lathrop determined to be of assistance to the poor victims of this serious malady, which was not understood. She received three months' training in simple nursing techniques and in the care of cancer victims. Her next step was to hire a tenement in the slum sections where she could be closer to those patients who needed her.

In 1898, an artist friend of Rose's named *Alice Huber* joined her in her work. Large

[45]_____"Death in the First Person." *American Journal of Nursing*, February 1970.

quarters were needed to provide accommodations to make it easier to give nursing care when it was needed. They purchased a three-story brick building at 426 Cherry Street in New York City and over the door they placed the sign: "St. Rose's Free Home for Incurable Cancer," and the quotation: "I was sick and ye visited Me." Both Rose and Alice had become members of the Third Order of St. Dominic.

Gradually, the demand for more nurses became evident and Rose Hawthorne Lathrop became the foundress of the order of sisters called *Servants of Relief for Incurable Cancer*, which was a branch of the Dominican Order. The membership of her religious family grew, as did the hospitals that they built and the quality of care rendered to many more patients. Of her work Rose once wrote:

I am trying to serve the poor as a servant. I wish to serve the cancerous poor because they are avoided more than any other class of sufferers; and I wish to go to them as a poor creature myself, though able to help them through gifts from friends and relatives and public kindness. It is by humility and sacrifice alone that we feel the holy spirit of pity.

In *St. Christopher's Hospice* in Sydenham near London a woman directs a most remarkable program. Dr. Cecily Saunders, nurse, medical social worker and now a physician, is the motivating influence behind the project as well as its director.[46] It was her dream that a milieu could be created in which a person who was dying could be cared for in a very special way. Dr. Saunders has been planning such a project and her hope and dreams were described in the March 1965 *American Journal of Nursing* called "The Last Stages of Life." Her dreams have been brought to fruition and serve as a model for what can be achieved when people really believe in an ideal.

An extension of St. Christopher's Hospice is the out-patient plan to assist a patient to attain his desire of dying at home with his own family whenever possible. In this period service is provided to the patient and his family and readmission to the Hospice occurs readily whenever this procedure is needed. A relative knows that even in his own home, he isn't carrying the fear and worry alone, for the staff continues their concerned care to those within the Hospice or those within their own homes—giving total care—social, psychological and spiritual.

In this remarkable enterprise, a sense of community and mutual support is noted, "for there is a bond in suffering and in shared experience which is expressed in caring for and about one another." Patients have expressed that they "find reassurance in feeling cared for and loved by the staff.... There is comfort and strength in the knowledge that whatever your weakness or uncertainty of faith, those about you believe in the meaningfulness of life and in the essential value of each person."

Mrs. Florence Wald, former Dean of the School of Nursing at Yale University, has been directing "A Nurse's Study of the Care for Dying Patients." Her project is resulting in plans for a Hospice similar to St. Christopher's.

A psychiatrist, Elisabeth Kubler-Ross, has written a thought-provoking and informative book entitled, *On Death and Dying.*[47] The book focuses on the meaning of death to those who are dying and the five stages that a dying patient experiences before death occurs. It has been reviewed as a discourse on the art of human dialogue.

Much has been enunciated and experienced in assisting a person and his family in facing the last stages of life.

NURSING PRACTICE—LEADERSHIP IN ACTION

Many courageous individuals have delineated a non-traditional approach to the delivery of nursing care. Several of these persons who have dared to try something different in the hope of better care for a greater number of people will be considered. One such person was Sister Elizabeth Kenny.

President Roosevelt made the whole country conscious of the problem of infantile paralysis and stimulated people to make large contributions to its relief. *Sister Elizabeth Kenny* of Australia was known as a teacher of special forms of treatment in infantile paralysis. She is an example of a nurse who, in making a nursing diagnosis, gave an important

[46]_____"Christmas at St. Christopher's." *American Journal of Nursing*, Vol. 71, No. 12, December 1971, pp. 2325–2330.

[47]Kubler-Ross, Elisabeth: *On Death and Dying.* New York, The Macmillan Co., 1969.

contribution to the care of many patients. Her plan of nursing care was based on scientific principles while carefully considering the comfort of her patient. The heat treatments which she devised have been used for the relief of many patients and are known as the Kenny treatments. She accepted the challenge, not by purposeful design but as a response to a need which she alone could fulfill.

Another remarkable personage in this century is *Mother Teresa*, a Yugoslavian, who gave up a comfortable teaching position in favor of ministering to the needs of lepers, cripples, dying derelicts, abandoned children and starving adults in troubled, underprivileged Calcutta (Fig. 13–19). Mother Teresa and the members of the nursing order she founded, called the *Order of the Missionaries of Charity*, which was recognized as an order in 1960, are highly respected and loved. There are no religious barriers to the people for whom they care, as many patients are Moslem and Hindu in addition to the Christians. These sis-

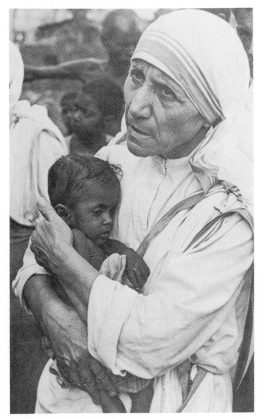

Figure 13–19. Mother Teresa shows loving concern for one of her precious patients.

ters are seen in a habit of a blue-edged white sari, modeled on the saris of the poor Indian women. They tend the poor in the streets, in their homes, in the hospices which they have opened to care for children, the destitute, the dying and the lepers. The plight of the poor in that country is reflected in the names given to the hospices: "Home for Dying Destitutes," and "Home for Sick, Crippled and Unwanted Children." Half of the patients have tuberculosis complicated by malnutrition. Life for these sisters is obviously precious, and its destruction by abortion or euthanasia is unacceptable.

Mother Teresa participated in a filmed interview by Malcolm Muggeridge for the B.B.C. in 1971. This former editor of the British humor magazine, *Punch,* is reputed to be a witty, sophisticated, sarcastic journalist and commentator. The data collected by Mr. Muggeridge appears in a book entitled *Something Beautiful for God.*[48] Of her he has said, "For me, Mother Teresa of Calcutta embodies Christian love in action. Her face shines with the love of Christ on which her whole life is centered, and her words carry that message to a world which never needed it so much."

Mother Teresa says to everyone, "Come do something for God," and she has hundreds of volunteers per day who assist her. Her community has expanded numerically and now has branches in Rome, Australia, Latin America and Holland.

Lydia Hall was the inspirational mover behind the philosophy and project of the *Loeb Center for Nursing and Rehabilitation* at Montefiore Hospital which opened in 1963. This institution provides professional nursing service in an institutional setting that bridges the general hospital and the home. At Loeb only professional nurses provide the nursing care. In the delivery of care, this nursing center at Loeb is comparable to an extension of a community nursing service in an institutional setting. Mrs. Hall stated that "the nurse is the chief therapeutic agent and the final effector in providing interrelated patient care. Medicine and allied fields offer ancillary therapy." It was her contention that "At Loeb, the presumption is that, as he needs less medical care, he needs not only more nursing care,

[48] Muggeridge, Malcolm: *Something Beautiful for God.* London, Harper and Row, 1971.

but more *professional* nursing care and teaching."

The patient, his family and the nurse analyze and solve those problems which must be tackled in order to achieve maximal health for the patient. The design of the building carries out the philosophy of the project and assists the most handicapped person while being comfortable and attractive. It reflects the desires of the staff: "We are with you in your efforts to gain health."[49]

Another experiment in this period of history is exemplified by the work of *M. Lucille Kinlein,* whose shingle outside her office in May of 1971 reflected a professional nurse who identifies herself as an *independent practitioner* of nursing. In addition to her independent practice, Miss Kinlein is a member of the faculty of Georgetown University School of Nursing and is also studying for her doctorate at Catholic University of America in Washington.

Many frustrations and "irreconcilables" prompted her to break with tradition, a prime one being the inability of her students to practice nursing within the structure of the scientific framework which they were taught and which they had designed. Miss Kinlein relates her objection to the perennial questions about why nurses need certain knowledge in order to function "as a nurse." She states: "There are never any boundaries to acquisition of knowledge in any field."[50]

Another area of concern was the lack of change from procedure-oriented treatment of patients within a medical regimen to the role of the nurse in assisting the return to an acceptable state of wellness. The insurmountable pressures within a hospital structure frequently prevented the ability to give the kind of nursing care that was needed or, if given, was achieved at a great physical and emotional cost. The lack of authority versus responsibility prompted the decision that responsibility for *nursing* should require "control over what I did to achieve my nursing goals."

These leaders have reflected in action what Rozella Schlotfeldt has emphasized: "Nursing is health care." It is her contention that the "goal of nursing as a field of professional endeavor is to help people attain, retain and regain health.... Nurses must take primary responsibility for health care." She summarizes her charge to leaders of nursing:

They must help students search for and find means to motivate persons to utilize their own resources to seek health—and these include teaching, counseling, stimulating, inquiring, and inspiring. Nurses must identify and explicate nursing therapies and teach their students to become proficient in sustaining, supporting, comforting, and helping persons during periods of infirmity, deprivation, disfigurement, changes in life style, crises, and periods of development and decline. Through compensating for an individual's inadequacies and adjusting his environmental circumstances, nurses must promote his motivation to seek health and his use of his own resources to attain, retain, or regain optimal health and function. Nursing, succinctly stated, is health care.[51]

RECOGNITION OF LEADERSHIP

Many nurses have been honored for their contributions to the health and welfare of others. One such person has been *Lillian D. Wald.* In reading of her outstanding accomplishments, it is gratifying to note and interesting to ponder the recognition she has received.

As early as 1912 Mount Holyoke College awarded her the degree of Doctor of Laws with the citation: "Lillian D. Wald, friend of those who need friends, originator of far-reaching municipal and national movements for the care of the sick and the poor and little children, a citizen of whom our greatest American city may be proud, we confer upon you the degree of Doctor of Laws and admit you to all its rights and privileges."

In 1913 she was awarded the medal of the National Institute of Social Sciences for "distinguished services rendered to humanity." In 1923 the Rotary Club of New York bestowed their first service medal "in recognition of her lifelong service to the world as sociologist, organizer and publicist." Miss Wald was referred to as a "student of the needs of the poor, organizer of agencies for better health, friend of the nurse, guardian and champion

---

[49] Hall, Lydia E.: "A Center for Nursing." *Nursing Outlook,* Vol. 11, No. 11, November 1963.

[50] Kinlein, M. Lucille: "Independent Nurse Practitioner." *Nursing Outlook,* Vol. 20, No. 1, January 1972, pp. 22–24.

[51] Schlotfeldt, Rozella M.: "This I Believe—Nursing is Health Care." *Nursing Outlook,* Vol. 20, No. 4, April 1972, pp. 245–246.

of the cause of childhood, and loving servant of needy humanity."

In 1926 *Better Times* magazine, a journal of sociology, presented her with a medal for distinguished social services because of her efforts in making public health nursing become "a vast city-wide, extra-mural hospital, the records of which constitute a valuable contribution to scientific knowledge."

Smith College, in 1930, awarded her an honorary degree of Doctor of Laws with the citation: "Lillian D. Wald, founder and head of the Henry Street Settlement, organizer of district nursing, originator of the work of the School Nurse and of the Federal Children's Bureau, active supporter of all enlightened effort for the welfare of the community, internationally known as an indomitable fighter for justice, mercy and freedom."

Even in the United States Congressional Record of 1934, Lillian Wald received commendation: "Her vision and courage have been largely responsible for the legislation resulting in minimum wage, workmen's compensation, the protection of women and children in factories, and the abolition of child labor."

Mayor La Guardia presented her in 1937 with the Certificate for Distinguished Service to the City of New York with the comment: "I would not have wanted to assume the responsibilities of my office in 1933 if Lillian Wald had not pioneered in 1893."

On September 12, 1971, Lillian D. Wald received the highest tribute among a distinguished list of awards when she joined other outstanding Americans in the *Hall of Fame for Great Americans.* Her bust and tablet will stand in the Colonnade at New York University. This accolade to a great person, a great leader and a great nurse can be shared by a profession of which she was proud.

NURSING PRACTICE—A NEW DEFINITION

Many states have been reexamining the definition of the practice of nursing. New York State amended their practice act on February 9, 1972 and enacted the following definition of the practice of professional nursing:

The practice of the profession of nursing as a registered professional nurse is defined as diagnosing and treating human responses to actual or potential health problems through such services as

casefinding, health teaching, health counseling and provision of care supportive to or restorative of life and well-being, and executing medical regimens prescribed by a licensed or otherwise legally authorized physician or dentist. A nursing regimen shall be consistent with and shall not vary any existing medical regimen.

The definitions used in the preceding are as follows:

"Diagnosing" in the context of nursing practice means that identification of and discrimination between physical and psychosocial signs and symptoms essential to effective execution and management of the nursing regimen. Such diagnostic privilege is distinct from a medical diagnosis.

"Treating" means selection and performance of those therapeutic measures essential to the effective execution and management of the nursing regimen, and execution of any prescribed medical regimen.

"Human Responses" means those signs, symptoms and processes which denote the individual's interaction with an actual or potential health problem.

States are currently considering the need for continuing education as a requisite for renewal of licensure.

NATIONAL COMMISSION FOR THE STUDY OF NURSING

Still another "study" of nursing and nursing education was undertaken in the 1960's. The National Commission for the Study of Nursing and Nursing Education was an independent group established by the American Nurses' Association and the National League for Nursing. Its objective was to conduct a comprehensive study of nursing education in the United States. In 1963 the Surgeon General's Consultant Group on Nursing, in their document *Toward Quality in Nursing,*[52] recommended an investigation of nursing education on a national basis, with special emphasis on the responsibilities and skills needed for a high level of nursing care.

In 1966 the Board of Directors of the American Nurses' Foundation voted a financial contribution to launch the study by the National Commission. Additional substantial

[52] U.S. Public Health Service: *Toward Quality in Nursing.* Report of the Surgeon General's Consultant Group on Nursing. Washington, D.C., Government Printing Office, 1963.

sums of money were contributed by the Avalon and Kellogg Foundations and an anonymous benefactor. The Commission functioned as an autonomous group with W. Allen Wallis, President of the University of Rochester, as president of the Commission. There were twelve members on the Commission, three of whom were nurses. Jerome P. Lysaught was appointed director of the project with Charles H. Russell as associate director.

In facing the magnitude of the assignment it was determined that the following essential problems needed to be scrutinized and solved: *the supply and demand for nurses, nursing roles and functions, the education of nurses* and *nursing careers.*

The final report with recommendations appeared in a book entitled *An Abstract for Action* referred to as the *"Lysaught Report."*[53] The Commission held that change in nursing could be visualized in terms of four basic priorities:

A. Increased research into the practice of nursing and the education of nurses;
B. Improved educational systems and curricula based on the results of that research;
C. Clarification of roles and practice conjointly with other health professions to ensure the delivery of optimum care; and
D. Increased financial support for nurses and for nursing to ensure adequate career opportunities that will attract and retain the number of individuals required for quality health care in the coming years.[54]

In their acknowledgments the staff paid tribute to two historic documents for assistance — Abraham Flexner's *Medical Education in the United States and Canada*, which was published in 1910, and Esther Lucile Brown's *Nursing For The Future* (1948). The important document of 1923 referred to as the *"Goldmark Report"* (*Nursing and Nursing Education in the United States*) received scant attention. It was reported that the decisions of Dr. Brown and this Commission were remarkably similar.

The Scope of Nursing Practice

In scrutinizing the characteristics, concepts and scope of the practice of nursing, the "shortage of nursing" was identified. After deliberation it was realized, as it has been so often in the past, that the shortage was not a quantitative but a qualitative one. Increasing numbers of persons carrying out fragments of the nursing role as well as non-nursing tasks at a moment in time when the delivery of health service reflects the enormous increase in scientific knowledge seemed unwise.

The misuse of nurses was noted while demands for increased clinical competency were emphasized. The obsolescence of traditional procedure-oriented skills was considered against the challenges of the needs of persons whose plan for care demanded utilization of newly acquired scientific and technological advances in health care delivery. It is the patient and the family who receive less than quality care when nurses are not properly prepared and cannot function in an acceptable patient-oriented nurse role.

This report recognized that nursing leaders and organized nursing groups have focused "on the intellectual demands placed on the nurse" and stressed "the growth in her decision-making responsibilities."[55] In addition, in contrast to the public's image of the nurse in white working in a hospital caring for a critically ill patient, this study designed a model less bound by the institutional setting. It identified that the nurse was "engaged in the community as well as in the hospital or nursing home." They saw "nursing practice separated into professional and technical components, with education as an entree to both, but with added knowledge required for professional decision-making and leadership." They realized that there had been a "determined effort by the profession to develop a science of nursing that will permit accurate prediction and control of the outcomes of nursing intervention."

It was felt that a controversial aspect was "the separation of the nursing role into professional and technical components" because the best-prepared nurse would be removed from patient care. The ingredients of nursing practice should be reflected in: "a keen sensitivity to the patient's wants, a comprehensive knowledge of procedures and technology, and a clear grasp of the behavioral and physical sciences that provide a basis for judgment."

---

[53] Lysaught, Jerome P.: *An Abstract for Action.* New York, McGraw-Hill Book Co., 1970.
[54] *Ibid.,* p. 155.

[55] *Ibid.,* p. 62.

The primary tasks of professional nursing include assessment, intervention and instruction. The growth of clinical specialization was noted and the Report stated that "the nurse clinician is the best hope to fill the professional gap in the health care system."[56]

Nursing Roles and Functions

Research in nursing has reflected a beneficial effect on the quality of nursing. The relationship of improved patient care can be observed also in the economics of patient care by reduction of cost to the patient.

Because of the crucial needs for an increase in research the following recommendations were made:

1. The Federal Division of Nursing, the National Center for Health Services Research and Development, other governmental agencies, and private foundations appropriate grant funds and/or research contracts to investigate the impact of nursing practice on the quality, effectiveness, and economy of health care.

2. Federal funds be supplied through the E.R.I.C. [Educational Research Information Center] program, or through the Division of Nursing, as well as private and state funds, to the American Nurses' Foundation so that it might become a national clearinghouse for the collection and dissemination of information about research and innovations in nursing.

3. The Division of Nursing, the National Center for Health Services Research and Development, and state and private funds allocate increased monies for applied research and demonstration grants that would examine new methods, procedures, settings, and personnel relationships for improved nursing practice. We further recommend that the following guidelines be used in expending funds:

a. Innovation and demonstration projects in patient care should be based on preceding research;

b. Innovations should be conceived and focused to improve methods of meeting patient needs, rather than designed primarily to answer professional problems;

c. All grants and contracts for applied research and demonstrations should include an allocation for the evaluation of results;

d. All innovations and demonstrations should be weighed against alternative courses of action that might produce similar results.

Both quality of care and comparative costs should be considered. It was felt that "nursing itself must assume responsibility to ensure that individuals undertake research."

In considering role articulation in health practice, it was felt that "nursing must be allowed—and required—to practice at its very highest capability."

Under the heading of Nursing Roles and Functions it would seem that history was repeating itself as one reads: "Because of the rising demands for health service, and because there are critical shortages among physicians as well as nurses, there have been many suggestions for basic reorganization of the nursing role. From the standpoint of many it makes sense to have the nurse take over as many functions from the doctor as she can capably handle."[57] Yet, there was recognition that nurses "cooperated with physicians in developing higher levels of treatment and intervention, but were adamant in maintaining a distinction between nursing and medical practice."

This Report referred to the suggestion made by the American Medical Association which encouraged thousands of nurses to practice medicine under the supervision of physicians. This enticement again attempts to lure the nurse into a subservient position.

The age-old plight which has confronted nursing was acknowledged when it was reported that the American Medical Association cleared the preceding "proposal with the American Hospital Association but... had not spoken... to their professional organization, the American Nurses' Association." Many nurses have inveighed against the idea of becoming a physician's assistant while welcoming the recognition by physicians of the professional nurse as a colleague.

The Commission recognized "that each profession has the right and responsibility to assess its own roles, but the critical need for joint action demands that congruent roles be articulated and planned among the professions." Several joint-conferences have been held on nurse-physician relationships by the American Nurses' Association and the American Medical Association. The Commission felt these have been successful and recommended that:

A national joint practice commission be established between medicine and nursing to discuss

---

[56]*Ibid.*, pp. 62–64.

[57]*Ibid.*, p. 5

and make recommendations concerning the congruent roles of the physician and the nurse in providing quality health care, with particular attention to the rise of the nurse master clinician; the introduction of the physician's assistant; the increased activity of other professions in areas long assumed to be the concern solely of the physician and/or the nurse.[58]

A counterpart joint practice commission on the state level was recommended as were joint discussions with health management executives, other professions and allied health personnel.

The nursing profession was challenged to provide "a sufficient number of nurses for a diversified health care delivery system while at the same time making a career in nursing practice more intrinsically rewarding."[59]

That many nurses desire to nurse and do it well was understood by this commission as many reporters, Esther Lucile Brown in particular, had discovered. In addition, it was recorded that the "more qualified the nurse, the more she desires independence and latitude of judgment. Optimum conditions should exist when nurses are able to concentrate on care activities and can rely on others to carry out related but non-nursing functions." It was the recommendation that nursing should design two basically related but variant career patterns for nursing practice:

a. One career pattern, episodic, would emphasize the nursing practice that is essentially curative and restorative, generally acute or chronic in nature and most frequently provided in the setting of the hospital or in-patient facility;

b. The second career pattern, distributive, would emphasize the nursing practice that is essentially designed for health maintenance and disease prevention. This is generally continuous in nature, seldom acute, and increasingly will take place in community or emergent institutional settings."[60]

This proposal suggests a dichotomy in the preparation for and practice of nursing which appears to be geared to the geographical setting in which one practices.

An emphasis was expressed in two recommendations upon the need for increasing depth of knowledge and competence in practice of one's field of expertise. A progression

was described from entry, through master clinician or specialist in the episodic form to master clinician or "highly capable generalist" in the distributive form of nursing.

As it has been recommended innumerable times in the past, the non-therapeutic clerical and technical functions should be performed by non-nursing personnel. The objective was to attempt to bring nurses back from the sheltering security of secretarial refuges which keep them from maintaining nursing control over the delivery of nursing care.

The importance of the leadership role for director of nursing practice on a colleague basis with medicine and health administration in policy making was reiterated. The need was expressed for nursing leadership in nursing education and nursing services to work more cooperatively even to the granting of joint appointments.

The rapidly changing scientific and technological influences upon the delivery of health care require the use of complex equipment and "the need for persons with new knowledge and the capacity to assume responsibility for individual action." It was recommended that nurses avail themselves of this technology:

a. to eliminate as much routine as possible, allowing them to achieve maximum personal contact with their charges;

b. to enlarge the monitoring and feedback systems that can supply information on individual conditions and reactions, thus facilitating further nursing intervention.[61]

The danger of providing a dehumanizing type of care was stressed when one became involved in the intricacies of the regimen while forgetting the human aspects of patient care. Because of this very real threat to the patient it was recommended that the *nurse* become the *coordinator of patient activities.* "It is in both the tradition and the particular capabilities of nursing to serve as this organizational link . . . to assure the continued humane concern for the indiviudal, and to provide for the coordination of professional intervention." This proposal anticipated "that the nurse will play the role of intermediary in future health care." The profession of nursing was reminded that it "is essential that the patient's personal feelings be taken into account and individual worth be recognized."

---

[58]*Ibid.*, p. 89.
[59]*Ibid.*, p. 90.
[60]*Ibid.*, pp. 91–92.

[61]*Ibid.*, p. 97

This aspect was sufficiently crucial that educators and practitioners of nursing were recommended to place *continuing* emphasis on this role. "On the nurse rests a major portion of the ultimate responsibility for seeing that health care is dispensed with dignity and concern."[62]

Nursing Education

In focusing upon the dilemma of nursing education the position taken by the American Nurses' Association in 1965 was recognized, but the study reported: "However, many nurses, and even more physicians and (hospital) administrators feel that there is much to commend the hospital school approach. . . ."[63]

In studying the reduction in the number of hospital-based schools of nursing, it was explained that societal trends, lack of qualified faculty, lack of qualified student applicants and the preference of students for programs that emphasized general education were instrumental in this change. The stance of this commission in placing nursing education within institutions of higher education was stressed by the following recommendations:

Each state have, or create, a master planning committee that will take nursing education under its purview, such committees to include representatives of nursing, education, other health professions, and the public, to recommend specific guidelines, means for implementation, and deadlines to ensure that nursing education is positioned in the mainstream of American educational patterns with its preparatory programs located in collegiate institutions.[64]

Another unusual recommendation suggested that:

Those hospital schools that are strong and vital, endowed with a qualified faculty, suitable educational facilities, and motivated for excellence be encouraged to seek and obtain regional accreditation and degree granting power.[65]

It has not been the custom for service agencies which maintain educational programs to receive regional accreditation from general educational bodies nor to be empowered to award degrees.

All other hospital schools of nursing were recommended to "move systematically and with dispatch to effect interinstitutional arrangements with collegiate institutions." Junior and senior collegiate institutions were encouraged to work cooperatively to develop programs with these hospital schools.

It was recommended that:

The state master planning committees be charged with drawing up a plan for each state to determine the number and minimum size of institutions to receive institutional and individual student aid; [and that]

Small programs be terminated or consolidated into larger programs in order to reduce the per unit costs of education and in order to make better allocation of qualified faculty.

Recommendations were made for the provision of financial assistance to nursing education, such that:

Nursing education institutions be encouraged and given federal and state awards and support grants proportional to the number of students enrolled, such moneys to be used to defray the expenses of operation and expansion, and to provide salary support for qualified faculty.

Federal and state grants for building and construction of facilities be sharply increased to update and enlarge laboratory and classroom areas. There should, however, be an effort made at each institution having multiple preparatory programs to encourage and plan joint, cooperative use of building, laboratories, etc.

Both state and regional committees explore the possibilities of sharing and increasing scarce faculty resources. A state, for example, might employ faculty through its university system to serve at several institutions for nursing education, while both state and regional associations could develop programs for the professional advancement of current and future faculty personnel.[66]

The need for reexamination of accreditation of educational programs was studied. It was recommended that a national committee of the American Nurses' Association and the National League for Nursing study and make recommendations for future accrediting of programs in nursing.

In consideration of curricular needs, joint planning between the junior and senior collegiate level was recommended to delineate "appropriate levels of general and specialized learning for the different types of educational institutions." It was stressed further that education is an open-ended process and the op-

---

[62]*Ibid.*, p. 98
[63]*Ibid.*, p. 6.
[64]*Ibid.*, p. 107.
[65]*Ibid.*, p. 109

[66]*Ibid.*, p. 112.

portunity to broaden one's education is a right of every individual.

In the area of graduate study and faculty development there should be adequate numbers of quality programs with permission withheld for the inauguration or expansion of weak ones. Graduate programs that prepared for positions in administration and education were less pertinent in today's society than those providing a clinical specialty.

Three specific types of preparation should receive priority in the provision of financial assistance for graduate programs in nursing: for those individuals intending to teach nursing, those preparing for the master clinician role, and those wishing to participate in the organization and delivery of nursing. It was recommended that Congress continue to expand such programs as the Health Manpower Act to:

a. Provide educational loans to nurses pursuing graduate degrees with provision for part or whole forgiveness based on subsequent years of teaching;

b. Provide postmaster and postdoctoral fellowships and traineeships for nursing faculty and master clinicians to permit added professional development and continuing reorientation to changing practice and developing health care delivery systems;

c. Provide earmarked funds for faculty members of schools of nursing to enable them to obtain additional formal academic preparation equal to that required for regular appointment to faculty posts in collegiate institutions. These funds should have similar forgiveness features based on years of continuing service.[67]

The desire for seeking innovative techniques to enhance learning effectiveness and efficiency resulted in the recommendation that Federal, state, and private funds be made available to nursing institutions:

a. In the form of small research grants or contracts to assess and evaluate the effectiveness of new media and technology for nursing education and to disseminate the results;

b. In the form of grants and stipends to support short-term workshops to acquaint faculty members with new media and instructional materials;

c. In the form of institutional grants or matching funds to permit the purchase and installation of media systems and the required technicians to maintain and operate them;

d. In the form of demonstration grants to develop a limited number of centers so that faculty members may visit and have "actual" experience with these new media and materials.[68]

A true profession enlarges the body of knowledge it uses and improves its education and service through research. It was incumbent upon this commission to recommend that:

Federal, state, and private funds be extended to support a limited number of institutions to establish or expand doctoral programs in nursing science. These programs should focus on developing research capabilities for the study of nursing practice and nursing education, and should undertake the specification and development of nursing theory and knowledge.

The Federal Division of Nursing, the National Center for Health Services Research and Development, other governmental agencies, and private foundations provide research funds and contracts for basic and applied research into the nursing curriculum, articulation of educational systems, instructional practices, facilities design, etc., so that the most functional, effective, and economic approaches are taken in the education and development of future nurses.[69]

It was recommended that the admission procedures be studied as well as placement tests and achievement tests for ease in retention in academic progression. The realm of academic counseling and opportunities for individual programs of instruction received scrutiny. "Growing capacity to allow the student to learn at his own rate can mean acceleration for the talented as well as deceleration for the capable but less rapid learners."

Continuing education was studied and even though it was recognized that it is the nurse's responsibility for his or her own continual learning, provision for obtaining an enriched program of education was the obligation of the profession. Therefore it was recommended that:

The state master planning committee for nursing education identify one or more institutions to be responsible for regional coverage of continuing education programs for nurses within that area, and further that:

a. Federal and state funds be utilized to plan and implement continuing education programs for nursing on either a statewide or broader basis (as suggested by the current interstate compacts for higher education); and

---

[67]*Ibid.*, p. 118.

[68]*Ibid.*, p. 119.

[69]*Ibid.*, p. 120.

b. In the face of changing health roles and functions, and the interdependence of the health professions, vigorous efforts be taken to have continuing education programs jointly planned and conducted by interdisciplinary teams.[70]

Attention was focused upon *in-service education* and the commission recommended that:

Health care facilities, including hospitals, nursing homes, and other institutions, either individually or collectively through joint councils, provide professional training staffs to supervise and conduct in-service training and provide released time, facilities, and organizational support for the presentation of in-service nursing education as well as that for other occupations.[71]

In order to implement the various recommendations, the commission encouraged that:

Federal, regional, state, and local governments adopt measures for the increased support of nursing research and education. Priority should be given to construction grants, institutional grants, advanced traineeships, and research grants and contracts. Further, we recommend that private funds and foundations support nursing research and educational innovations where such activities are not publicly aided. We believe that a useful guide for the beginnings of such a financial aid program would be in the amounts and distribution of funds authorized by Congress for fiscal 1970, with proportional increases from other public and private agencies.[72]

Nursing Careers

Nursing as a rewarding and satisfying career was examined. It was acknowledged that there have been two traditional solutions to the problem, namely the constant onrush of campaigning to increase the number of students of nursing as well as increasing markedly the categories of helping personnel such as practical nurses, nurse aides, attendants and orderlies. The commission reiterated that "the profession must evaluate the current emphasis on quantity of nursing service to the near exclusion of quality considerations. The competency required of today's nurse practitioners makes it mandatory that prospective students be recruited through

careful screening. Health personnel are not mere hands; and the growing complexity of care should serve to deemphasize our concern with numbers alone."

The commission perceived a lack of input by nurses in planning operations for health. "Until recently, the National Advisory Commission on Health Manpower had not a single nurse among its members, and only one nurse on any of its seven specialized panels." The American Hospital Association has now acquiesced to the request of nurse leadership, and nurses have "a voice in all areas of its activities."

It is imperative that nurses assume an active role in the planning and action programs involving health care. Nurses must realize that all aspects of care and their changes such as new buildings, staffing patterns, and treatments have a direct influence on nurse activities. Nurses must have a voice in the determination of those things that effect nursing care. The commission recommended that "Nurses be appointed to and hold membership in, groups involved in health manpower planning at all governmental and regional levels."

Concern for the retention of qualified practitioners was expressed. The unhappiness and dissatisfaction of nurses was examined as were the many factors responsible for the loss of members from the profession. Career satisfaction seemed to be directly proportional to the ability to carry out the nursing care role. The impact on financial inequities between levels of nursing and between beginning and experienced practitioners was acknowledged. In order to retain capable nurse practitioners and to entice inactive but skilled nurses back into service, adequate financial reward and nursing care function incentive must be realized.

In order "to provide greater recognition for those who pursue a career in nursing service, and, just as importantly, to improve the quality of care by retaining expert practitioners in their specialty," the commission recommended that "health management administrators and clinical directors of nursing service build on current improvements in starting salaries to create a strong reward system for remaining in clinical practice by developing schedules of substantially increasing salary levels for experienced nurses functioning in advanced capacities."

In appreciation of the view that "the

---

[70]*Ibid.*, p. 122.
[71]*Ibid.*, p. 123.
[72]*Ibid.*, p. 124.

present undifferentiated approach to clinical nursing skill should be revised," it was recommended that:

Personnel policies in all health care facilities should be so designed that they:
a. Differentiate levels of responsibility in accord with the concepts of staff nurse, clinical nurse, and master clinician with appropriate intermediate grades. These levels should be designed according to the content of the position and the clinical proficiency required for competent performance;
b. Provide for promotion granted on the basis of acquisition of the knowledge and demonstrated competence to perform in a given position.[73]

That nurses will be ensured "the opportunity to provide the highest quality of patient care," a "redirection of health care practices" must be effected. This would relieve nurses of non-nursing activities and permit concentration on the nursing functions. To this end, it was recommended that:

Health management administrators and clinical directors of nursing service establish conditions to promote optimum opportunity for excellence in nursing practice by providing such elements as sufficient staff to develop and execute a personal care plan for each individual, the opportunity to discharge appropriate nursing functions in client teaching, counseling, and rehabilitation, and the surveillance and evaluation of the nursing plan for care.[74]

It was verified that "full excellence in the humane delivery of health care" will be achieved if and when *qualified personnel* are given the *time* to function as they desire and are prepared to do.

Well-prepared nurses will be retained or will return much more readily when programs in continuing education as well as in-service preparation are provided.

Provision for on-going continuance of professional nurse membership revolves around the recruitment of students of nursing. The challenge of contemporary nursing should be publicized. A clear and correct interpretation should be presented. The need for the profession to disseminate accurate information to guidance counselors resulted in the recommendation that "state nurses' associations and state leagues for nursing undertake more effective dissemination of information to high school guidance counselors on the changing status of nursing, the opportunities for expanded clinical practice, the improving salary levels, and other career aspects of the profession."

The scientific expansion of the base of nursing with its influence on the new therapeutic treatments requires knowledgeable practitioners. The public must be assured of competency and therefore licensure came under scrutiny. Although all states issue licenses, in eight states there is no mandatory licensure requirement. The commission recommended that "all remaining states without mandatory licensure laws for registered nurses immediately adopt appropriate regulation to this effect."

In addition to initial licensure the question of renewal of licensure to assure continued professional competency was considered. States are considering requiring individuals to present documented evidence of participation in continuing education. The commission recommended that "all state licensure laws for nursing be revised to require periodic review of the individual's qualifications for practice as a condition for license renewal."

As the levels of nursing become more visible the question of multiple licensure or certification will need delineation. "Health professions have held to the tradition of basic licensure followed by recognition of advanced levels through examination or review by professional bodies." For example, the specialties of medicine have specialty boards which attest to the special knowledge and skill that permit the physician to be declared a fellow of the American College of the specialty in question.

The American Nurses' Association has for some time been considering the inception of an Academy of Nursing which might act in a similar capacity for nursing.

In order to function effectively, to truly represent nursing, the commission recommends that:

The national nursing organizations press forward in their current study of functions, structures, methods of representation, and interrelationships in order to determine:
a. Areas of overlap or duplication that could be eliminated;
b. Areas of need that are currently unmet; and
c. Areas or functions that could be transferred

---

[73] *Ibid.*, p. 134.
[74] *Ibid.*, p. 135.

from one organization to another in light of changing systems and practices.[75]

Their plea for unified support by nurses is recognized in the recommendation that "individual nurses make a professional commitment to their organizations by joining and supporting one or more of them, at the same time ensuring that the organizations become more surely representative and more truly the designated spokesmen for nurses."

Implementation of Report

The emphasis of the Commission on Nursing and Nursing Education turned from investigation to implementation. Although change had been noted after each of the preceding "studies" of nursing, the noticeable effects were not proportional to the input of significant data and the pertinence of the suggestions for improvement. The Commission felt a strong motivation to launch a plan to enforce their recommendations. It has been noted that heat and light can be generated after the publishing of the results of a study but eventually lethargy and inertia conquer. The members of this Commission felt that "change is absolutely necessary to realize the potential contribution of nursing to the solution of our many health problems."

The implementation phase placed emphases on the following:

1. The development and expansion of nursing practice together with a reexamination of role relationships among the health professions;
2. The repatterning of educational systems in nursing to meet current exigencies and provide a foundation for innovation; and
3. The emergence of an unambiguous profession that would, in fact, be a full partner in shaping health policy and in serving the needs of our people."[76]

Dr. Leroy E. Burney, former U.S.P.H.S. Surgeon General and currently president of the Milbank Memorial Fund, assumed the presidency of the Commission. There were replacements in membership on this Commission. Of the twenty members five were nurses.

Funds were supplied from the Kellogg Foundation with contributions from N.L.N. and A.N.A.

A tangible aspect of implementation was noted in the establishment of a National Joint Practice Commission. Their assignment was to discuss, study and make recommendations concerning the related roles of the nurse and physician in providing quality care. Approval for this project was received from both the A.N.A. Board of Directors and the A.M.A. Board of Directors.

The following members serve on this Commission:

Nurse Practitioners

Genrose J. Alfano, New York
Patricia Devine, Kansas
Marilyn J. Howe, Ohio
Nancy Melvin, Arizona
Anna B. Sherlock, Arizona
Shirley Smoyak, New Jersey
Virginia Stone, North Carolina
Barbara B. Taylor, Massachusetts

Medical Practitioners

Thomas F. Dillon, New York
A. Allan Fischer, Indiana
Robert A. Hoekelman, New York
Joseph W. Marshall, Idaho
William H. Muller, Jr., Virginia
Robert A. Murray, Texas
Otto C. Page, Oregon
James W. Walker, Florida

The continued efforts will be directed in three areas, that of joint practice, statewide planning and dissemination.

Appraisal of the "Lysaught Report" has been forthcoming. The Report has been viewed as not without fault. Perusal of primary historical documentation appeared to be nonexistent and many inaccuracies in historical viewpoint and content occur. Constructive criticism of the study has been published, and the weaknesses in basing the fruits of such a study upon such an inexact foundation have been identified.[77]

In the content of the Report many studies of nursing have been referred to as attesting "to the persistence of problems in the nursing profession" rather than those faced by the nursing profession.

---

[75]*Ibid.*, p. 144.

[76]Lysaught, Jerome: "From Abstract into Action." *Nursing Outlook*, March 1972, Vol. 20, No. 3, p. 173.

[77]Cristy, Teresa E., Poulin, Muriel A., and Hover, Julie: "An Appraisal of An Abstract for Action." *American Journal of Nursing*, Vol. 71, No. 8, August 1971, pp. 1574–1581.

Research by Nurses

The first two criteria of a profession as identified by the Bixlers in their article on the professional status of nursing were:

1. A profession utilizes in its practice a well defined and well organized body of specialized knowledge which is on the intellectual level of higher learning.
2. A profession constantly enlarges the body of knowledge it uses and improves its technics of education and service by the use of the scientific method.[78]

Recognition of the need for research in nursing has been documented in articles in the American Journal of Nursing and by action of Boards of Directors of the American Nurses' Association.

Due to the efforts of the Association of Collegiate Schools of Nursing, the journal *Nursing Research* was launched in 1952. In the first issue Helen L. Bunge's editorial described the dual purpose of the journal which was: "To inform members of the nursing profession and allied professions of the results of scientific studies in nursing, and to stimulate research in nursing."[79]

The inception of the American Nurses' Foundation, Inc. was to fulfill the desire of encouraging research studies. In 1955 the American Nurses' Association gave $100,000 to this new organization to be used for studies of nursing functions.

A concerted effort began to emerge by nurse leadership to encourage the formation of a body of knowledge, nursing science, while concomitantly stimulating the much-needed research studies in nursing care.

In recent years there has been a commitment by nurses to enhance the care of people through research aimed at achievement of wholeness and wellness of man. Martha Rogers has stated:

Man is a unified phenomenon subject to natural laws and characterized by a complex electrodynamic field.... Man's consciousness and creativity are integral dimensions of man's wholeness.

Nursing's age-old commitment to human health and welfare has taken on new dimensions. The fundamental assumptions on which nursing knowledge and nursing practice rest are being rewritten by the very terms of man's existence. People are at the center of nursing's purpose. The descriptive, explanatory and predictive principles that direct professional nursing practice are rooted in a fundamental concept of the wholeness of life.[80]

In reflecting on the *science of nursing*, Rogers asserted that: "The science of nursing is not a summation of facts and principles drawn from other sources. Nursing's science is an emergent—a new product. The unifying principles and hypothetical generalizations basic to nursing seek to describe, explain, and predict about the phenomenon central to nursing's purpose—man."

The science of nursing evolves from a body of abstract knowledge which was obtained from scientific research and translated into the education of nurses and the practice of nursing. There have been many studies of research in nursing practice recorded in the literature as well as in unpublished doctoral dissertations.

The national Academy of Nursing has been established and the Board of Directors of the American Nurses' Association in January, 1973 elected 36 nationally prominent nurses to become charter fellows of the Academy. At the time of the announcement it was stressed that "nursing is in the front ranks of the health field, particularly in the realm of practice, as well as in the areas of research and education."

In retrospect, the nurse has been an important, dynamic force in the history of mankind. Nursing has been prominent in the struggle to assist all people in saving lives, in preventing illness, and even in achieving maximum health potential. The area of operation for nursing service has been man's place of existence: in homes, schools, offices, factories, farms, hospitals, clinics, extended care facilities, on ships, in the air, on battlefields and in remote places of the earth. The nurse faces enormous challenges today.

The knowledge explosion and its impact on the health profession has been summed up by Dr. Robert Morison, Director of Medical and Natural Sciences of The Rockefeller Foundation:

[78]Bixler, G. K. and Bixler, R. W. "The professional Status of Nursing." *American Journal of Nursing*, Sept. 1945.

[79]Bunge, Helen L., Editorial. "A Cooperative Venture." *Nursing Research*. June 1952, p. 5.

[80]Rogers, Martha: *An Introduction to the Theoretical Basis of Nursing*. Philadelphia, F. A. Davis Company, 1970, p. 34.

The explosion of knowledge is bound to continue; we know not for exactly how long, but it is already well beyond the grasp of single individuals. We have touched on three possible ways of coping with it. In the first place, we must learn to separate the significant from the insignificant—to save our effort for what really counts. Second, like it or not, we must continue to split knowledge up into manageable segments by the process known as specialization, but let us always remain alert to the dangers of specializing just for the sake of being a specialist. Finally, we must grasp confidently and firmly the opportunity offered by machines with far greater capabilities to learn, store, compare and recall than we have ourselves. Some may already fear that this path will inevitably lead to a domination of man by the machine and by the knowledge he has created.

But there is another, more attractive, and for me a more likely possibility: we can look upon our machines, and on our knowledge as means for freeing us from traditional labors and ancient fears. We should then have freedom to cultivate those human capabilities the machine can never know—how to share the sorrows of another person, to share with him our joys and pleasures, to see and appreciate the beauty of the world and perhaps even to add some new beauty to it.

Historically many well-qualified, articulate leaders in nursing have reported and recorded a message of progress despite innumerable obstacles; only the future can know how well they have been understood and appreciated. One can only speculate and reflect on Ruskin's remark: "Every noble life leaves the fiber of it, interwoven forever in the work of the world."

REFERENCE READINGS

Brainard, Annie M. *The Evolution of Public Health Nursing.* Philadelphia, W. B. Saunders Company, 1922.

Breckinridge, Mary. *Wide Neighborhoods,* New York, Harper and Brothers, 1952.

Brown, Amy F. *Research in Nursing.* Philadelphia, W. B. Saunders Co., 1958.

Chayer, Mary Ella. *School Nursing.* New York, G. P. Putnam's Sons, 1937.

Duffus, R. L. *Lillian Wald, Neighbor and Crusader.* New York, The Macmillan Company, 1938.

Gardner, Mary S. *Public Health Nursing.* 3rd ed., New York, The Macmillan Company, 1936.

Gilbert, Ruth. *The Public Health Nurse and Her Patient.* New York, The Commonwealth Fund, 1940.

Goostray, Stella. *Fifty Years, A History of the School of Nursing, The Children's Hospital, Boston.* Boston, Alumnae Association of the Children's Hospital School of Nursing, 1940.

Leahy, Kathleen and Cobb, M. Marguerite. *Fundamentals of Public Health Nursing.* New York, McGraw-Hill Book Company, 1966.

McGrath, Bethel J. *Nursing in Commerce and Industry.* New York, The Commonwealth Fund, 1946.

Morrissey, A. B. *Rehabilitation Nursing.* New York, G. P. Putnam's Sons, 1951.

Poole, Ernest. *Nurses on Horseback.* New York, The Macmillan Company, 1933.

Rogers, Martha E. *An Introduction to the Theoretical Basis of Nursing.* Philadelphia, F. A. Davis Company, 1970.

Russell, William Logie. *The New York Hospital—A History of the Psychiatric Service, 1771–1936.* New York, Columbia University Press, 1945.

Simmons, Leo W., and Henderson, Virginia. *Nursing Research.* New York, Appleton-Century-Crofts, 1964.

Stewart, Isabel M. and Austin, Anne L. *A History of Nursing.* New York, G. P. Putnam's Sons, 1962.

Struthers, Lina Rogers. *The School Nurse.* New York, G. P. Putnam's Sons, 1917.

———. *The Public Health Nursing Curriculum Guide.* Prepared by a joint committee of the National Organization for Public Health Nursing and the U.S. Public Health Service, 1942.

Tinkham, Catherine and Voorhees, Eleanor. *Community Health Nursing—Evolution and Process.* New York, Appleton-Century-Crofts, 1972.

Wald, Lillian D. *The House on Henry Street.* New York, Henry Holt and Company, 1915.

Wales, Marguerite. *The Public Health Nurse in Action.* New York, The Macmillan Company, 1969.

Waters, Ysabella. *Visiting Nursing in the United States.* New York, Charities Publication Committee, 1909.

Index

Page numbers in *italics* refer to illustrations.